Integrating Psychotherapy into Nursing Practice

Kübra Gülırmak Güler
Ondokuz Mayıs University, Turkey

IGI Global
Scientific Publishing
Publishing Tomorrow's Research Today

Vice President of Editorial | Melissa Wagner
Director of Acquisitions | Mikaela Felty
Director of Book Development | Jocelynn Hessler
Production Manager | Mike Brehm
Cover Design | Jose Rosado

Published in the United States of America by
IGI Global Scientific Publishing
701 East Chocolate Avenue
Hershey, PA, 17033, USA
Tel: 717-533-8845 | Fax: 717-533-7115
Website: https://www.igi-global.com E-mail: cust@igi-global.com

Library of Congress Cataloging-in-Publication Data

LCCN: 2025949691 (CIP Data Pending)
ISBN13: 9798337365268
Isbn13Softcover: 9798337365275
EISBN13: 9798337365282
British Cataloguing in Publication Data
A Cataloguing in Publication record for this book is available from the British Library.

Table of Contents

Detailed Table of Contents

The increasing complexity of patient needs demands that the integration of psychotherapy skills and principles become an essential component of high-quality, comprehensive, and equitable patient-centered care. For the Psychiatric Mental Health Advanced Practice Nurse (PMH APN), psychotherapy is a foundational and mandated role, requiring policy support to ensure they practice to the full scope of their license in integrated systems. Across specialties, specialized interventions are validated: CBT is adapted for effective use in medical settings, and Dignity Therapy (DT) provides a brief psychotherapeutic approach for end-of-life care, relieving existential distress and generating a legacy document. Holistic care requires viewing the patient-caregiver dyad as the unit of care, utilizing joint interventions to reduce caregiver stress and improve patient symptoms. Furthermore, equitable care demands trauma-informed support that recognizes how intersectionalities of influence—such as race, gender, and citizenship—profoundly affect the health outcomes of marginalized populations.

In an era of increasing globalization, migration, and social change, cultural competence has emerged as a fundamental pillar of modern psychotherapeutic nursing. This chapter emphasizes that mental health care must transcend biological and psychosocial boundaries to incorporate a holistic understanding of a client's cultural identity, values, and belief systems. Because culture fundamentally shapes how individuals perceive illness and express distress, the nurse's ability to provide culturally sensitive care is the determining factor in building trust and ensuring treatment adherence. Central to this practice are the theoretical frameworks of Campinha-Bacote, which highlights the importance of self-awareness and cultural desire, and Leininger, which posits cultural congruence as the heart of care quality. Ultimately, cultural competence requires more than just external knowledge; it demands that nurses confront their own biases to foster ethical, empathic, and effective therapeutic relationships in an increasingly diverse healthcare landscape.

Cognitive Behavioral Therapy (CBT) in nursing practice is an evidence-based and patient-centered approach that helps nurses address the relationship between thoughts, emotions, and behaviors influencing health outcomes. By incorporating CBT principles into daily care, nurses can assist patients in recognizing maladaptive thinking patterns, developing effective coping strategies, and improving self-management skills in various clinical settings. CBT-informed nursing interventions enhance therapeutic communication, reduce psychological distress, and support adherence to treatment plans. This approach aligns with the holistic nursing perspective by integrating psychological and physical care, contributing to improved patient well-being, resilience, and overall quality of life.

This chapter examines the theoretical foundations and clinical applications of mindfulness- and acceptance-based approaches within contemporary psychosocial intervention frameworks. Core processes such as present-moment awareness, acceptance, cognitive defusion, self-as-context, values, and committed action are outlined to demonstrate how these mechanisms enhance psychological flexibility. Evidence supporting Mindfulness-Based Stress Reduction and Acceptance and Commitment Therapy is reviewed, with emphasis on their relevance to emotional regulation, chronic illness management, and holistic nursing practice.

This study explores the theoretical framework and clinical application of Positive Psychotherapy (PPT) and Strengths-Based Interventions, emphasizing the shift from a pathology-centered to a resource-oriented paradigm in healthcare. Developed by Nossrat Peseschkian, PPT integrates humanistic and psychodynamic elements,

Trauma is defined as a deep emotional wound that emerges when an individual is exposed to events that threaten their life or cause serious psychological harm. In recent years, events such as natural disasters, wars, and sexual abuse have increased the number of individuals in society who are exposed to trauma (Nievergelt et al., 2024). Posttraumatic stress disorder (PTSD) is one of the primary psychological consequences of traumatic experiences. In addition to PTSD, it has been observed that individuals may develop dissociative symptoms after traumatic events, that is, a sense of alienation from oneself or one's surroundings (APA, 2015). In this chapter, the definition of trauma, its common symptoms and effects, the role and importance of stabilization in trauma treatment, the principles of trauma-informed care, and psychiatric nursing practices with individuals who have experienced trauma are discussed.

The evolution of nursing in digital environments represents a profound transformation in healthcare delivery, professional practice, education, and patient engagement. The integration of digital technologies—such as electronic health records (EHRs), telehealth systems, artificial intelligence (AI), wearable sensors, and mobile health (mHealth) applications—has redefined the roles, responsibilities, and competencies of nurses in the 21st century. This digital transformation has enabled nurses to transcend traditional clinical boundaries, providing care that is more data-driven, patient-centered, and accessible. In the early stages, nursing's interaction with technology was largely administrative, focusing on documentation and record-keeping. However, as digital health infrastructures matured, the scope of nursing practice expanded dramatically, aligning with global movements toward digital health transformation. The modern nurse now operates in a hybrid environment that combines human compassion with technological precision.

This study examines the evolving role of mental health and psychiatric nursing, focusing on the authority and boundaries of advanced practice nursing in psychotherapy. Within a comparative legal framework, the transition from Peplau's interpersonal process

Preface

Nursing is not merely the provision of care; it is bearing witness to human vulnerability, remaining present with suffering, and accompanying the quiet steps of healing. In this sense, nursing is inherently a therapeutic profession. However, within modern healthcare systems, this therapeutic essence is often rendered invisible amid heavy workloads, biomedical priorities, and time constraints. Yet nurses are the healthcare professionals who maintain the longest and closest contact with patients—those who respond to urgent calls for care, perceive what remains unspoken, recognize anxiety in a glance, and remain closest to the emotional world of individuals. The book *Integrating Psychotherapy into Nursing Practice* has been prepared with the aim of making this profound and frequently overlooked dimension of nursing visible once again. The fundamental premise of the book is that psychotherapy is not an application confined to specific disciplines; rather, it is an integral, complementary, and empowering component of nursing care. Accordingly, this volume explores how psychotherapeutic perspectives, attitudes, and skills can be integrated into nursing practice in an ethical, evidence-based, and sustainable manner.

ABOUT THIS BOOK

The structure of the book has been intentionally designed to guide the reader through a conscious and holistic conceptual flow. The opening chapters address the conceptual foundations of psychotherapy in nursing, offering an integrative framework across diverse nursing specialties, families, and populations. Building on this foundation, the subsequent chapters examine core psychotherapeutic approaches—such as cognitive behavioral therapy, mindfulness- and acceptance-based approaches, positive psychotherapy, and supportive and interpersonal psychotherapy—discussed alongside their application within nursing-specific roles.In the following sections, the book focuses on the contributions of psychotherapeutic sensitivity to nursing care in clinical contexts that require multidisciplinary approaches, such as oncology, as well as in settings where trauma-informed approaches are essential. It then turns to the rapidly digitalizing healthcare landscape, addressing digital interventions, telepsychotherapy applications, and the emerging therapeutic roles assumed by nurses in digital environments. The final section provides a comprehensive conclusion by focusing on authority, boundaries, and professional responsibilities in psychotherapeutic nursing practice through the lenses of clinical education, ethical responsibility, and legal frameworks. All chapters included in this volume reflect an interdisciplinary perspective that builds bridges between psychotherapy and nursing. By bringing together theoretical foundations and clinical experience, the contributing authors aim to offer readers not only a conceptual framework but also a practice-oriented perspective to guide clinical application.

It is my hope that this book will serve not only as a reference source for nursing students, clinical nurses, academics, and mental health professionals, but also as a companion that reminds readers of the humane and therapeutic essence of nursing. I firmly believe that integrating psychotherapy into nursing practice strengthens not only the well-being of those receiving care, but also nurses' professional satisfaction, sense of meaning, and psychological resilience.

With the hope that this work—reminding us that healing is possible not only through treatment, but through *being understood*—will open new horizons for nursing practice and education.

Editor

Dr. Kübra Gülirmak Güler

Chapter 1
Broadening Horizons Integrating Psychotherapy Across Nursing:
Specialties, Families, and Diverse Populations

Yogita Kalra
https://orcid.org/0009-0009-5136-9098
Lovely Professional University, India

Prabhjyot Kour
https://orcid.org/0009-0009-4430-7593
Lovely Professional University, India

Bhawna Verma
Vardhman Mahavir Medical College, India & Safdarjung Hospital, India

ABSTRACT

The increasing complexity of patient needs demands that the integration of psychotherapy skills and principles become an essential component of high-quality, comprehensive, and equitable patient-centered care. For the Psychiatric Mental Health Advanced Practice Nurse (PMH APN), psychotherapy is a foundational and mandated role, requiring policy support to ensure they practice to the full scope of their license in integrated systems. Across specialties, specialized interventions are validated: CBT is adapted for effective use in medical settings, and Dignity Therapy (DT) provides a brief psychotherapeutic approach for end-of-life care, re-

DOI: 10.4018/979-8-3373-6526-8.ch001

lieving existential distress and generating a legacy document. Holistic care requires viewing the patient-caregiver dyad as the unit of care, utilizing joint interventions to reduce caregiver stress and improve patient symptoms. Furthermore, equitable care demands trauma-informed support that recognizes how intersectionalities of influence—such as race, gender, and citizenship—profoundly affect the health outcomes of marginalized populations.

INTRODUCTION

Figure 1. Nursing's New Mandate: Integrating Psychotherapy for Holistic Care

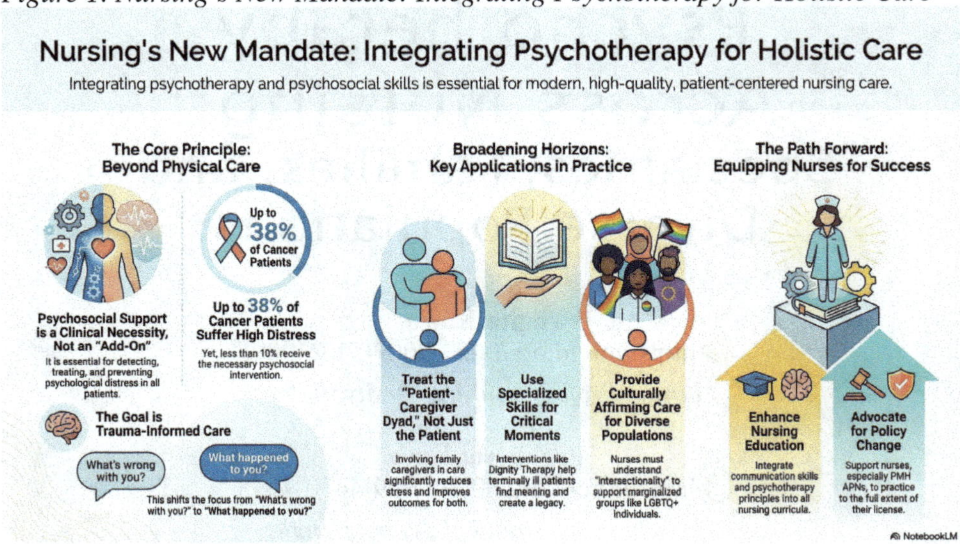

Nursing's New Mandate: Integrating Psychotherapy for Holistic Care
Integrating psychotherapy and psychosocial skills is essential for modern, high-quality, patient-centered nursing care.
The Core Principle: Beyond Physical Care
Up to 38% of Cancer Patients
Psychosocial Support is a Clinical Necessity, Not an "Add-On"
It is essential for detecting, treating, and preventing psychological distress in all patients.
Up to 38% of Cancer Patients Suffer High Distress
Yet, less than 10% receive the necessary psychosocial intervention.
The Goal is Trauma-Informed Care
What's wrong with you?
What happened to you?
This shifts the focus from "What's wrong with you?" to "What happened to you?"
Broadening Horizons: Key Applications in Practice
Treat the "Patient-Caregiver Dyad," Not Just the Patient
Involving family caregivers in care significantly reduces stress and improves outcomes for both.
Use Specialized Skills for Critical Moments
Interventions like Dignity Therapy help terminally ill patients find meaning and create a legacy.
Provide Culturally Affirming Care for Diverse Populations
Nurses must understand "intersectionality" to support marginalized groups like LGBTQ+ individuals.
The Path Forward: Equipping Nurses for Success
Enhance Nursing Education
Integrate communication skills and psychotherapy principles into all nursing curricula.
Advocate for Policy Change
Support nurses, especially PMH APNs, to practice to the full extent of their license.
NotebookLM

Source: Adapted from NotebookLM (2024).

The contemporary healthcare environment is defined by complexity, marked by the increasing prevalence of psychosocial and mental health challenges across all patient populations, coupled with a shifting paradigm toward holistic and patient-centered care (K. R. Delaney et al., 2017; Kaas, 2020; Kague, n.d.). This chapter, titled "Broadening Horizons: Integrating Psychotherapy Across Nursing Specialties, Families, and Diverse Populations," argues that the integration of psychotherapy skills and principles is an essential component of high-quality, comprehensive, and equitable nursing care. Nurses serve as the pivotal frontline healthcare providers, often spending more time with patients than any other clinician and acting as a primary point of communication (Estes & Karten, 2014; Kaas, 2020; Kague, n.d.; Lyu et al., 2024, 2024). Consequently, their capacity to address the psychological, emotional, and existential needs of patients and their families is critical to achieving positive health outcomes (Banerjee et al., 2017; Travado, 2015).

Historically, while nursing prides itself on providing balanced physical and emotional care, in practice, physical care often dominates (Suzuki, n.d.). However, the rising visibility of psychological distress (PD)—a universal clinical phenomenon—necessitates a formal and systematic approach to psychosocial care that goes beyond mere "comfort care" or "handholding stuff" (Suzuki, n.d.). Psychosocial care, aimed at the detection, diagnosis, treatment, and prevention of psychological distress, is now recognized as a crucial component of quality care delivery (Suzuki, n.d.; Travado, 2015). The central purpose of this chapter is to illustrate the diverse applications of psychotherapy within nursing and advocate for the necessary educational and policy changes required to equip the entire nursing workforce to deliver comprehensive psychosocial care effectively to individuals, their families, and diverse, marginalized populations.

The Foundational Imperative: Psychotherapy and the Nursing Role

The role of the nurse demands a relational approach, as the relationship between the client and the clinician is recognized as a profound therapeutic factor (Horvath et al., 2011) (Norcross & Lambert, 2018). This healing alliance is consistently associated with positive treatment outcomes across various contexts (Horvath et al., 2011; Norcross & Lambert, 2018). However, nurses often report difficulties communicating effectively with patients, especially in high-stakes environments, leading to potential increases in patient uncertainty, anxiety, dissatisfaction, and poorer quality of life (Banerjee et al., 2017).

For Psychiatric Mental Health Advanced Practice Nurses (PMH APNs), particularly the Psychiatric Mental Health Nurse Practitioner (PMHNP), the practice of psychotherapy is an intrinsic and foundational role (K. R. Delaney et al., 2017). PMH APN programs are required to cover a minimum of two psychotherapy modalities for certification (K. R. Delaney et al., 2017). PMH APNs are valuable assets in integrated care models, providing comprehensive mental health services, including both pharmacotherapy and psychotherapy, and are crucial for wellness initiatives that help clients develop self-management plans by increasing self-efficacy and empowerment (K. R. Delaney et al., 2017; K. R. Delaney & Vanderhoef, 2019). PMH Advanced Practice Registered Nurses (APRNs) are educated at the masters or doctoral level, and their scope of practice explicitly includes providing psychotherapy, diagnosing, managing, prescribing for, and treating mental health problems (K. R. Delaney et al., 2017). This contrasts with PMH Registered Nurses (RNs), who practice under a scope that allows them to assess, address, and manage behavioral health issues (K. R. Delaney et al., 2017; K. R. Delaney & Vanderhoef, 2019).

Despite the clear mandates for PMH APNs to practice psychotherapy, challenges exist, such as the scarcity of psychiatrists, a dearth of preceptors, and market pressures that often prioritize medication management over psychotherapy due to higher reimbursement rates (K. R. Delaney et al., 2017). Addressing these workforce issues and fully leveraging the capabilities of PMH nurses is essential for the expansion of team-based integrated care and increasing access to mental health services, particularly in underserved areas (Corso & Gage, 2016; Durbin et al., 2016).

This need for integrated expertise extends beyond specialized PMH roles. Across the profession, providing psychosocial care is fundamentally recognized as nursing work (Suzuki, n.d.). However, traditional nursing practice frequently lacks reflection on the clinical significance of psychosocial care. Nurses' descriptions of psychosocial care often vary widely, including subjective terms like "an area of nursing," "going above and beyond," or "touchy feely" nursing, which may reflect confusion or ambivalence toward the role, or even "role abdication" when compared to the rigorous approach taken toward physical care (Kague, n.d.; Suzuki, n.d.). A key insight is that increasing nurses' understanding of the **clinical significance** of psychosocial care, particularly its link to preventing psychological distress and improving health outcomes (e.g., academic performance or quality of life), is critical for fostering greater nurse involvement (Suzuki, n.d.).

BROADENING PSYCHOSOCIAL INTEGRATION ACROSS SPECIALTIES

The demand for integrating psychosocial care and psychotherapeutic skills is evident across major nursing specialties.

Oncology Nursing and High-Stakes Communication

In oncology, nurses are vital throughout the cancer journey, supporting patients and families through complex decisions and intense emotions. Psychological distress (PD) is prevalent, with up to 38% of cancer patients experiencing high levels of distress, yet often less than 10% receive the necessary psychosocial intervention due to various barriers (Banerjee et al., 2017; Suzuki, n.d.). The goal of psychosocial care in oncology is the detection, diagnosis, and treatment of PD.

Specific communication skills training (CST) programs have been proven feasible and acceptable for oncology nurses (Banerjee et al., 2017, 2017; Buckley et al., n.d.; Canivet et al., 2014). These programs focus on crucial skills such as:

- Responding empathically to patients (Banerjee et al., 2017).
- Discussing death, dying, and end-of-life goals of care.
- Responding to challenging interactions with families.
- Clarifying skills, which showed significant improvement post-training.

The largest gains observed in CST programs are typically found in empathy skills, which are highly significant for oncology nursing practice (Banerjee et al., 2017). Effective communication and relational skills are deemed crucial for achieving positive patient outcomes in this high-stakes setting (Banerjee et al., 2017; Canivet et al., 2014). Nurses must be equipped to handle difficult family dynamics and provide comprehensive psychosocial support, recognizing that the clinical practice guidelines expect nurses to assess, monitor, discuss, and document psychosocial care as a component of integrated care (Dionne-Odom et al., 2018; Suzuki, n.d.).

Pediatric Nursing and Comprehensive Mental Health Care

Mental health challenges among children and adolescents, ranging from anxiety and depression to ADHD and trauma-related disorders, are increasing, with an estimated 10-20% of children and adolescents worldwide experiencing mental health disorders (George, 2023; Kague, n.d.). Pediatric nurses, as frontline providers, must adopt a comprehensive and multidimensional approach to care.

Pediatric mental health nursing requires distinct considerations compared to adult care, demanding tailored approaches due to the unique developmental needs and vulnerabilities of young patients (Kague, n.d.). Effective strategies include:

- **Early identification and assessment:** Nurses must recognize early signs and symptoms through comprehensive assessments, careful observation, and utilizing standardized screening tools appropriate for developmental stage and cognitive abilities (Kague, n.d.).
- **Interdisciplinary collaboration:** Pediatric nurses must work with mental health professionals, educators, and social workers to form a holistic and coordinated approach (Kague, n.d.).
- **Evidence-based interventions:** Nurses must be knowledgeable about interventions like cognitive-behavioral therapy (CBT), play therapy, and family-centered approaches (Kague, n.d.).
- **Creating a therapeutic environment:** Establishing a safe, supportive, child-friendly atmosphere that promotes trust and open communication is paramount (Kague, n.d.).

The role of the pediatric nurse extends beyond traditional tasks to encompass assessment, early detection, prevention, and intervention strategies.

The Relational Core of Care: Families and Existential Dimensions

The integration of psychotherapy extends necessarily to the patient's context, mandating the involvement of family and caregivers (Dionne-Odom et al., 2018). Research strongly indicates that interventions delivered jointly to patients and caregivers can significantly reduce caregiver stress, improve their coping skills, knowledge, and quality of life, and even decrease patient symptoms, thus improving physical and mental health (K. R. Delaney et al., 2017; Dionne-Odom et al., 2018; Northouse et al., 2012). Family caregivers, especially of patients with serious illnesses like cancer, frequently experience high levels of stress, psychological impairment, sleep disturbances, and physical health changes (Northouse et al., 2012). It is critical to view the patient-caregiver dyad as the unit of care and to provide timely support and resources (Dionne-Odom et al., 2018; Northouse et al., 2012). Caregivers with high depressive or anxiety symptoms often express significantly higher interest in formal support services like therapy or counseling and assistance from national organizations compared to the general caregiver population (Banerjee et al., 2017). Identifying caregivers who may have pre-existing emotional concerns or serious illness themselves is vital (Ferrell & Wittenberg, 2017).

Existential and Meaning-Centered Approaches

For patients facing serious illness or end-of-life care, nursing must incorporate existential care, which requires a relational, strengths-based approach (Tarbi et al., 2023). Existential suffering, particularly at the last stage of life, can be transformed into a foundation for healing and well-being through an approach known as Existential Positive Psychology (PP 2.0) (Ferrell & Wittenberg, 2017). PP 2.0 focuses on transcending and transforming suffering and cultivating spiritual and existential capabilities to achieve personal growth and flourishing (Wong & Yu, 2021).

Nurses can integrate these principles into daily practice by:

1. **Maintaining a strengths-based orientation:** Assessing personal resources developed over a lifetime (ways of coping and growing amidst struggle) that can be leveraged during distress (Tarbi et al., 2023).
2. **Grounding care firmly in relationships:** Recognizing relationships as a therapeutic cornerstone, advocating for patient connection, and fostering authentic relationships where vulnerability and existential oscillations (between suffering

and growth) are welcomed and witnessed (Ferrell & Wittenberg, 2017; Tarbi et al., 2023).

3. **Responding moment to moment:** Specific psychotherapeutic interventions exist that nurses, particularly in palliative care, can apply or assist in administering. Dignity Therapy (DT) is a novel psychotherapeutic intervention designed to address psychosocial and existential distress in terminally ill patients (Chochinov et al., 2005; George, 2023; Martínez et al., 2017). DT invites patients to discuss issues that matter most, resulting in a "generativity document" they can bequeath to family or friends (Chochinov et al., 2005). DT focuses on dignity conservation tasks such as settling relationships, sharing words of love, and preparing legacies of memory and shared values (George, 2023). Nurses are considered strong candidates for administering DT due to their holistic focus on care, inclusive of spirituality, although workload concerns must be addressed (George, 2023). Meaning-Centered Psychotherapy (MCP) is another scientifically validated, meaning-centered therapy for advanced cancer, aiming to sustain and enhance a sense of meaning in the face of existential crisis (Wong & Yu, 2021). This approach is structured around specific themes of meaning relevant to cancer patients, such as historical context, attitudinal values, and creative values (Wong & Yu, 2021).

ADDRESSING DIVERSITY AND TRAUMA: CULTURAL SENSITIVITY AND AFFIRMING PRACTICES

A foundational principle of integrating psychotherapy is the imperative for culturally sensitive and affirming care, especially for diverse and marginalized populations (Barker & Buchanan-Barker, 2011; Clarke, n.d.; Guruge & Khanlou, 2004; Yamada & Brekke, 2008). Nurses must be aware of and respectful of gender diversity, promote equality, and implement inclusive practices (Barker & Buchanan-Barker, 2011; Clarke, n.d.; Guruge & Khanlou, 2004).

Trauma-Informed Care (TIC)

Trauma is a pervasive public health problem with long-lasting negative impacts on physical and mental health (Antebi-Gruszka & Scheer, 2021; Levenson et al., 2023). Trauma-informed approaches shift the focus from "What's wrong with you?" to "What happened to you?" by realizing trauma's widespread impact, recognizing its signs and symptoms, integrating knowledge into practice, and actively resisting re-traumatization (Goldstein et al., 2024). Organizational trauma-informed practice s (which should precede clinical changes) involve creating a safe environment, training all staff, and preventing secondary traumatic stress (Antebi-Gruszka & Scheer, 2021; Goldstein et al., 2024; Levenson et al., 2023).

TIC, when applied within an LGBTQ+ affirmative practice framework, is essential for supporting resilience and healing in these populations (Levenson et al., 2023). LGBTQ+ individuals are at higher risk for bias, discrimination, harassment, and violence, leading to unique traumagenic experiences (Levenson et al., 2023). Affirming TIC practices involve:

- Fostering psychological safety and establishing safe, consistent, and non-shaming relationships (Levenson et al., 2023).
- Demonstrating a proactive affirming stance by using gender-affirming language and appropriate pronouns, and ensuring intake forms are inclusive of diverse identities (Levenson et al., 2023).
- Promoting collaboration and mutuality, recognizing the inherent power imbalance in mental health services, which can feel threatening to LGBTQ+ individuals (Levenson et al., 2023).
- Acknowledging historical trauma and the complex intersectionality of sexual, gender, racial, and ethnic diversity (Levenson et al., 2023).

Serving SGM Forced Migrants

For sexual and/or gender minority (SGM) forced migrants, the lack of dedicated research into their mental health and acculturation needs is significant (Clarke, n.d.). These individuals often face unique compounding challenges, including traumatic experiences, discrimination, cultural barriers, and difficulties in identity reconstruction and trauma recovery (Clarke, n.d.).

When working with this population, practitioners must:

- Avoid pathologization (Clarke, n.d.).
- Recognize that central concepts of Western mental health discourse (e.g., depression, anxiety, PTSD) may not have direct equivalents in non-Western cultures (Clarke, n.d.).
- Understand the "intersectionalities of influence"—how multiple social identity dimensions (e.g., race, gender, citizenship) intersect to affect health (Hermaszewska et al., 2022). An ecosystemic framework is helpful here, situating individual issues within familial, community, and societal realms (Barker & Buchanan-Barker, 2011; Guruge & Khanlou, 2004).

Culturally responsive care involves actively listening to community needs, valuing community expertise, and, where possible, I ncorporating cultural rituals or traditions into mental health programs (Yamada & Brekke, 2008).

PEDAGOGICAL AND POLICY CHALLENGES: EQUIPPING THE NURSING WORKFORCE

To realize the vision of integrated psychotherapy across specialties, major changes in nursing education, policy, and organizational support are required.

Psychotherapy Integration in Training

The movement toward psychotherapy integration—the process of learning from different therapeutic viewpoints to enhance efficacy and efficiency (Aafjes-van Doorn et al., 2018)—is common globally (Aafjes-van Doorn et al., 2018). However, training in psychotherapy integration lacks empirical support and coherence. The debate persists over whether an integrative approach should be taught from the outset of training or encouraged later, once expertise in one specific model (e.g., Cognitive Behavioral Therapy or psychodynamic therapy) has been established (Aafjes-van Doorn et al., 2018).

Regardless of timing, training in psychotherapy integration should include didactic and experiential elements, supervision, and readings. The current low quantity and quality of empirical studies on training efficacy illustrate a significant gap. It is critical to raise awareness of psychotherapy integration as an essential part of clinical and academic training to inform clinical practice guidelines. This lack of training extends to fundamental psychosocial skills. Oncology nurses, for example, have reported a lack of psychology knowledge and communication skills (Aafjes-van Doorn et al., 2018; Lyu et al., 2024).

Organizational and Policy Action

The systematic integration of psychotherapy requires policy-level changes, especially concerning the acceptance and remuneration of nurses providing this care (Suzuki, n.d.). Recommendations include:

- **Enhanced Nursing Education:** Undergraduate curricula must ensure greater nurse involvement in psychosocial care. This includes providing skills training in therapeutic verbal and nonverbal communication (Goldstein et al., 2024).

- **Integrated Care Models:** Integrated care, defined as the systematic coordination of general and behavioral health care, is essential. Nurses' self-perceptions may become barriers unless they are educated to see themselves as "essential players" in this model. PMH APNs are key leaders in designing patient-centered cultures of care within integrated systems (K. R. Delaney et al., 2017; Dionne-Odom et al., 2018).
- **Policy Advocacy:** Nurses must advocate for equitable access to mental health care, including parity laws that mandate mental health services be covered at the same level as physical health services. There is also a need to advocate for policies that ensure psychosocial care and services are included in national cancer plans and comprehensive treatment programs (Lyu et al., 2024; Travado, 2015).

This concludeda that the future of high-quality, patient-centered healthcare hinges upon nursing's adoption of robust psychotherapy principles and skills across all specialties, recognizing and addressing the needs of families and diverse, traumatized populations (Levenson et al., 2023). By focusing on enhanced education, supporting the patient-caregiver dyad, applying strengths-based existential models like Dignity Therapy, and implementing trauma-informed, culturally affirming practices, nursing can fulfill its holistic mandate and significantly improve patient outcomes globally (Chochinov et al., 2005; Martínez et al., 2017; Suzuki, n.d.). The chapters that follow will delve into the practical strategies and policy implications necessary to enact this vital transformation.

REVIEW OF LITRATURE

The literature supports the imperative for greater integration of psychosocial interventions in nursing, addressing professional role complexity, specialized care needs (oncology, palliative care), family dynamics, and culturally sensitive care for diverse populations.

The Foundation of Psychotherapy Integration in Nursing

The integration of psychotherapy and psychosocial care is viewed as an essential component of high-quality, patient-centered care. Nurses are pivotal members of healthcare teams, often spending the most time with patients and serving as a primary source of communication. However, suboptimal communication frequently occurs in high-stakes environments, leading to increased patient anxiety, non-compliance, dissatisfaction, and poorer quality of life.

Psychotherapy and Advanced Practice Nursing: The practice of psychotherapy is intrinsically mandated within the role of the Psychiatric Mental Health Advanced Practice Nurse (PMH APN). PMH APN programs must cover a minimum of two psychotherapy modalities for certification. PMH Advanced Practice Registered Nurses (APRNs) are educated at the master's or doctoral level, allowing them to provide psychotherapy, as well as diagnose, manage, prescribe for, and treat mental health issues (K. R. Delaney et al., 2017). Despite their capacity, PMH nurses' capabilities in integrated care environments often have little visibility to federal mental health agencies (K. R. Delaney et al., 2017; K. R. Delaney & Vanderhoef, 2019).

Integration Models and Training: Psychotherapy integration, defined as looking beyond the confines of single therapeutic approaches to enhance efficacy and efficiency, is common practice globally (Aafjes-van Doorn et al., 2018). This integration can take different forms, including assimilative, theoretical, or common factors integration (Aafjes-van Doorn et al., 2018). The existing literature on the efficacy of training in psychotherapy integration is limited in quantity and quality, underscoring the need for continued research and development of evidence-based training methods (Aafjes-van Doorn et al., 2018). All nurses, regardless of specialty, require knowledge, skill, and judgment to competently practice therapeutic interactions, necessitating ongoing reflection on their practice and learning needs (Psychotherapy and the controlled act component of psychotherapy – CNO).

Psychosocial Care in Specialized Settings (Oncology and Palliative Care)

The literature extensively documents the need for psychosocial interventions across the disease continuum, particularly in oncology and palliative care (Suzuki, n.d.; Travado, 2015).

Addressing Psychological Distress: Psychosocial care is fundamentally aimed at the detection, diagnosis, and treatment of Psychological Distress (PD). This care involves assessing needs, coordinating biomedical and psychosocial care, assisting with coping, and systematically following up on plans (Suzuki, n.d.).

Nurse Role Beliefs and Barriers: While nurses perceive providing psychosocial care as a fundamental nursing activity and a dimension of holistic care, significant barriers exist (Suzuki, n.d.). Previously reported structural barriers include lack of time, heavy workload, and inadequate education/skills (Suzuki, n.d.). Focus group data indicates nurses also experience internal barriers, such as personal stress, lack of interest, and nurse motivation, sometimes leading to hesitancy or "role abdication" regarding holistic care. Nurses' awareness of the clinical significance of psychosocial care is considered key to increasing their systematic involvement in providing this care (Suzuki, n.d.).

Evidence-Based Interventions in Medical Settings: Cognitive Behavioral Therapy (CBT) is an empirically supported treatment widely reviewed through meta-analyses (Valente, 2017; Wong & Yu, 2021, p.). CBT has demonstrated efficacy in reducing cancer-specific thought intrusions and anxiety symptoms in breast cancer patients (Melton, PhD, Abpp, 2017). It is also effectively applied to manage fatigue in cancer survivors (Aafjes-van Doorn et al., 2018; Dionne-Odom et al., 2018; Drew, 2014; Guruge & Khanlou, 2004; Hermaszewska et al., 2022; Kaas, 2020). The delivery of CBT in medical settings necessitates adaptations, often shifting the focus from full symptom recovery to improved functioning and emphasizing a multidisciplinary approach (Magidson & Weisberg, 2014).

Palliative and End-of-Life Existential Support: In palliative care, advanced interventions address existential suffering (Tarbi et al., 2023; Wong & Yu, 2021). Existential Positive Psychology (PP 2.0) emphasizes transforming suffering as a foundation for wellbeing and cultivating spiritual capabilities to achieve personal growth and flourishing (Tarbi et al., 2023; Wong & Yu, 2021).

- **Dignity Therapy (DT):** DT is a novel, brief psychotherapeutic intervention for patients near the end of life, designed to relieve psychological and existential distress (Chochinov et al., 2005; Fitchett et al., 2015; George, 2023; Martínez et al., 2017). It encourages patients to discuss what matters most and results in a "generativity document" they can bequeath to family (Chochinov et al., 2005). Research suggests DT is beneficial, particularly showing efficacy in reducing anxiety and depression scores in patients with high levels of baseline psychological distress (Martínez et al., 2017).
- **Integrative Meaning Therapy (IMT):** IMT, a form of dialectical palliative counseling, seeks to guide clients to a deeper understanding of their problems from a larger perspective and discover their true identity and place in the world, facilitating resilience (Wong & Yu, 2021). Life review or reminiscence is a helpful component for palliative care patients (Wong & Yu, 2021).

Supporting Families and Caregivers

The emotional and psychological strain on family caregivers (FCGs) is significant, with many surpassing clinical cut-offs for depression and anxiety symptoms (Banerjee et al., 2017; Dionne-Odom et al., 2018).

Caregiver Needs and Interventions: Family caregivers of older adults with cancer are often underprepared and demonstrate a strong interest in receiving formal support services, particularly education/training and assistance from organizations

(Dionne-Odom et al., 2018). For cancer caregivers, therapeutic interventions generally fall into three categories: psychoeducational (64%), skills training (22%), and therapeutic counseling (15%) (Ferrell & Wittenberg, 2017). Psychoeducational interventions have been shown to positively impact caregivers' knowledge and capacity to provide care, as well as improve psychological correlates of burden (e.g., depressive and anxious symptoms) (K. R. Delaney et al., 2017). Care for the patient-caregiver dyad is essential, as integrated interventions, like telephone Interpersonal Counseling, have resulted in significant decreases in depression and anxiety symptoms for both patients and informal caregivers (Dalirirad et al., 2021; K. R. Delaney et al., 2017; Northouse et al., 2012).

Culturally Sensitive, Affirming, and Trauma-Informed Care

Trauma-Informed Care (TIC): Trauma is a pervasive public health problem requiring nurses to adopt a Trauma-Informed Care approach (Guest & Miller, 2024). Key TIC principles involve incorporating trauma screening, training staff in trauma-specific treatments, and ensuring patient involvement (Goldstein et al., 2024; Levenson et al., 2023). Universal trauma precautions, which involve routinely anticipating that individuals have a history of trauma, are recommended in nursing practice (Guest & Miller, 2024). The implementation of TIC strategies, such as focusing on engagement, involvement, and cross-sector collaboration, has been shown to improve patient and system outcomes across diverse settings, including oncology and mental health (Goldstein et al., 2024).

Serving Sexual and Gender Minority (SGM) and Forced Migrant Populations: There is a significant lack of research exploring the mental health and acculturation needs of sexual and/or gender minority (SGM) forced migrants (Clarke, n.d.). These individuals face severe stressors throughout their lives, including pervasive violence, discrimination, economic exclusion, and barriers to healthcare access (Hermaszewska et al., 2022).

- **Culturally Affirming Practice:** Counselling psychologists are encouraged to avoid pathologization of non-Western mental health concepts and use culturally adapted tools. Affirmative SGM practice requires inclusive facilities, appropriate staff training, and inclusive materials. Trauma-Informed and Affirmative Mental Health Practices are necessary for working with LGBTQ+ clients (Levenson et al., 2023).
- **Intersectionality:** The concept of "intersectionalities of influence" highlights how multiple social identities (e.g., race, gender, citizenship) intersect to affect health outcomes, necessitating an ecosystemic framework for under-

standing individual issues within familial, community, and societal realms (Guruge & Khanlou, 2004).

- **Culturally Competent Care:** Delivering culturally competent nursing care, community partnerships, and advocacy efforts is essential to address mental health disparities in underserved populations, including LGBTQ+ individuals and racial/ethnic minorities (Yamada & Brekke, 2008). Effective care requires treatment models to be culturally adapted to align with the expectations, needs, and goals of the specific cultural group, as interventions normed on one population may not be equally effective with others (Chochinov et al., 2005; Kague, n.d.; Yamada & Brekke, 2008).

The goal of broadening horizons in nursing practice and education is to empower nurses to address holistic patient needs, promote resilience, and mitigate suffering in a complex and diverse world.

METHODOLOGY

The methodology for this book chapter is like an architect designing a specialized hospital wing. Instead of relying on a single blueprint (one study type), the architect uses systematic geological surveys (meta-analyses) to confirm the foundation's strength (therapeutic alliance and core CBT efficacy), focus group interviews with future staff (qualitative studies) to understand their workflow needs and barriers (nurse role beliefs and systemic issues), and detailed blueprints from various specialized builders (implementation frameworks like TIC and SCAP) to ensure the specialized rooms (different care settings, e.g., palliative, diverse populations) are functional, integrated, and ready for training new employees. The final output is a cohesive, functional structure designed to improve patient outcomes.

I. Overall Approach and Conceptual Framework

The chapter utilizes a synthesis methodology, grounding its arguments in several distinct yet convergent conceptual frameworks:

1. **Psychotherapy Integration Perspective:** The chapter adopts the perspective that psychotherapy integration is now common practice globally, aiming to look beyond single therapeutic approaches to enhance efficacy and efficiency. This includes exploring different types of integration, such as assimilative, theoretical, and common factors integration (Aafjes-van Doorn et al., 2018).

2. **Nursing and Professional Competency Focus:** The methodology centers on the nurse's role, particularly in identifying and overcoming barriers to providing psychosocial care. This involves examining nurses' self-efficacy, role beliefs, and the need for competency development in therapeutic interactions and integrated care approaches (Clarke, n.d.; Melton, PhD, Abpp, 2017; Suzuki, n.d.).
3. **Multilevel/Ecosystemic Context:** For diverse populations, the approach utilizes an ecosystemic framework to locate individual health issues within familial, community, and social realms (Guruge & Khanlou, 2004). This includes considering the "intersectionalities of influence" that affect health outcomes among marginalized groups (Guruge & Khanlou, 2004).

II. Data Sources and Review Strategies

The methodology relies on systematically reviewing and synthesizing empirical evidence from diverse fields:

A. Systematic Literature Review and Meta-Analytic Synthesis

The chapter employs findings from high-level synthesis methods, similar to those used in the source material, to establish the empirical foundation for various interventions.

- **Psychotherapy Integration Training:** The chapter draws on systematic reviews examining the efficacy of training in psychotherapy integration, noting the typical methods include longer (at least 12 weeks) group trainings that incorporate experiential, didactic, and supervision elements (Aafjes-van Doorn et al., 2018).
- **Therapeutic Relationship/Alliance:** The methodology incorporates meta-analytic reviews of the therapeutic relationship, specifically the alliance in individual psychotherapy, confirming its substantial and consistent contribution to outcomes independent of the specific treatment type (Horvath et al., 2011; Norcross & Lambert, 2018).
- **Evidence-Based Interventions (EBI):** Synthesis includes empirically supported treatments like Cognitive Behavioral Therapy (CBT), especially its adaptations for use in medical settings (e.g., psycho-oncology) (Magidson & Weisberg, 2014; Melton, PhD, Abpp, 2017; Travado, 2015). This approach requires balancing specialization with generalization and adapting outcomes to improved functioning rather than full symptom recovery (Magidson & Weisberg, 2014).

- **Caregiver Interventions:** The methodology synthesizes studies on interventions for informal cancer caregivers (ICs), categorizing them into: psychoeducation (the largest category), problem-solving/skills building, supportive therapy, family/couples therapy, CBT, interpersonal therapy (IPT), complementary and alternative medicine (CAM), and existential therapy (Applebaum & Breitbart, 2013; K. R. Delaney et al., 2017).

B. Qualitative Research and Needs Assessment

The methodology integrates findings from qualitative studies to understand contextual realities, professional perceptions, and implementation barriers:

- **Nurse Role Beliefs and Barriers (Oncology):** This involves incorporating findings from qualitative descriptive designs using focus group methodology (Suzuki, n.d.). Key research questions guiding this area include what nurses believe their role is in psychosocial care, and what is required for nurses to take on a greater role (e.g., training, support). Data analysis relies on methods such as thematic content analysis (e.g., Burnard's 14 steps) and the use of key codes and field notes to capture nurse narratives (Suzuki, n.d.).
- **Existential and Palliative Care:** It utilizes qualitative and mixed-methods research detailing specialized brief psychotherapeutic interventions like Dignity Therapy (DT) (Chochinov et al., 2005; Martínez et al., 2017) and Integrative Meaning Therapy (IMT) (Wong & Yu, 2021). For DT, data collection involves a manualized protocol using semi-structured interviews (30–60 minutes) to create a "generativity document" (Chochinov et al., 2005; Martínez et al., 2017).
- **Diverse Populations (SGM Forced Migrants):** The methodology integrates findings from qualitative studies and systematic reviews focused on the lived experiences of sexual and/or gender minority (SGM) forced migrants, often employing paradigms like Constructivist Grounded Theory (CGT), reflective practice, and a qualitative systematic review (meta-ethnography) to develop theoretical models (Clarke, n.d.; Hermaszewska et al., 2022).

C. Implementation and Training Models:

The chapter draws heavily on pedagogical and organizational implementation frameworks to propose practical next steps:

- **Trauma-Informed Care (TIC) Implementation:** The approach synthesizes systematic reviews on TIC implementation, using frameworks like

SAMHSA's 10 TIC implementation domains (e.g., engagement, collaboration) to map successful strategies and outcomes (Goldstein et al., 2024).

- **Cultural Competence Assessment:** The methodology requires referencing tools and approaches like the Sociocultural Assessment Protocol (SCAP), which is designed to identify and respond to key sociocultural issues (e.g., stigma, social support, self-identity) across different populations and settings (Yamada & Brekke, 2008).
- **Training Development:** The methodology supports the development of standardized curricula, such as for CBT in medical settings, using techniques like identifying a parsimonious set of common techniques that cut across clinical presentations and disease management issues (Magidson & Weisberg, 2014). For Psychiatric Mental Health Advanced Practice Registered Nurses (PMH APRNs), the methodological foundation includes workforce analysis and identifying critical content gaps in education, such as in integrated care, child mental health, and telehealth (K. R. Delaney & Vanderhoef, 2019; Travado, 2015).

III. Dissemination and Future Directions

The final component of the methodology involves translating research findings into actionable recommendations for nursing practice, education, and policy (Aafjes-van Doorn et al., 2018; Norcross & Lambert, 2018). This includes:

- **Practice Recommendations:** Offering practical advice to nurses (e.g., advanced practitioners in oncology) on how to use specific techniques (e.g., relaxation, thought stopping) within their defined scope of practice (Melton, PhD, Abpp, 2017).
- **Training Implications:** Highlighting the need to integrate these findings into nursing curricula, such as training medical staff in psychosocial and communication skills (Banerjee et al., 2017; Travado, 2015).
- **Policy Advocacy:** Using the accumulated evidence base to advocate for the inclusion of psychosocial care as a specific area of service provision in health policies and cancer plans (Travado, 2015).

The methodology employed ensures that the proposed book chapter is grounded in diverse evidence, reflective of professional challenges, and oriented toward measurable, integrated clinical practice improvements.

RESULTS

The evidence synthesized across nursing specialties, family care, and diverse populations overwhelmingly supports the necessity of integrating psychotherapeutic and psychosocial interventions into core nursing practice. Key findings across the four main areas of this chapter include:

Psychotherapy in Specialized Nursing (Oncology)

Communication Skills Training (CST) programs for oncology nurses are feasible and acceptable. These programs significantly impact nurses' self-efficacy and lead to the uptake of empathic communication and clarifying skills (Banerjee et al., 2017).

Effective communication is linked to improved patient recovery rates, better pain control, adherence to treatment, enhanced psychological functioning, and overall quality of life (QOL) (Banerjee et al., 2017). Specifically, trained nurses demonstrate improved ability to ask patients about emotions and cognitions associated with pain and use fewer paternalistic statements regarding pain management (Canivet et al., 2014).

Dignity Therapy (DT) is an empirically validated, brief psychotherapeutic intervention designed to address psychosocial and existential distress in terminally ill patients. It invites patients to discuss issues important for their legacy, resulting in a "generativity document" (Chochinov et al., 2005; Martínez et al., 2017).

DT demonstrates high patient satisfaction (91–93%) and is associated with a heightened sense of dignity, purpose, and meaning (Chochinov et al., 2005; Fitchett et al., 2015; Martínez et al., 2017). It shows efficacy in reducing suffering and depressive symptoms, particularly in patients experiencing high baseline psychological distress (Martínez et al., 2017).

The Foundational Role of the PMH APN

The practice of psychotherapy is intrinsically mandated within the scope of practice for the Psychiatric Mental Health Advanced Practice Nurse (PMH APN). PMH APN programs are required to cover a minimum of two psychotherapy modalities for certification (H. Delaney & Casey, 2022; K. R. Delaney et al., n.d., 2017; K. R. Delaney & Vanderhoef, 2019).

PMH APRNs are educated at the graduate level (masters or doctoral) to provide the full range of mental health services, including diagnosis, treatment, pharmacotherapy, and psychotherapy.

PMH APNs are valuable partners in integrated care models and wellness initiatives, helping clients with serious mental illness (SMI) develop self-management plans by increasing their self-efficacy and empowerment (K. R. Delaney & Vanderhoef, 2019).

However, the effective utilization of PMH APRNs is hampered by misinformation about their scope of practice in federal reports and market pressures that often limit post-graduation practice to medication management, despite their extensive training in psychotherapy (K. R. Delaney et al., 2017).

Focus on the Patient-Caregiver Dyad

Family caregivers (FCGs) experience substantial stress and are at risk for psychological impairment, sleep disturbances, and physical health changes. FCGs report a high interest in receiving formal support, especially education or training (Applebaum & Breitbart, 2013; Dionne-Odom et al., 2018).

It is crucial to consider the patient-caregiver dyad as the unit of care. Interventions delivered jointly to patients and caregivers can significantly reduce negative effects, improve caregiver coping, knowledge, and quality of life, and may lead to decreases in patient symptoms (Dionne-Odom et al., 2018; Ferrell & Wittenberg, 2017; Smith-Coggins et al., 2006).

Oncology nurses frequently encounter difficult family dynamics, confirming the need for communication skills that effectively extend to family interactions. DT is one example of an intervention that benefits both the patient and the family by providing a legacy document (Chochinov et al., 2005; Smith-Coggins et al., 2006).

Addressing Diverse Populations

There is a significant lack of research exploring the mental health and acculturation needs of sexual and/or gender minority (SGM) forced migrants. This population faces extreme hostility, pervasive violence, discrimination, and barriers to healthcare (Clarke, n.d.; Hermaszewska et al., 2022).

The asylum process itself can be re-traumatizing, and isolation and loneliness impede successful acculturation (Clarke, n.d.).

An ecosystemic framework is necessary to understand how "intersectionalities of influence" (e.g., race, gender, citizenship) affect the health outcomes of marginalized groups (Barker & Buchanan-Barker, 2011; Guruge & Khanlou, 2004).

Affirmative practice requires inclusive facilities, staff training, and attention to the unique needs of transgender individuals, who are often the most marginalized segment of the SGM community (Hermaszewska et al., 2022).

DISCUSSION AND IMPLICATIONS

The convergence of clinical research and professional role analyses indicates that the future of high-quality nursing hinges upon a renewed commitment to integrated psychosocial care.

The Mandate for Patient-Centered Care: The findings unequivocally establish that effective psychosocial support is not an optional add-on but a fundamental, mandated dimension of high-quality patient-centered care (Corso & Gage, 2016; Kaas, 2020). The success demonstrated by CST in enhancing patient outcomes, such as improving pain control and adherence (Canivet et al., 2014), elevates communication and psychosocial skill development to a core clinical competency (Banerjee et al., 2017). While nurses generally consider psychosocial care a fundamental nursing activity, greater emphasis must be placed on communicating the clinical significance of this care to ensure systematic involvement (Suzuki, n.d.). Failing to provide formalized, systematic psychosocial care, which includes assessment, monitoring, and referral, leaves patients in a precarious position given the risks of psychological distress (PD) (Harker et al., 2016; Suzuki, n.d.).

Overcoming Professional Barriers: The reliance on individual nurse volition to provide psychosocial care, irrespective of specialty, must be challenged through institutional clarity and policy. Nurses' role beliefs are critical to clinical practice, yet structural barriers (lack of time, workload, lack of accountability) persist (K. R. Delaney et al., 2017; K. R. Delaney & Vanderhoef, 2019; Valente, 2017). Policy implications are particularly strong for the PMH APN workforce, whose capabilities are often obscured from federal health agencies. Advocating for policies that allow PMH APNs to practice to the full extent of their license, including independent authority for psychotherapy, is necessary to mitigate mental health provider shortages, especially in rural and underserved areas. When nurses are educated, confident, and their role is clearly supported to include providing psychosocial care, clinical practice will reflect that appraisal (Suzuki, n.d.).

Holistic Care and Family Inclusion: The necessity of addressing the patient-caregiver dyad as the primary unit of care is a defining feature of holistic practice (Dionne-Odom et al., 2018; Given & Given, n.d.; Martínez et al., 2017). Interventions must actively engage family members to reduce caregiver burden and improve outcomes for both parties (Ferrell & Wittenberg, 2017). Nurse leaders need to promote competency in complex family interactions (Banerjee et al., 2017). Specialized interventions like Dignity Therapy illuminate how psychosocial care can intrinsically benefit the family unit by extending the patient's legacy and fostering a heightened sense of meaning and purpose that lessens patient suffering (Canivet et al., 2014; Chochinov et al., 2005). This dual benefit underscores why family inclusion is inseparable from true holistic nursing care.

Implementing Culturally Affirming Practice: For the chapter's vision of broadening horizons to be equitable, nursing practice must move beyond basic competence toward culturally sensitive and affirming care (Yamada & Brekke, 2008). This requires nurses to adopt an ecosystemic framework to understand individual difficulties within familial, community, and societal realms, recognizing how "intersectionalities of influence" create profound vulnerabilities for marginalized populations (Guruge & Khanlou, 2004). Affirmative practice necessitates specific changes: avoiding the pathologization of non-Western concepts (Clarke, n.d.), implementing Trauma-Informed Care (TIC) strategies (Goldstein et al., 2024; Hermaszewska et al., 2022), and ensuring inclusive facilities and staff trained on the unique mental health needs of SGM individuals, especially transgender forced migrants who face pervasive violence and discrimination (Hermaszewska et al., 2022).

CONCLUSION AND FUTURE DIRECTIONS

The successful integration of psychotherapy across nursing specialties, with robust attention to families and diverse populations, is not merely an enhancement but an essential component of high-quality, patient-centered care. The evidence confirms that effective communication and specialized psychosocial interventions significantly impact patient physical and psychological outcomes, arguing against the dominance of the biomedical model.

Nursing leadership, educators, and policymakers must advocate for enhanced nursing education and policy changes to support integrated care. Key actions include:

Consolidating general communication skills training with specific modules tailored to clinical challenges, such as cancer pain management, to maximize efficacy.

Developing and implementing systematic frameworks for Trauma-Informed Care across clinical settings to improve patient engagement and outcomes.

Ensuring PMH APNs are supported to practice to the full scope of their license, including providing psychotherapy, to address critical workforce gaps.

Establishing systems for documentation and accountability for formalized, systematic psychosocial care, which is currently often volitional and underreported.

FUTURE RESEARCH

Future research must address significant gaps in knowledge, particularly for the most marginalized populations. Research is urgently needed to:

Explore the mental health and acculturation needs of SGM forced migrants, including the specific barriers and facilitators to help-seeking.

Investigate the impact of CST programs on relevant patient outcomes (beyond intermediate outcomes like nurse self-efficacy).

Clarify nurses' conceptual understanding and operational definition of "formalized, systematic psychosocial care" versus "comfort care" to reduce professional confusion and inconsistency in practice.

Support cost-analysis studies on efficient staffing models and the contributions of PMH RNs and APNs within integrated care teams to inform wider implementation.

By broadening horizons in nursing practice and education, we empower nurses to address holistic patient needs, promote resilience, mitigate suffering, and significantly improve health outcomes in an increasingly complex and diverse world.

REFERENCES

Aafjes-van Doorn, K., Klinar Alfaro, D., Fialová, M., & Kamsteeg, C. (2018). Psychotherapy integration training around the globe: A personal and empirical perspective. *Journal of Psychotherapy Integration*, *28*(4), 505–520. DOI: 10.1037/int0000135

Antebi-Gruszka, N., & Scheer, J. R. (2021). Associations Between Trauma-Informed Care Components and Multiple Health and Psychosocial Risks Among LGBTQ Survivors of Intimate Partner Violence. *Journal of Mental Health Counseling*, *43*(2), 139–156. DOI: 10.17744/mehc.43.2.04

Applebaum, A. J., & Breitbart, W. (2013). Care for the cancer caregiver: A systematic review. *Palliative & Supportive Care*, *11*(3), 231–252. DOI: 10.1017/S1478951512000594

Banerjee, S. C., Manna, R., Coyle, N., Penn, S., Gallegos, T. E., Zaider, T., Krueger, C. A., Bialer, P. A., Bylund, C. L., & Parker, P. A. (2017). The implementation and evaluation of a communication skills training program for oncology nurses. *Translational Behavioral Medicine*, *7*(3), 615–623. DOI: 10.1007/s13142-017-0473-5

Barker, P. J., & Buchanan-Barker, P. (2011). Mental Health Nursing and the Politics of Recovery: A Global Reflection. *Archives of Psychiatric Nursing*, *25*(5), 350–358. DOI: 10.1016/j.apnu.2011.03.009

Buckley, C., Radhakrishnan, A., Boran, L., Brennan, M., & Travers, Á. (n.d.). Barriers and Facilitators of Help-Seeking for LGBTQ+ Survivors of Sexual Violence. *Systematic Reviews*.

Canivet, D., Delvaux, N., Gibon, A.-S., Brancart, C., Slachmuylder, J.-L., & Razavi, D. (2014). Improving communication in cancer pain management nursing: A randomized controlled study assessing the efficacy of a communication skills training program. *Supportive Care in Cancer*, *22*(12), 3311–3320. DOI: 10.1007/s00520-014-2357-2

Chochinov, H. M., Hack, T., Hassard, T., Kristjanson, L. J., McClement, S., & Harlos, M. (2005). Dignity Therapy: A Novel Psychotherapeutic Intervention for Patients Near the End of Life. *Journal of Clinical Oncology*, *23*(24), 5520–5525. DOI: 10.1200/JCO.2005.08.391

Clarke, T. (n.d.). *Exploring the mental health and acculturation needs of sexual and/or gender minority forced migrants*.

Corso, K. A., & Gage, D. (2016). Nurses and Psychologists Advancing the Patient-Centered Medical Home Model. *Nursing Administration Quarterly*, *40*(3), 192–201. DOI: 10.1097/NAQ.0000000000000176

Dalirirad, H., Seyedfatemi, N., & Najafi, T. (2021). Effect of an Educational Support Programme on Caregiver Burden Among the Family Members of Patients Undergoing Coronary Artery Bypass Graft Surgery. *Sultan Qaboos University Medical Journal*, *21*(2), e266–e274. DOI: 10.18295/squmj.2021.21.02.016

Delaney, H., & Casey, C. (2022). The promise of a four-day week? A critical appraisal of a management-led initiative. *Employee Relations: The International Journal*, *44*(1), 176–190. DOI: 10.1108/ER-02-2021-0056

Delaney, K. R., Cooper, J. L., & Nshemerewire, S. (n.d.). *THE PRACTICE OF CHILD MENTAL HEALTH NURSES.*

Delaney, K. R., Naegle, M. A., Valentine, N. M., Antai-Otong, D., Groh, C. J., & Brennaman, L. (2017). The Effective Use of Psychiatric Mental Health Nurses in Integrated Care: Policy Implications for Increasing Quality and Access to Care. *The Journal of Behavioral Health Services & Research*. Advance online publication. DOI: 10.1007/s11414-017-9555-x

Delaney, K. R., & Vanderhoef, D. (2019). The Psychiatric Mental Health Advanced Practice Registered Nurse Workforce: Charting the Future. *Journal of the American Psychiatric Nurses Association*, *25*(1), 11–18. DOI: 10.1177/1078390318806571

Dionne-Odom, J. N., Applebaum, A. J., Ornstein, K. A., Azuero, A., Warren, P. P., Taylor, R. A., Rocque, G. B., Kvale, E. A., Demark-Wahnefried, W., Pisu, M., Partridge, E. E., Martin, M. Y., & Bakitas, M. A. (2018). Participation and interest in support services among family caregivers of older adults with cancer. *Psycho-Oncology*, *27*(3), 969–976. DOI: 10.1002/pon.4603

Drew, B. L. (2014). The Evolution of the Role of the Psychiatric Mental Health Advanced Practice Registered Nurse in the United States. *Archives of Psychiatric Nursing*, *28*(5), 298–300. DOI: 10.1016/j.apnu.2014.07.002

Durbin, A., Durbin, J., Hensel, J. M., & Deber, R. (2016). Barriers and Enablers to Integrating Mental Health into Primary Care: A Policy Analysis. *The Journal of Behavioral Health Services & Research*, *43*(1), 127–139. DOI: 10.1007/s11414-013-9359-6

Estes, J. M., & Karten, C. (2014). Nursing Expertise and the Evaluation of Psychosocial Distress in Patients With Cancer and Survivors. *Clinical Journal of Oncology Nursing*, *18*(5), 598–600. DOI: 10.1188/14.CJON.598-600

Ferrell, B., & Wittenberg, E. (2017). A review of family caregiving intervention trials in oncology. *CA: a Cancer Journal for Clinicians*, *67*(4), 318–325. DOI: 10.3322/caac.21396

Fitchett, G., Emanuel, L., Handzo, G., Boyken, L., & Wilkie, D. J. (2015). Care of the human spirit and the role of dignity therapy: A systematic review of dignity therapy research. *BMC Palliative Care*, *14*(1), 8. DOI: 10.1186/s12904-015-0007-1

George, D. A. S. (2023). *Addressing India's Healthcare Worker Shortage: Evaluating Strategies to Improve Medical Education and Retention*. https://doi.org/DOI: 10.5281/ZENODO.8370878

Given, B., & Given, C. W. (n.d.). *WHAT KNOWLEDGE AND SKILLS DO CAREGIVERS NEED?* Goldstein, E., Chokshi, B., Melendez-Torres, G., Rios, A., Jelley, M., & Lewis-O'Connor, A. (2024). Effectiveness of Trauma-Informed Care Implementation in Health Care Settings: Systematic Review of Reviews and Realist Synthesis. *The Permanente Journal*, *28*(1), 135–150. DOI: 10.7812/TPP/23.127

Guest, H., & Miller, C. L. (2024). Trauma-Informed Care in Nursing Curricula: Development of a Simulation-Based Educational Framework to Guide Health Professions. *Nursing Education Perspectives*, *45*(5), 271–275. DOI: 10.1097/01.NEP.0000000000001313

Guruge, S., & Khanlou, N. (2004). *Intersectionalities of Influence: Researching the Health of Immigrant and Refugee Women. 36*(3).

Harker, R., Pidgeon, A. M., Klaassen, F., & King, S. (2016). Exploring resilience and mindfulness as preventative factors for psychological distress burnout and secondary traumatic stress among human service professionals. *Work (Reading, Mass.)*, *54*(3), 631–637. DOI: 10.3233/WOR-162311

Hermaszewska, S., Sweeney, A., Camminga, B., Botelle, R., Elliott, K., & Sin, J. (2022). Lived experiences of transgender forced migrants and their mental health outcomes: Systematic review and meta-ethnography. *BJPsych Open*, *8*(3), e91. DOI: 10.1192/bjo.2022.51

Horvath, A. O., Del Re, A. C., Flückiger, C., & Symonds, D. (2011). Alliance in individual psychotherapy. *Psychotherapy (Chicago, Ill.)*, *48*(1), 9–16. DOI: 10.1037/a0022186

Kaas, M. J. (2020). Will We Be Ready? Preparing Psychiatric-Mental Health Nurses for Future Practice. *Journal of the American Psychiatric Nurses Association*, *26*(1), 112–119. DOI: 10.1177/1078390319878767

Kague, J. (n.d.). *Addressing Mental Health Challenges in Pediatric Nursing: Strategies for Comprehensive Care*.

Levenson, J. S., Craig, S. L., & Austin, A. (2023). Trauma-informed and affirmative mental health practices with LGBTQ+ clients. *Psychological Services*, *20*(Suppl 1), 134–144. DOI: 10.1037/ser0000540

Lyu, X.-C., Jiang, H.-J., Lee, L.-H., Yang, C.-I., & Sun, X.-Y. (2024). Oncology nurses' experiences of providing emotional support for cancer patients: A qualitative study. *BMC Nursing*, *23*(1), 58. DOI: 10.1186/s12912-024-01718-1

Magidson, J. F., & Weisberg, R. B. (2014). Implementing Cognitive Behavioral Therapy in Specialty Medical Settings. *Cognitive and Behavioral Practice*, *21*(4), 367–371. DOI: 10.1016/j.cbpra.2014.08.003

Martínez, M., Arantzamendi, M., Belar, A., Carrasco, J. M., Carvajal, A., Rullán, M., & Centeno, C. (2017). 'Dignity therapy', a promising intervention in palliative care: A comprehensive systematic literature review. *Palliative Medicine*, *31*(6), 492–509. DOI: 10.1177/0269216316665562

Melton, L. (2017). Brief introduction to cognitive behavioral therapy for the advanced practitioner in oncology. *Journal of the Advanced Practitioner in Oncology*, *8*(2), 188. DOI: 10.6004/jadpro.2017.8.2.6

Norcross, J. C., & Lambert, M. J. (2018). Psychotherapy relationships that work III. *Psychotherapy (Chicago, Ill.)*, *55*(4), 303–315. DOI: 10.1037/pst0000193

Northouse, L., Williams, A., Given, B., & McCorkle, R. (2012). Psychosocial Care for Family Caregivers of Patients With Cancer. *Journal of Clinical Oncology*, *30*(11), 1227–1234. DOI: 10.1200/JCO.2011.39.5798

Smith-Coggins, R., Howard, S. K., Mac, D. T., Wang, C., Kwan, S., Rosekind, M. R., Sowb, Y., Balise, R., Levis, J., & Gaba, D. M. (2006). Improving Alertness and Performance in Emergency Department Physicians and Nurses: The Use of Planned Naps. *Annals of Emergency Medicine*, *48*(5), 596–604.e3. DOI: 10.1016/j.annemergmed.2006.02.005

Suzuki, K. (n.d.). *COLLEGE OF SOCIAL AND BEHAVIORAL SCIENCES*.

Tarbi, E. C., Broden, E. G., Rosa, W. E., Hayden, A., & Morgan, B. E. (2023). Existential Care in Daily Nursing Practice. *AJN. The American Journal of Nursing*, *123*(10), 42–48. DOI: 10.1097/01.NAJ.0000979092.39243.d4

Travado, L. (2015). *The Role and Challenges of Psycho-Oncology in Improving Cancer care*. Unpublished. https://doi.org/DOI: 10.13140/RG.2.1.2076.8086

Valente, S. M. (2017). Managing Professional and Nurse–Patient Relationship Boundaries in Mental Health. *Journal of Psychosocial Nursing and Mental Health Services*, *55*(1), 45–51. DOI: 10.3928/02793695-20170119-09

Wong, P. T. P., & Yu, T. T. F. (2021). Existential Suffering in Palliative Care: An Existential Positive Psychology Perspective. *Medicina*, *57*(9), 924. DOI: 10.3390/medicina57090924

Yamada, A.-M., & Brekke, J. S. (2008). Addressing mental health disparities through clinical competence not just cultural competence: The need for assessment of sociocultural issues in the delivery of evidence-based psychosocial rehabilitation services. *Clinical Psychology Review*, *28*(8), 1386–1399. DOI: 10.1016/j.cpr.2008.07.006

KEY TERMS AND DEFINITIONS

CBT (Cognitive Behavioral Therapy): An evidence-based intervention and empirically supported treatment. It has demonstrated efficacy in medical settings, such as reducing anxiety symptoms in breast cancer patients and managing fatigue in cancer survivors.

Dignity Therapy (DT): A novel, brief psychotherapeutic intervention designed specifically for terminally ill patients to address psychosocial and existential distress. It results in a "generativity document" (a legacy document) that patients can bequeath to family or friends.

Ecosystemic Framework: A conceptual approach utilized for diverse populations that helps locate individual health issues within familial, community, and societal realms.

Intersectionalities of Influence: The concept that highlights how multiple social identity dimensions (e.g., race, gender, citizenship) intersect to affect the health outcomes of marginalized groups.

Patient-Caregiver Dyad: Refers to the patient and their family caregiver, which is critical to view as the unit of care. Interventions delivered jointly to the dyad can significantly reduce caregiver stress, improve coping skills, and decrease patient symptoms.

Patient-Centered Care: A shifting paradigm in the contemporary healthcare environment. Effective psychosocial support is identified as a fundamental, mandated dimension of high-quality, comprehensive, and equitable patient-centered care.

PMH APN (Psychiatric Mental Health Advanced Practice Nurse): An advanced practice nurse (educated at the masters or doctoral level) for whom the practice of psychotherapy is an intrinsic and foundational role. They are trained to provide the full range of mental health services, including diagnosis, treatment, pharmacotherapy, and psychotherapy, and are key leaders in integrated care models.

Psychological Distress (PD): A universal clinical phenomenon that is highly prevalent (e.g., up to 38% of cancer patients experience high levels of distress). Psychosocial care is fundamentally aimed at the detection, diagnosis, treatment, and prevention of PD.

Psychosocial Care: A systematic approach to care that is aimed at the detection, diagnosis, treatment, and prevention of psychological distress. It is fundamentally recognized as nursing work, although often lacks formal reflection or systematic application.

Psychotherapy Integration: The process of learning from different therapeutic viewpoints to enhance efficacy and efficiency, often looking beyond the confines of single therapeutic approaches. This practice is common globally.

Trauma-Informed Care (TIC): An approach that shifts the clinical focus from "What's wrong with you?" to "What happened to you?". TIC principles involve realizing trauma's widespread impact, recognizing its signs and symptoms, integrating knowledge into practice, and actively resisting re-traumatization.

Chapter 2
Cultural Competence in Psychotherapeutic Nursing Practice

Kübra Tan
https://orcid.org/0000-0002-7591-8436
Artvin Coruh University, Turkey

ABSTRACT

In an era of increasing globalization, migration, and social change, cultural competence has emerged as a fundamental pillar of modern psychotherapeutic nursing. This chapter emphasizes that mental health care must transcend biological and psychosocial boundaries to incorporate a holistic understanding of a client's cultural identity, values, and belief systems. Because culture fundamentally shapes how individuals perceive illness and express distress, the nurse's ability to provide culturally sensitive care is the determining factor in building trust and ensuring treatment adherence. Central to this practice are the theoretical frameworks of Campinha-Bacote, which highlights the importance of self-awareness and cultural desire, and Leininger, which posits cultural congruence as the heart of care quality. Ultimately, cultural competence requires more than just external knowledge; it demands that nurses confront their own biases to foster ethical, empathic, and effective therapeutic relationships in an increasingly diverse healthcare landscape.

INTRODUCTION

Cultural competence is a core component of modern nursing practice. Today, healthcare services contain more cultural diversity than ever before as a result of migration, globalization, wars, social change, and the impact of communication

DOI: 10.4018/979-8-3373-6526-8.ch002

technologies. This diversity requires nurses to adopt a holistic approach, not only in biological and psychosocial terms but also in cultural terms. In psychotherapeutic nursing, the client's emotional, cognitive, and behavioral processes, as well as their cultural identity, belief system, values, and way of life, determine the direction of the therapeutic process.

While psychotherapeutic nursing aims to support mental well-being, it cannot overlook the individual's interaction with their environment, social roles, and cultural norms. Culture directly affects how a person defines illness, how they express psychological distress, and their help-seeking behaviors. Therefore, the nurse's ability to adopt an approach that is sensitive to cultural differences is a determining factor in establishing and maintaining therapeutic relationships. The absence of cultural sensitivity may lead to misunderstandings, ethical dilemmas, and non-adherence to treatment.

Cultural competence does not only refer to the nurse "knowing" different cultures, but also to becoming aware of their own cultural biases and using this awareness effectively in professional relationships. Campinha-Bacote's model explains this process in five fundamental dimensions: awareness, knowledge, skill, encounters, and desire. Leininger's transcultural nursing approach, on the other hand, places culture at the heart of nursing care and emphasizes that cultural congruence is directly related to the quality of care.

This chapter discusses the importance of cultural competence in psychotherapeutic nursing practice from both theoretical and practical perspectives. The aim is to strengthen nurses' ability to establish trust-based, empathic, and ethical therapeutic relationships with individuals from diverse cultural backgrounds. The chapter elaborates on the theoretical foundations of cultural competence, its reflections in the psychotherapeutic process, its ethical dimensions, and the educational and institutional strategies for its development.

1. THE CONCEPT OF CULTURAL COMPETENCE AND THEORETICAL FOUNDATIONS

1.1. The Concept of Cultural Competence

Cultural competence refers to the capacity of healthcare professionals to provide effective, respectful, and sensitive care to individuals from diverse cultural backgrounds. In nursing, this concept is not limited to cultural awareness alone; it also requires understanding individuals' values, beliefs, communication styles, and health behaviors and integrating these into the care process (Jeffreys, 2015). In psychotherapeutic nursing, cultural competence ensures that the therapeutic relationship is built on trust, empathy, and mutual understanding. When working with individuals who hold different cultural values, it is critically important for the success of the therapeutic process that the nurse is aware of their own biases, accepts the client's way of life without judgment, and communicates with cultural sensitivity (Campinha-Bacote, 2002). Today, cultural competence is recognized as an ethical obligation in the nursing profession in the United States. The International Council of Nurses (ICN, 2021) defines cultural competence as an inseparable component of the quality of professional care. A culturally competent nurse organizes the care plan in a meaningful and respectful manner, considering the individual's cultural values.

1.2. Components of Cultural Competence

Cultural competence is not a static field of knowledge but a dynamic learning process (Campinha-Bacote, 2011). Campinha-Bacote defines cultural competence through five key components: cultural awareness, knowledge, skill, encounters, and desire.

- **Cultural awareness** is the recognition of one's own cultural biases.
- **Cultural knowledge** involves understanding the health beliefs and behaviors of different cultures.
- **Cultural skill** is the ability to consider cultural differences in assessments and interventions.
- **Cultural encounters** are experiences gained through interactions with individuals from different cultures.
- **Cultural desire** refers to the internal motivation to become culturally competent (Campinha-Bacote 2002).

These components support nurses' development at both the cognitive and emotional levels. In psychotherapeutic nursing, cultural awareness and skills enhance the effectiveness of therapeutic communication and increase clients' trust (Douglas et al., 2014).

1.3. Theoretical Foundations and Models

1.3.1. Leininger's Transcultural Nursing Theory

Leininger emphasized that culture constitutes the essence of nursing care and developed the "Transcultural Nursing Theory" (Leininger & McFarland, 2006). According to this theory, care cannot be considered independently of the cultural context. Leininger's Sunrise Model evaluates the individual's culture together with elements such as belief systems, social structure, family organization, economy, technology and values. In psychotherapeutic nursing, this approach enables the nurse to understand the client's mental state not only within an individual framework but also within social and cultural frameworks. In this way, nurses can relate clients' sources of stress and coping styles to their cultural values (McFarland & Wehbe-Alamah, 2015).

1.3.2. Campinha-Bacote's Model of the Process of Cultural Competence

Campinha-Bacote (2002) describes cultural competence as "an ongoing developmental process rather than a goal." This model encourages nurses to learn through cultural interactions and continuously evaluate their own level of competence. In psychotherapeutic practice, this approach helps nurses correctly interpret clients' cultural expressions and narratives of psychological distress. For instance, when a client explains their emotional pain using cultural terms such as "being affected by the evil eye" or "fate," these expressions should be understood as part of a cultural meaning system. Interpreting these expressions without confusing them with medical pathologies is an indicator of culturally sensitive nursing.

1.3.3. Purnell's Model for Cultural Competence

Purnell (2016) proposed a holistic model that addresses cultural competence at both the individual and institutional levels. This model consists of 12 cultural domains, such as communication, family structure, religion, health beliefs, nutrition, and biological differences. In this respect, it enables the nurse to understand the patient not only from a biomedical perspective but also from a cultural perspective. In psychotherapeutic nursing, this approach provides guidance, particularly in issues such as the expression of emotions, privacy, social roles, and shame culture (Jeffreys, 2015).

1.4. The Importance of Cultural Competence in Psychotherapeutic Nursing

In psychotherapeutic nursing, cultural competence is essential for nurses to establish a trust-based, empathetic, and respectful relationship with clients. A nurse with a high level of cultural sensitivity does not focus solely on the symptoms of an illness; they also evaluate the meaning of these symptoms within their cultural context. Thus, misunderstandings and communication breakdowns are prevented (Papadopoulos 2006). A culturally insensitive approach may weaken the therapeutic process, undermine the client's trust, and reduce treatment participation (Douglas et al., 2014). In contrast, culturally competent nurses strengthen both mental recovery and the effectiveness of psychotherapeutic interventions by accepting the individual's cultural value system. Cultural competence in psychotherapeutic nursing is not only an ethical requirement but also a prerequisite for effective care. Leininger's culture-based care framework, Campinha-Bacote's process model of cultural competence and Purnell's holistic approach provide nurses with guidance to enhance their cultural awareness and diversify their practices. A culturally competent nurse incorporates the client's system of beliefs and values into the care process; thus, both clinical effectiveness and the depth of the therapeutic relationship increase.

2. THE IMPACT OF CULTURE ON THE PSYCHOTHERAPEUTIC PROCESS

2.1. The Relationship Between Culture, Identity and Mental Health

Culture is one of the primary determinants of an individual's identity; it shapes values, beliefs, behavioral patterns, and emotional expressions. In the psychotherapeutic process, culture is a significant factor that determines how individuals perceive themselves and their psychological distress (Kirmayer, 2012). Mental health is not only a product of biological or individual psychological processes but also of social norms, religious values, family roles, and cultural meaning systems. Therefore, in evaluating the factors that influence the therapeutic process, nurses must consider the client's cultural identity. In some cultures, individualism, personal expression, and autonomy are highly valued, whereas in collectivist cultures, community, family approval, and harmony are prioritized (Triandis, 2018). This difference can directly affect how the client expresses emotions during the therapeutic process and the nature of the trust relationship established with the nurse. In psychotherapeutic nursing practices, cultural identity is critically important for understanding how clients make sense of their psychological distress and how help-seeking behaviors are shaped (Bhugra & Bhui, 2018).

2.2. The Effect of Culture on Illness Perception and Help-Seeking Behavior

Culture determines how individuals perceive illness, interpret symptoms, and shape their help-seeking behaviors. For example, in some cultures, depression is regarded as a biological disorder, while in others, psychological distress may be interpreted as "lack of faith," "social nonconformity" or "a test of fate" (Kleinman, 1988). This may lead to misassessments and mismatches in interventions during the psychotherapeutic nursing process. The access of migrants or individuals with minority status to mental health services may be further restricted by additional cultural and linguistic barriers. For instance, a study published in 2024 reported that factors such as language barriers, trust issues, and stigma reduce the rates at which migrants seek mental health services (Soares, Cameira, Abreu & Pereira, 2024). In this context, a culturally sensitive nursing approach should aim to open up help-seeking pathways by respecting clients' cultural world of meaning. A culturally competent nurse does not evaluate these behaviors as wrong or irrational; instead, they understand the client's cultural framework and structure the therapeutic process accordingly.

2.3. Reflections of Cultural Differences on Therapeutic Communication

In psychotherapeutic nursing, communication is the cornerstone of therapeutic relationships. However, communication styles vary considerably from culture to culture. Verbal statements, silence, body language, use of personal space, and eye contact all carry cultural meanings (Hall, 1976). For example, in some Asian societies, eye contact is seen as disrespectful, whereas in Western societies, it is viewed as a sign of trust and sincerity. Similarly, in some cultures, an individual who expresses their emotions openly may be viewed as "honest and healthy," while in others such behavior may be seen as "a lack of self-control" (Wing Sue & Sue, 2008). A meta-study published in 2024 showed that nurses who received cultural competence training experienced significant improvements in their communication skills and established trust relationships with clients more rapidly (Osmancevic et al., 2025). This finding reveals the importance of reconstructing communication in psychotherapeutic nursing practices within a cultural context. A nurse who can communicate with cultural sensitivity increases the client's trust and strengthens the therapeutic alliance. Culturally competent communication involves not only linguistic but also emotional, cognitive, and contextual awareness (Jeffreys, 2015). For this reason, nurses must interpret clients' nonverbal cues (gestures, facial expressions, posture, silence) within their cultural context.

2.4. Expression of Emotions, Silence and Social Roles

The expression of emotion is a culturally learned behavior. Western cultures generally encourage emotional expression, whereas in Eastern societies, the suppression of emotions is regarded as a sign of maturity (Markus & Kitayama, 2014). In the therapeutic process, these differences can affect nurses' empathic understanding and interpretations. Simultaneously, the concept of power distance is reflected in the therapeutic relationship. Power distance refers to the extent to which less powerful members of a society accept and expect an unequal distribution of power. In cultures with high power distance, individuals may prefer to establish hierarchical relationships with healthcare professionals, making it difficult to develop an egalitarian relationship in therapy (Hofstede, 2001). Cultures such as Malaysia and Mexico, which have high power distance, tend to accept hierarchical structures in which authority is rarely questioned and decision-making is concentrated at the top. In cultures with low power distance, such as Denmark and New Zealand, people prefer flatter organizational structures and expect leaders to be accessible and open to contributions. For example, in a workplace with a high power distance, employees may not object to their managers' decisions even if they disagree with them. In this context, nurses need to reshape their communication style within the client's cultural perception of power. For example, in collectivist cultures such as Japan or Turkey, a client's silence may not indicate resistance or lack of interest; instead, it may be a sign of respect or thoughtfulness (Wing Sue & Sue, 2008). Therefore, interpretations made without awareness of the cultural context may lead to misunderstandings in therapeutic communications. Gender roles are also important cultural factors that affect the psychotherapeutic process. In some societies, women are not welcomed to express their emotions openly, while men are expected to avoid emotional behaviors that might be perceived as signs of weakness (Papadopoulos, 2021). This requires nurses to consider cultural expectations when evaluating clients' emotion regulation patterns.

2.5. Cross-Cultural Power Distance and the Therapeutic Relationship

Culture determines not only individual communication but also the balance of power between the client and nurse. Hofstede's concept of "power distance" explains the level at which societies relate to authority figures (Hofstede, 2001). In societies with a high power distance, individuals tend to accept healthcare professionals without question. This may cause nurses to experience difficulties in bringing the therapeutic relationship onto an egalitarian plane. In cultures with low power distance, individuals prefer to engage in open dialogue with health care professionals. In psychotherapeutic nursing, awareness of this difference affects how the client expresses themselves, participates in decision-making, and plays an active role in the treatment process (Bhugra & Bhui, 2018). Culture is an unseen yet crucial aspect of the psychotherapeutic process. It shapes an individual's identity, emotional expression, illness perception, and participation in the therapeutic relationship.

Therefore, it is not only a clinical skill but also an ethical responsibility for nurses to develop cultural awareness.

2.6. Cultural Appropriateness in Clinical Assessment and Interventions

In psychotherapeutic nursing, assessment and intervention processes require consideration of cultural meanings. For example, in some cultures, psychological distress is expressed somatically; therefore, focusing solely on psychological symptoms in the assessment process would be an incomplete approach (Sakai et al., 2025). In addition, the increasing number of culturally sensitive studies confirms this necessity (Lyons et al., 2025). In therapeutic nursing, intercultural sensitivity is a critical factor in terms of service accessibility and treatment effectiveness. A culturally sensitive nurse structures the therapeutic process by interpreting the client's behaviors not from their own cultural perspective but from the client's cultural context. In this way, nurses can strengthen empathy, reduce misunderstandings, and adopt a cross-culturally inclusive care approach.

3. THERAPEUTIC APPROACHES SENSITIVE TO CULTURAL DIVERSITY

3.1. Establishing a Therapeutic Relationship Based on Cultural Sensitivity

Establishing a therapeutic relationship with cultural sensitivity is not merely a technical skill in nursing care; it is also an ethical, communicative, and contextual approach. One study emphasized that culturally sensitive psychotherapy is not limited to technical adaptations; the therapist must also develop cultural awareness, humility, and a reflective attitude (Stingl & Hanewald, 2025). From the nurse's perspective, this approach requires reviewing one's own cultural biases and assumptions when communicating with the client, understanding the client's cultural world, and shaping the therapeutic process accordingly. Furthermore, nonverbal forms of communication (eye contact, personal space, and silence) carry different meanings in different cultures; being sensitive to these nuances strengthens the therapeutic relationship (Kittler et al., 2011; Son et al., 2025). The quality of the therapeutic alliance is directly related to the client's feeling of being understood by the therapist. Cultural sensitivity supports this process; conversely, cultural insensitivity may damage the relationship and lead the client to drop out of therapy early or to nonadherence to interventions (Osmancevic et al., 2025). In this context, the nurse's responsibilities include recognizing their own cultural identity and biases, gaining knowledge about the client's culture, accepting the client's way of life without judgment, and taking cultural needs into account throughout the therapeutic process.

3.2. Culture-Specific Psychotherapeutic Interventions

In today's multicultural societies, traditional psychotherapy models may not always be directly appropriate; therefore, culture-specific adaptations are required in psychotherapeutic nursing. For example, one study showed that a short-term, culturally adapted intervention called "Value-Based Counseling (VBC)" applied to immigrant and refugee populations significantly increased resilience and perspective-taking ability (Orang et al., 2023). Such strength-based approaches focus not on pathology but on the client's cultural resources and resilience. In addition, a positive psychology program developed for migrant and refugee groups, BAMBOO for Refugees, is a five-week, group-based, culturally adapted, strength-based intervention (Hendriks et al., 2024). These examples demonstrate the feasibility and effectiveness of culturally adapted psychotherapeutic interventions in nursing settings. Within culture-specific interventions, the following strategies are important: using materials that are appropriate to the client's language and communication style, reorganizing metaphors and narratives in a way that is culturally congruent, developing group work or community-based support models, and using intercultural interpreters or cultural mediators (Theodosopoulos et al., 2024). Nurses should also consider the individual's cultural identity and migration experiences that may influence trauma and help-seeking when preparing an intervention plan.

3.3. Working with Migrant, Refugee and Minority Groups

Migrant and refugee individuals face multiple barriers, such as language, culture, lack of knowledge about the system, stigma, and access to healthcare (Theodosopoulos et al., 2024; Liu et al., 2025). A review study revealed that migrants encounter barriers such as language, lack of cultural mediators, and poor system coordination during care transitions (e.g., from refugee clinics to the general healthcare system) (Liu et al., 2025).

Therefore, nurses must develop strategies at both systemic and individual levels when working with migrant and refugee clients. The following points are important in practice.

- Using interpreter or cultural mediator services
- Implementing empowerment-focused interventions in the context of the client's migration or refugee experience

- Developing sensitivity to stigma and discrimination in minority groups
- Integrating community-based support models and peer-support groups
- Ensuring that the nurse is familiar with institutional systems of cultural integration and referral (e.g., processes of access to services, referral mechanisms)

These approaches increase the effectiveness of psychotherapeutic nursing practices and improve the care experience of migrant and refugee clients. In summary, working with migrant, refugee, and minority groups requires not only individual therapeutic skills but also the development of cultural sensitivity, systemic awareness, and community-based approaches.

3.4. The Nurse's Role and Responsibilities in Cultural Competence

The active role of nurses is crucial for the success of therapeutic approaches that are sensitive to cultural diversity. Nurses should engage in continuous professional development by evaluating their cultural identity and assumptions, participate in cultural competence training within the team, and promote cultural sensitivity within their institution (Osmancevic et al., 2025). Furthermore, nurses should take a cultural history to clarify the client's cultural and migration experiences, create cultural care plans with the client, and adapt the therapeutic process to the client's culture. From an ethical perspective, they must respect the client's cultural values, avoid stereotyping, and remain aware of power relations (Son et al., 2025). At the institutional level, interpreter services, cultural mediators, and multilingual support materials should be readily available within the system. Therapeutic approaches sensitive to cultural diversity involve specific strategies related to the therapeutic relationship, intervention design, and client populations. These approaches should focus not only on the question "what to do if the client is from a different culture" but also on "how to actively integrate the client's cultural identity into the therapy process." Cultural sensitivity in psychotherapeutic nursing care is an indispensable component of therapeutic effectiveness and quality of care.

4. ETHICAL DIMENSIONS AND PROFESSIONAL RESPONSIBILITIES

4.1. Cultural Bias, Stereotyping and Ethical Dilemmas

In psychotherapeutic nursing practices, approaches that are insensitive to cultural differences frequently lead to ethical violations and damage the therapeutic process.

Cultural bias and stereotyping can negatively affect the therapeutic relationship between nurses and clients (Papadopoulos, 2006). Stereotypes involve making generalizations by assuming that individuals belonging to a particular culture share homogeneous characteristics. This can lead nurses to overlook the individuality of the client and make biased decisions (Dewing, 2020). From an ethical standpoint, such approaches violate the principles of respect, justice, non-maleficence, and autonomy. A culturally competent nurse acknowledges that clients may have different values and belief systems, makes decisions with this awareness, and avoids judgmental attitudes. The absence of cultural sensitivity can create a condition referred to as "ethical blindness," particularly when working with refugee, minority, or migrant individuals. In this case, the nurse may unintentionally cause harm by failing to recognize the patient's cultural needs (Kump & Scholz, 2022). For example, disregarding the request of a female client who refuses to be examined by a male nurse for religious reasons constitutes cultural insensitivity and ethical violation.

4.2. The Balance Between Cultural Sensitivity and Patient Autonomy

Autonomy, a fundamental ethical principle, defines an individual's right to make their own decisions freely. However, cultural differences can alter the interpretation of autonomy (Beauchamp & Childress, 1994). In individualistic cultures, autonomy is associated with individual decision-making, whereas in collectivist cultures, decision-making within the family or community is considered more appropriate (Kağıtçıbaşı, 2005). In psychotherapeutic nursing, this difference is particularly important in processes such as treatment consent, confidentiality, and information sharing. For example, although clients have the right to make their own decisions, they may not wish to participate in therapy without obtaining family approval. In such cases, nurses must maintain a careful balance between respecting cultural values and preserving the individual's autonomy (Ličen & Prosen, 2023). According to the ICN (2021) Code of Ethics, nurses must respect each individual's right to make decisions in accordance with their value system; however, these decisions must not harm others. The balance between cultural sensitivity and ethical principles depends on the nurse's professional judgment and ethical awareness throughout the therapeutic process.

4.3. Confidentiality, Privacy and Conflicts of Cultural Values

Privacy and confidentiality form the basis of ethical care in psychotherapeutic processes. However, perceptions of confidentiality are also influenced by cultural differences (Jeffreys 2015). In some cultures, it is considered natural for family members to be informed about the patient, whereas in others, the individual's privacy is prioritized (Wing Sue & Sue, 2008). In community-based cultures, families directly participate in individuals' health decisions, which requires confidentiality boundaries to be redefined within the therapeutic process (Son et al., 2025). Ethically, nurses should not share information without the client's consent; however, the cultural expectation of family involvement may require a flexible evaluation of this boundary. At this point, the nurse must establish a delicate balance between preserving the client's trust and respecting cultural value. A culturally sensitive approach requires discussing the issue of confidentiality openly with the client, determining boundaries together by considering cultural values, and carrying out the process transparently.

4.4. Professional Boundaries and Power Imbalances

The therapeutic relationship must be established within professional boundaries. However, cultural differences can influence these power dynamics. In societies with high power distance, nurses may be perceived as "authority figure," leading clients to feel passive (Hofstede, 2001). This may harm the egalitarian nature of the therapeutic relationship and limit the client's participation. A culturally competent nurse recognizes this power imbalance, encourages the client's participation in the decision-making process, and creates a trust-based environment (Bhugra & Bhui, 2018). In addition, with the rise of digitalization, the protection of professional boundaries in online psychotherapeutic nursing practice has introduced new ethical challenges (Wies et al., 2021). Nurses must also be sensitive to confidentiality, professional distance, and cultural misunderstandings on online platforms.

4.5. Ethics-Sensitivity Training and Institutional Responsibility

Ethical sensitivity is a fundamental competence that enables nurses to recognize potential ethical problems early, identify value conflicts, and make decisions that prioritize patient benefits. In nursing, ethical decisions are based not only on individual values but also on institutional structures and professional standards. The ICN's 2021 Code of Ethics for Nurses outlines the framework of ethical behavior under headings such as nurse–patient relationship, professional practice, the profession, and global health; this provides a reference for institutions to structure ethics education systematically. Educational interventions can strengthen ethical sensitivity and cultural competence. A systematic review published in 2024 showed that ethical sensitivity is a fundamental component of professional competence among nursing students and that ethical knowledge and participation in clinical/learning environments increase sensitivity. This finding indicates that ethics education should be supported by permanent and practice-based curriculum modules (Shadi et al., 2024).

Cultural competence training also indirectly supports ethical decision-making, as culturally sensitive communication facilitates the concretization of autonomy and justice principles. An umbrella review that combined the effects of programs aimed at improving the cultural competence of both nurses and students summarized educational components, teaching methods, and impact domains, providing evidence-based design principles for institutions. It also showed that cultural competence interventions increased competence levels among nurses; this increase provides a critical basis for recognizing ethical dilemmas and strengthening patient-centered decision-making (Lee et al., 2025). Institutional strategies should not be limited to one-off training sessions; they must incorporate continuity and a structured approach. In addition to curriculum-based courses, in-service training, case-based simulations, reflective practice sessions, ethics consultation/supervision lines, and interpreter–cultural mediator services should be integrated. An educational study conducted in Türkiye in 2024 demonstrated that a semester-long transcultural nursing curriculum significantly improved students' cultural communication and competence scores, and qualitative findings also indicated an enhanced perception of safe/ethical care (Tosun et al., 2024). Such structured programs increase preparedness for ethical dilemmas at the institutional level.

Finally, practice guidelines provide institutions with roadmaps. Practical guiding principles for the implementation of transcultural nursing care offer direction regarding cultural assessment, communication, interpreter use, and the alignment of institutional policies with the ethical framework. When used in conjunction with the ICN Code of Ethics, these guidelines make ethical sensitivity sustainable at the institutional level. In psychotherapeutic nursing, ethical dimensions are intertwined with cultural differences. Cultural biases, stereotyping, perceptions of privacy, autonomy, and power balance determine the ethical boundaries of the therapeutic process. A culturally competent nurse views ethical principles not as abstract rules but as dynamic guides that must be reinterpreted within each client's cultural context. This understanding protects individual dignity and forms the basis of inclusive, respectful, and fair psychotherapeutic care.

5. EDUCATIONAL AND INSTITUTIONAL STRATEGIES THAT STRENGTHEN THERAPEUTIC APPROACHES SENSITIVE TO CULTURAL DIVERSITY

5.1. The Necessity of Nursing Education Sensitive to Cultural Diversity

On a global scale, increasing migration movements, refugee crises, and multicultural social structures show that sensitivity to cultural diversity in nursing education is no longer an optional topic but an essential professional competence. Education sensitive to cultural diversity aims to enable nurses to provide respectful, equitable, and effective therapeutic care to individuals from different ethnic origins, religious beliefs, and lifestyles (Ličen & Prosen, 2023). Recent studies have indicated that nursing students often experience difficulties in communication, building trust, and making ethical decisions when they encounter migrant and refugee individuals in clinical settings (Theodosopoulos et al., 2024). Therefore, education sensitive to cultural diversity in nursing should not be limited to "introducing different cultures"; it should also cover practical themes such as trauma-informed care, intercultural communication, interpreter use, and the reflection of religious and social differences in clinical practice.

5.2. Educational Models for Working with Migrant, Refugee and Minority Groups

The most effective forms of training to increase cultural sensitivity are learning methods based on simulation, case analysis, and cultural interaction. A mixed-method study conducted in 2024 demonstrated that cultural competence training focused on working with migrant and refugee individuals led to significant increases in nursing students' empathy and ethical awareness (Raval et al., 2024).

Such training should focus particularly on the following:

- Recognition of post-traumatic stress and culturally shaped psychological symptoms
- The ability to establish therapeutic communication according to cultural differences
- Managing religious, linguistic and gender-based barriers
- Sensitivity to stigma and discrimination in minority individuals

These modules should be implemented not only for students but also as in-service training for actively practicing nurses.

5.3. Institutional Policies: Ethical and Inclusive Services for Migrant and Refugee Individuals

The continuity of therapeutic care sensitive to cultural diversity depends on the systematic support mechanisms established by institutions. Healthcare institutions should develop interpreter services, cultural mediators, multilingual information materials, and trauma-informed care protocols to facilitate refugees and migrants' access to healthcare services (Liu et al., 2025). Furthermore, institutions' provision of regular ethics and cultural awareness training for staff helps employees act more consciously to prevent discriminatory and bias-based behaviors (Theodosopoulos et al., 2025). At the level of institutional leadership, cultural inclusivity should be visible not only in policy documents but also in performance indicators and in quality evaluation systems.

5.4. Community-Based Collaborations and Multidisciplinary Approaches

Working with migrant and refugee individuals should be addressed not only at the clinical level but also through community-based approaches. In culturally sensitive therapeutic care, collaboration between different disciplines, such as psychiatrists, psychologists, social workers, community health nurses, interpreters, and cultural mediators, is important. Culturally adapted group-based interventions, such as BAMBOO for Refugees (Hendriks et al., 2024), enhance individual resilience and bolster social recovery by fostering cultural bonds. Inspired by this model, collaboration between nurses and community centers, migrant support organizations, and non-governmental organizations can facilitate access to services and reinforce the client's social support system.

5.5. Cultural Safety and Institutional Sustainability

Cultural safety describes a care environment in which the individual feels valued, respected, and protected from discrimination. This concept is a key ethical framework, particularly when working with minority and migrant groups (Douglas et al., 2014). Institutions are recommended to use patient feedback systems, staff awareness surveys, and cultural safety indicators to evaluate cultural safety. In addition, the development of ethical leadership models sensitive to cultural diversity by nurse leaders can help establish a sustainable culture of inclusivity within institutions.

6. FUTURE PERSPECTIVES

Global migration, increasing cultural diversity, and social inequalities have transformed the nursing profession into a field of responsibility that is not only clinical but also psychosocial and cultural. In this context, cultural competence is not just a skill but an ethical, professional, and therapeutic necessity. The data reviewed show that cultural awareness, self-reflection, empathic communication, and a sense of social justice are at the center of psychotherapeutic nursing practices (Bhugra & Bhui, 2018; Ličen & Prosen, 2023). Cultural competence does not merely mean "showing respect for different cultures"; it requires viewing the individual's cultural background, lived traumas, and value system as active components of the therapeutic process. This understanding allows for the reinterpretation of the principles of trust, respect, empowerment, and inclusivity in nursing care. Especially when working with migrant, refugee, and minority groups, culturally sensitive approaches increase both patient safety and treatment adherence (Theodosopoulos et al., 2024; Liu et al., 2025).

6.2. Effects of Cultural Competence in Psychotherapeutic Nursing

Culturally competent psychotherapeutic nursing practices yield outcomes at multiple levels:

- **At the individual level,** a culturally sensitive therapeutic process enables the client to feel understood and accepted. This strengthens the therapeutic alliance, increases trust, and facilitates engagement in treatment (Wing Sue & Sue, 2008).
- **At the clinical level,** culturally competent nurses assess phenomena such as post-traumatic stress, identity loss, or migration-related depression more accurately and recognize cultural symbols without misinterpretation (Orang et al., 2023).
- **At the institutional level,** cultural awareness contributes to a reduction in communication errors and ethical violations and an increase in equity of access to services (Theodosopoulos et al., 2025). Cultural safety also supports staff retention and job satisfaction (Pirhofer et al., 2022).

Therefore, cultural competence is not only an individual skill but also an indicator of quality and safety for the entire system (Douglas et al., 2014).

6.3. Priorities in the Nursing Education of the Future

Looking ahead, nursing education should adopt an interdisciplinary and experiential model that places cultural diversity sensitivity at its core. In the period after 2025, the spread of cultural competence training on digital platforms will increase accessibility but will also bring ethical and privacy issues to the fore. Therefore, digital cultural simulations, gamified ethical decision modules, and trauma-informed e-learning systems can be considered new pedagogical domains (Osmancevic et al., 2025). Additionally, digital refugee stories or art-based reflective sessions can enhance students' empathy and cultural awareness (Baysal et al., 2025). To measure the impact of these innovative methods in education, culturally competent and ethical sensitivity scales adapted to digital environments must be developed (Yava et al., 2023).

6.4. Institutional Policies and Global Responsibility

The sustainability of culturally competent care depends more on institutional commitment than on individual effort. Healthcare institutions must establish cultural consultancy units, interpreter services, and multilingual information systems. A report issued by the WHO in 2024, the *Global Competency Standards for Refugee and Migrant Health Workers*, defines cultural sensitivity not merely as an "educational goal" but as an institutional quality standard. In addition, the psychological resilience and secondary trauma awareness of nurses working in migrant and refugee health should be supported, and supervision and reflective sessions should be included in institutional protocols (Hendriks et al., 2024). Viewing cultural diversity not as a "difference to be managed" but as a richness that contributes to healthcare services forms the basis of future ethical nursing understanding.

6.5. Recommendations for Research and Policy

- **Measuring Cultural Competence:** Localized versions of valid and reliable assessment tools should be developed for different cultural contexts (Campinha-Bacote, 2011).
- **Impact Analysis of Educational Interventions:** The long-term effects of simulation-based, trauma-informed, and strength-based training aimed at working with migrant and refugee groups should be monitored (Raval et al., 2024).
- **Policy Alignment:** Cultural safety should be an integral part of the national nursing curriculum standards.

- **Interdisciplinary Collaboration:** Collaboration should be strengthened among psychiatrists, social workers, psychologists, cultural mediators, and community leaders.
- **Global Solidarity and Ethical Sharing:** Knowledge-sharing networks in the field of migrant health (e.g., the WHO Migration Health Network) should be supported.

Cultural competence is not merely an add-on to psychotherapeutic nursing; it is at the heart of person-centered care. In a world marked by migration, displacement, and cultural ruptures, nurses'sensitivity affects not only clinical outcomes but also social peace. Therefore, therapeutic approaches sensitive to cultural diversity are among the most powerful bridges that carry nursing practice toward an ethical, humane, and sustainable future.

7. REFLECTIONS ON CLINICAL PRACTICE, POLICY RECOMMENDATIONS AND FUTURE DIRECTIONS

7.1. Clinical Integration of Cultural Competence in Psychotherapeutic Nursing

Cultural competence should not remain solely at the level of education or awareness; it must be systematically integrated into clinical decision-making processes, care protocols, and team communication. This integration transforms the nurse's therapeutic role from a "technical practitioner" into a healthcare professional who acts as a cultural mediator. Trauma-informed care, cultural safety, and empathy-based models developed in recent years (Douglas et al., 2014; Orang et al., 2023; Liu et al., 2025) form the basis of this integration. For example:

- **Therapeutic communication protocols** should include exploring the patient's cultural context through questions ("Who makes health decisions in your family?" "Which beliefs comfort you in the treatment process?").
- **Assessment forms** should include variables such as cultural identity, language, religious practices, and migration history.
- **Care plans** should incorporate psychotherapeutic goals that do not conflict with cultural values.

In this way, cultural awareness becomes not only an "ethical" but also a clinically effective criterion in care.

7.2. Institutional Policies and Sustainability

Culturally diverse nursing practices are sustainable only through institutional support. Hospitals, community health centers, and mental health institutions should systematically implement the following steps:

- **Cultural Competence Committees:** Each institution should establish a body responsible for monitoring the cultural appropriateness of care protocols (Theodosopoulos et al., 2025).
- **In-Service Training Policy:** At least once a year, mandatory training on cultural competence, ethical sensitivity, and trauma-informed care should be organized for all nurses (Osmancevic et al., 2025).
- **Language and Mediation Services:** Institutions should collaborate with professional interpreters and authorize staff for "cultural mediation" (WHO, 2024).
- **Cultural Safety Indicators:** Indicators such as patient satisfaction, rate of ethical violations, and level of access to services should be measured regularly and included in quality reports (Douglas et al., 2014).

These steps ensure that nursing care is not only patient-centered, but also community-centered and justice-oriented.

7.3. National Policy and Educational Recommendations

1. **Curriculum Reform:** Cultural competence should be a compulsory course and clinical practice area in undergraduate nursing programmes. National authorities, such as higher-education councils, should incorporate cultural safety and ethical awareness standards into the accreditation criteria for nursing education.
2. **Accreditation and Continuing Education:** Ministries of Health and nursing associations may define nurses who have received cultural competence training as "certified therapeutic nurses." This increases both professional recognition and service quality (Yava et al., 2023).
3. **Migration and Mental Health Policies:** Special nursing units should be established to improve migrant and refugee access to mental health services, and training in cultural mediation and trauma-informed care should be mandatory (Liu et al., 2025).

7.4. Research Priorities and Scientific Gaps

- **Relationship Between Cultural Competence and Clinical Outcomes:** More longitudinal studies are needed to examine the effects of the level of cultural competence on patient safety, treatment adherence, and therapeutic alliance.
- **Cultural Simulation Technologies:** The use of virtual reality (VR) and AI-based scenarios in nursing education is a promising field for increasing cultural empathy (Baysal et al., 2024).
- **Experiences of Minority Nurses:** The ethical stress, microaggressions, and professional resilience levels of nurses who are culturally in the minority within institutions should be investigated (Pirhofer et al., 2022).
- **Policy Analysis:** The implementation levels and outcomes of cultural safety policies at the international level should be examined comparatively (WHO, 2024).

7.5. The Future of Psychotherapeutic Nursing: The Ethical Dimension of Cultural Transformation

In the 21st century, psychotherapeutic nursing is evolving into a discipline that deals not only with illness but also with culture, identity, trauma, and social justice. Cultural competence is both the ethical core and human compass of this transformation.

Working with migrant, refugee, and minority groups turns nurses into not only clinicians but also compassionate witnesses, cultural translators, and agents of social peace (Hendriks et al., 2024; Wing Sue & Sue, 2008). Therefore, cultural competence should be seen not just as "conscious awareness" but as an ethical imperative for building inclusive health policies and just societies. Culturally sensitive psychotherapeutic nursing will be at the center of "healing dialogue" in future health systems. Unless an integrated understanding of cultural competence is developed at the levels of individual awareness, institutional policy, and social collaboration, healthcare services can be neither fully ethical nor equitable. Cultural competence in nursing is not only about respecting differences; it is the shared language of humanity's healing.

8. NEW HORIZONS: CULTURAL TRANSFORMATION, DIGITAL THERAPEUTIC SPACES AND DECOLONIAL NURSING PERSPECTIVES

Cultural diversity has transformed contemporary nursing from being merely a clinical profession into an ethical, political, and technological field of action. Phenomena such as migration, digitalization, artificial intelligence, and social media have redefined the nature of the "therapeutic relationship" in nursing. Psychotherapeutic nursing is no longer limited to the psychological healing of individuals; it is becoming a practice that also aims to restore cultural identity, narrative, and belonging (Bhugra & Bhui, 2018). This transformation brings themes such as digital inclusivity, decolonial ethics, intercultural resilience, and community-based renewal to the forefront, especially in working with migrant, refugee, and minority groups.

8.1. Digital Cultural Therapeutic Spaces: New Opportunities and Risks

Digital mental health practices, which rapidly expanded in the post-pandemic period, have removed borders and globalized intercultural counseling and nursing services. However, this has also raised new questions: How is culture represented in digital environments? How is empathy established on a screen? How is privacy protected in the context of cultural differences? Yang and Jang (2025) emphasized that the most important ethical dilemmas in digital psychotherapeutic nursing involve confidentiality, privacy, and cultural misunderstanding. According to the OECD (2023) report, *Artificial Intelligence and the Health Workforce*, the rapid spread of digital health technologies can create new inequalities in access to healthcare, especially in low-resource settings. Therefore, nurses must develop not only technical skills but also digital inclusivity and cultural awareness-based competencies; they must learn to establish "culturally meaningful communication" in AI-supported and online care environments while considering patients' cultural and linguistic diversity (OECD, 2023). The concept of *digital cultural safety* comes to the fore here: the language used, visual materials, case scenarios, and simulations must be cleansed of cultural bias; digital care systems should be designed so as not to exclude different cultural identities (Crawford et al., 2022). This approach can transform the digital sphere from a "cold technology" into a new face of human connection in the future of psychotherapeutic nursing care.

8.2. Cultural Resilience: From Trauma to Empowerment

Cultural resilience is the capacity of a community or individual to recover after trauma by drawing on cultural values, social networks, and belief systems (Ungar, 2021). Migrant and refugee groups carry not only trauma but also repertoires of cultural resilience: intra-community support, religious beliefs, traditional healing practices, storytelling, and collective hope are powerful tools of psychosocial recovery (Panter-Brick & Eggerman, 2011). Recognizing these elements in psychotherapeutic nursing means accepting that the individual is not merely a "victim" but an active subject of recovery. The nurse can incorporate the client's cultural strengths into the therapy process, such as prayer, ritual, community-based solidarity, music, or art. These approaches are not only culturally sensitive but also resilient-building strategies.

8.3. Decolonial Nursing and Cultural Liberation

Discussions on cultural competence have long relied on Western-centric concepts. In recent years, decolonial nursing has begun to question the colonial traces of knowledge production and care practice. This approach argues that nursing science is based not only on "modern" biomedical models but also on the knowledge systems of Indigenous, migrant, and minority communities, which should be accepted as equally valuable sources of knowledge (Abiri et al., 2024). Decolonial nursing defines cultural differences not as "knowledge to be learned" but as an equal domain of knowledge. This perspective implies transforming power relations in psychotherapeutic nursing: the nurse is not a "teacher" but a witness and facilitator of a shared healing process. For example, mental health practices among Inuit communities in Canada are built on individuals sharing life stories and community members participating in these experiences through "silent witnessing." This process is both cultural and therapeutic in nature. Moreover, the decolonial approach treats cultural competence not only as an individual behavioral pattern but also as a matter of institutional justice and representation. According to this perspective, health systems must recognize the knowledge, experiences, and leadership contributions of minority groups and ensure their greater visibility in decision-making mechanisms (Abiri et al., 2024).

8.4. Community-Based Therapeutic Spaces: Participatory and Shared Healing

Culturally sensitive psychotherapeutic nursing should extend beyond individual counseling rooms to create community-based healing spaces. Group-based initiatives, such as BAMBOO for Refugees (Hendriks et al., 2024), enable individuals to regain meaning through cultural solidarity. Culturally sensitive psychotherapeutic nursing comes to life not only in individual therapy rooms but also in the healing spaces of communities. Community-based therapeutic spaces are participatory environments in which individuals experience psychological reconstruction through collective solidarity, storytelling, and cultural rituals. These spaces transform nurses into professionals who not only provide care but also heal and learn with the community. The World Health Organization (WHO) has highlighted two important group-based interventions with proven feasibility in low-resource settings for mental health work with refugee and migrant communities: Self-Help Plus (SH+) and Problem Management Plus (PM+). The SH+ program is a method developed to reduce symptoms of stress, anxiety, and depression, and its effectiveness among adult refugee and migrant communities has been demonstrated (Tol et al., 2020; WHO, 2023). Various studies have found that SH+ reduces anxiety and increases psychological resilience (Epping-Jordan et al., 2016). Similarly, the PM+ intervention offers an effective recovery model for conditions such as post-traumatic stress, depression, and functional impairment. Randomized controlled trials conducted in countries such as Pakistan and Jordan have shown that PM+ significantly reduces psychological distress (Dawson et al. 2015; Rahman et al. 2019). These interventions reflect the healing power of shared experiences in nursing practice: participants reduce feelings of loneliness by interacting with individuals with similar life stories, developing mutual trust, and rebuilding a sense of resilience.

9. CULTURAL REPAIR AND COMMUNITY RESILIENCE

Community-based approaches do not only target psychological symptoms; they also contribute to the processes of cultural repair and identity reconstruction. Culturally meaningful activities (e.g., music, handicrafts, sharing traditional foods, prayer, or community stories) strengthen individuals' sense of belonging, repair social connections, and reinterpret healing within a cultural context (Vindevogel, 2025; Siddiq et al., 2023). This demonstrates that cultural competence in nursing is based not only on knowledge but also on lived experiences. In such interventions, nurses assume flexible roles: sometimes as facilitators, sometimes as participants, and sometimes as observers. The aim is not to establish a hierarchical care relationship but to create a healing space based on mutual learning and trust. This approach centers the concept of "shared recovery." The recovery process is no longer a structure managed solely by professionals; it becomes a collective transformation experienced by the community (UNHCR 2024).

10. INSTITUTIONAL PERSPECTIVE: THE UNHCR AND IOM FRAMEWORK

International organizations, particularly the United Nations High Commissioner for Refugees (UNHCR) and the International Organization for Migration (IOM), define community-based mental health and psychosocial support (MHPSS) programs as integral to refugee health. Within this framework, nurses must act not only as providers of individual care but also as cultural mediators who strengthen communities' collective resilience and cultural endurance (UNHCR, 2024; IOM, 2023). Cultural safety is not merely an institutional procedure; it is an experience lived through mutual witnessing, respect, and shared meaning-making within the community. Thus, community-based healing spaces are one of the most concrete and humane forms of culturally sensitive nursing care. Community-based therapeutic spaces represent the future of psychotherapeutic nursing, based on cultural sensitivity. This approach transcends the boundaries of individual therapy and redefines healing in terms of social solidarity, cultural belonging, and ethical responsibility. In this process, nurses play roles not only as healthcare workers but also as cultural witnesses, builders of solidarity, and members of healing communities. Culturally sensitive psychotherapeutic nursing will shape the future not only as a care practice but also as a practice of intercultural dialogue. Working with migrant, refugee, and minority individuals should provide nurses with not only clinical skills but also cultural wisdom, digital ethics, environmental awareness, and political sensitivity. Approaches such as decolonial perspectives, cultural liberation, digital cultural safety, community-based healing, and ecotherapy are paradigms that are redefining nursing in the 21st century. From this perspective, cultural competence is no longer "knowledge that is learned" but an ethical way of life that is lived, shared, and constantly evolving.

REFERENCES

Abiri, A., Ferere, A. H., Jordan, J., & Kinuthia, W. (2024). Decolonizing Nursing Education: Promoting Curricula for Community Engagement. In *Transforming Social Determinants to Promote Global Health: Achieving Health Equity through Lived Experiences* (pp. 421–433). Springer Nature Switzerland.

Baysal, E., Rodriguez-Arrastia, M., & Roman, P. (2025). Innovative Game-Based Teaching Methods for Promoting Nursing Students' Cultural Competence and Attitudes Toward Refugees: An Explanatory Sequential Mixed Study. *Journal of Transcultural Nursing*, *36*(3), 290–302. PMID: 39543903

Beauchamp, T. L., & Childress, J. F. (1994). *Principles of biomedical ethics*. Edicoes Loyola.

Bhugra, D., & Bhui, K. (Eds.). (2018). *Textbook of cultural psychiatry*. Cambridge University Press.

Campinha-Bacote, J. (2002). The process of cultural competence in the delivery of healthcare services: A model of care. *Journal of Transcultural Nursing*, *13*(3), 181–184. PMID: 12113146

Campinha-Bacote, J. (2011). Delivering patient-centered care in the midst of a cultural conflict: The role of cultural competence. *Online Journal of Issues in Nursing*, *16*(2), 1–8. PMID: 22088154

Crawford, A., Richardson, L., Simmonds, E., Wiljer, D., & Strudwick, G. (2022). Digital compassion, health equity, and cultural safety: from the therapeutic relationship to the organization of virtual care. In *Virtual Mental Health Care for Rural and Underserved Settings* (pp. 55–67). Springer International Publishing.

Dawson, K. S., Bryant, R. A., Harper, M., Tay, A. K., Rahman, A., Schafer, A., & Van Ommeren, M. (2015). Problem Management Plus (PM+): A WHO transdiagnostic psychological intervention for common mental health problems. *World Psychiatry; Official Journal of the World Psychiatric Association (WPA)*, *14*(3), 354. PMID: 26407793

Dewing, J. (2020). Privilege and the call of the appeal.

Douglas, M. K., Rosenkoetter, M., Pacquiao, D. F., Callister, L. C., Hattar-Pollara, M., Lauderdale, J., & Purnell, L. (2014). Guidelines for implementing culturally competent nursing care. *Journal of Transcultural Nursing*, *25*(2), 109–121. PMID: 24549502

Epping-Jordan, J. E., Harris, R., Brown, F. L., Carswell, K., Foley, C., García-Moreno, C., & van Ommeren, M. (2016). Self-Help Plus (SH+): A new WHO stress management package. *World Psychiatry; Official Journal of the World Psychiatric Association (WPA), 15*(3), 295. PMID: 27717271

Hendriks, T., de Jong, J., Hassankhan, A., & van Woerkom, M. (2024). BAMBOO for Refugees—A culturally sensitive positive psychology intervention: A protocol for a pilot randomized controlled trial. *International Journal of Applied Positive Psychology*, *9*(2), 553–582.

Hofstede, G. (2001). *Culture's consequences: Comparing values, behaviors, institutions and organizations across nations*. Sage publications.

ICN. (2021). The ICN Code of Ethics for Nurses: Revised 2021. In International Council of Nurses. International Council of Nurses. https://www.icn.ch/sites/default/files/inline-files/2012_ICN_Codeofethicsfornurses International Council of Nurses. (2021). ICN code of ethics for nurses. ICN.

Jeffreys, M. R. (2015). *Teaching cultural competence in nursing and health care: Inquiry, action, and innovation*. Springer Publishing Company.

Kirmayer, L. J. (2012). Cultural competence and evidence-based practice in mental health: Epistemic communities and the politics of pluralism. *Social Science & Medicine*, *75*(2), 249–256. PMID: 22575699

Kittler, M. G., Rygl, D., & Mackinnon, A. (2011). Special Review Article: Beyond culture or beyond control? Reviewing the use of Hall's high-/low-context concept. *International Journal of Cross Cultural Management*, *11*(1), 63–82.

Kleinman, A. (1988). *Rethinking psychiatry: from cultural category to personal experience The Free Press*.

Kump, B., & Scholz, M. (2022). Organizational routines as a source of ethical blindness. *Organization Theory*, *3*(1), 26317877221075640.

Leininger, M. M., & McFarland, M. R. (2006). *Culture care diversity and universality: A worldwide nursing theory*. Jones & Bartlett Learning.

Ličen, S., & Prosen, M. (2023). The development of cultural competences in nursing students and their significance in shaping the future work environment: A pilot study. *BMC Medical Education*, *23*(1), 819. DOI: 10.1186/s12909-023-04800-5

Liu, A., Yazdani, Y., Elias, M., Patel, K., Budzi, D., Saad, A., & Pottie, K. (2025). Transition in care interventions for Refugee, Immigrant and other Migrant (RIM) populations: A health equity-oriented scoping review. *Globalization and Health, 21*(1), 25. PMID: 40307839

Lyons, P., Edwardes, A., Bladon, L., & Abel, K. M. (2025). Culturally sensitive mental health research: A scoping review. *BMC Psychiatry, 25*(1), 190. PMID: 40033264

Markus, H. R., & Kitayama, S. (2014). Culture and the self: Implications for cognition, emotion, and motivation. In *College student development and academic life* (pp. 264–293). Routledge.

McFarland, M. R., & Wehbe-Alamah, H. B. (2015). *Leininger's culture care diversity and universality: A worldwide nursing theory*. Jones & Bartlett Publishers.

OECD. (2023). *Artificial Intelligence and the Health Workforce*. OECD Publishing., DOI: 10.1787/9a31d8af-

Orang, T. M., Missmahl, I., Gardisi, M., & Kluge, U. (2023). Rethinking mental health care provided to migrants and refugees; a randomized controlled trial on the effectiveness of Value Based Counseling, a culturally sensitive, strength-based psychological intervention. *PLoS One, 18*(3), e0283889. PMID: 37000817

Osmancevic, S., Steiner, L. M., Großschädl, F., Lohrmann, C., & Schoberer, D. (2025). The effectiveness of cultural competence interventions in nursing: A systematic review and meta-analysis. *International Journal of Nursing Studies*, •••, 105079.

Panter-Brick, C., & Eggerman, M. (2011). Understanding culture, resilience, and mental health: The production of hope. In *The social ecology of resilience: A handbook of theory and practice* (pp. 369–386). Springer New York.

Papadopoulos, I. (Ed.). (2006). *Transcultural health and social care: development of culturally competent practitioners*. Elsevier Health Sciences.

Pirhofer, J., Bükki, J., Vaismoradi, M., Glarcher, M., & Paal, P. (2022). A qualitative exploration of cultural safety in nursing from the perspectives of Advanced Practice Nurses: Meaning, barriers, and prospects. *BMC Nursing, 21*(1), 178. PMID: 35787799

Purnell, L. D. (2016). The Purnell model for cultural competence. In *Intervention in mental health-substance use* (pp. 57–78). CRC Press.

Rahman, A., Khan, M. N., Hamdani, S. U., Chiumento, A., Akhtar, P., Nazir, H., & van Ommeren, M. (2019). Effectiveness of a brief group psychological intervention for women in a post-conflict setting in Pakistan: A single-blind, cluster, randomised controlled trial. *Lancet, 393*(10182), 1733–1744. PMID: 30948286

Raval, V. V., Gopal, B., Aggarwal, P., Mohan, M. P., Padmakumari, P., Thomas, E., & Hay, M. C. (2024). Training in Cultural Competence for Mental Health Care: A Mixed-Methods Study of Students, Faculty, and Practitioners from India and USA. *Culture, Medicine and Psychiatry*, *48*(4), 699–730. PMID: 38954183

Sakai, S., An, J., Kang, M., & Kwak, H. (2025). Somatic in the East, Psychological in the West?: Investigating Clinically-Grounded Cross-Cultural Depression Symptom Expression in LLMs. arXiv preprint arXiv:2508.03247.

Shadi, A. Z., Zohreh, V., Eesa, M., & Anoshirvan, K. (2024). Moral sensitivity of nursing students: A systematic review. *BMC Nursing*, *23*(1), 99. PMID: 38321462

Siddiq, H., Elhaija, A., & Wells, K. (2023). An integrative review of community-based mental health interventions among resettled refugees from Muslim-majority countries. *Community Mental Health Journal*, *59*(1), 160–174. PMID: 35751790

Soares, M. R., Cameira, M. P., Abreu, P., & Pereira, M. (2024). Cultural Diversity and Mental Health Care: A Case Study. *European Psychiatry : the Journal of the Association of European Psychiatrists*, *67*(S1), S522–S522.

Son, C., Forsgren, E., Öhlén, J., & Sawatzky, R. (2025). Person-centred care for migrants: A narrative review of health care literature. *Frontiers in Health Services*, *5*, 1573813. PMID: 40740479

Stingl, M., & Hanewald, B. (2025). Culturally sensitive psychotherapy-technique or attitude? *Frontiers in Psychology*, *16*, 1599855. PMID: 41112539

Theodosopoulos, L., Fradelos, E. C., Panagiotou, A., Dreliozi, A., & Tzavella, F. (2024). Delivering culturally competent care to migrants by healthcare personnel: A crucial aspect of delivering culturally sensitive care. *Social Sciences*, *13*(10), 530.

Tol, W. A., Leku, M. R., Lakin, D. P., Carswell, K., Augustinavicius, J., Adaku, A., & van Ommeren, M. (2020). Guided self-help to reduce psychological distress in South Sudanese female refugees in Uganda: A cluster randomised trial. *The Lancet. Global Health*, *8*(2), e254–e263. PMID: 31981556

Tosun, B., Yılmaz, E. B., Dirgar, E., Şahin, E. B., Hatipoğlu, K. P., & Yava, A. (2024). Evaluating the effectiveness of a new curriculum for transcultural nursing education: A mixed-method study. *BMC Nursing*, *23*(1), 813. PMID: 39511551

Triandis, H. C. (2018). *Individualism and collectivism*. Routledge.

Ungar, M. (Ed.). (2021). *Multisystemic resilience: Adaptation and transformation in contexts of change*. Oxford University Press.

UNHCR. (2024). Community-based Mental Health and Psychosocial Support (MHPSS) approaches for refugees and migrants.

Vindevogel, S., Boumahdi, Y., Alabbas, F., & Magerman, J. (2025). Transcultural mental health and psychosocial support in asylum reception centres: A Delphi review of guidelines for the frontline workforce. *International Journal of Migration, Health and Social Care*.

WHO. (2023). *Self-Help Plus (SH+) and Problem Management Plus (PM+) Implementation Guidance*. World Health Organization.

WHO/Europe. (2024). *Global competency standards for health workers providing care to refugees and migrants*. World Health Organization Regional Office for Europe.

Wies, B., Landers, C., & Ienca, M. (2021). Digital mental health for young people: A scoping review of ethical promises and challenges. *Frontiers in Digital Health, 3*, 697072. PMID: 34713173

Wing Sue, D., & Sue, D. (2008). *Counseling the culturally diverse: Theory and practice*. John Wiley & Sons, Inc.

Yang, H. M., & Jang, Y. E. (2025). Ethics of nursing in the digital age: Perceptions and challenges among Korean nursing students. *BMC Medical Ethics*, *26*(1), 143. PMID: 41107902

Yava, A., Tosun, B., Papp, K., Tóthová, V., Şahin, E., Yılmaz, E. B., & Leyva-Moral, J. M. (2023). Developing the better and effective nursing education for improving transcultural nursing skills cultural competence and cultural sensitivity assessment tool (BENEFITS-CCCSAT). *BMC Nursing*, *22*(1), 331. DOI: 10.1186/s12912-023-01476-6

Chapter 3

Cognitive Behavioral Therapy (CBT) in Nursing Practice:

The Role of Psychiatric Nurses in Applying Cognitive and Behavioral Interventions

Elif Güzide Emirza
https://orcid.org/0000-0003-3652-2428
Ondokuz Mayıs University, Turkey

ABSTRACT

Cognitive Behavioral Therapy (CBT) in nursing practice is an evidence-based and patient-centered approach that helps nurses address the relationship between thoughts, emotions, and behaviors influencing health outcomes. By incorporating CBT principles into daily care, nurses can assist patients in recognizing maladaptive thinking patterns, developing effective coping strategies, and improving self-management skills in various clinical settings. CBT-informed nursing interventions enhance therapeutic communication, reduce psychological distress, and support adherence to treatment plans. This approach aligns with the holistic nursing perspective by integrating psychological and physical care, contributing to improved patient well-being, resilience, and overall quality of life.

DOI: 10.4018/979-8-3373-6526-8.ch003

1. INTRODUCTION

Cognitive Behavioral Therapy (CBT) is a psychotherapy approach based on the reciprocal relationships between emotions, thoughts, and behaviors, aiming to understand and change psychological problems, supported by strong scientific evidence (Dobson & Dozois, 2021; Türkçapar, 2019; Beck & Dozois, 2011). In recent years, it has been demonstrated that CBT techniques can be effectively used not only in psychotherapy but also in nursing, psychiatry, chronic disease management, rehabilitation, palliative care, and general medical practice. Therefore, integrating CBT-based approaches into patient care supports patients' psychological well-being and enhances treatment compliance, quality of life, and care outcomes (Yotulmaz & Dirik, 2023). This section will cover CBT and its fundamental principles, followed by a systematic discussion of how nurses can adapt CBT techniques to clinical care processes and case formulations.

2. BASIC PRINCIPLES OF PSYCHOTHERAPY AND COGNITIVE THERAPY

Psychotherapy can be likened to learning a new language in the internal experience domain, which encompasses an individual's feelings, thoughts, and behavioral patterns regarding themselves, others, and the world in the psychological realm. This analogy is particularly evident in cognitive behavioral therapy, where the client's acquisition of new cognitive frameworks, emotion regulation skills, and behavioral strategies is a structured, systematic, and instructive process, much like the step-by-step acquisition of a foreign language (Beck & Dozois, 2011). People typically learn a new language by first understanding it, then producing it; they progress through stages of selecting the right expressions, repeating them, practicing, and eventually using the language in everyday life. Similarly, in therapy, individuals first learn to recognize their automatic thoughts, schemas, and emotion-behavior relationships; then they begin to develop more adaptive cognitive and behavioral responses by restructuring these patterns (Dobson & Dozois, 2021; Beck & Dozois, 2011).

Just as repetition, exposure, and use in natural contexts are critical for gaining fluency in a new language, regular homework assignments, behavioral experiments, emotion regulation practices, and the process of trying out new strategies in daily life are equally important for consolidating the skills learned in therapy (Gumport et al., 2015). Therefore,

Psychotherapy is not only a process of gaining insight, but also of acquiring a new 'psychological language' and applying this language in various life contexts (Dobson & Dozois, 2021).

If there is no factor driving the individual to learn a new language; or if, despite such a reason existing, the person is unwilling to make an effort or put in the work; or if there is a mismatch between the learning method and the person's own desires and expectations, or between the teaching method and the instructor, then expecting that person to learn the "new language" is largely unrealistic. Here, the "driving factor" is not merely superficial motivation; it is a form of willingness that accepts setting aside time for learning, taking risks, and coping with processes that require repetition and practice (Türkçapar, 2019; Özdel, 2015). The success of the learning process is not merely a matter of desire; consistency between the intention to learn and learning behaviors (regular study, practice, receiving feedback, and application) is also necessary. Furthermore, the alignment between the teaching method and the learner's learning style, expectations, and experiences significantly affects the speed and permanence of learning (Tzur et al., 2022).

In summary, psychotherapy is not a "passive intervention applied to the individual," but a jointly conducted process that requires the active participation of the individual. Therefore, specific prerequisites must be met for psychotherapy to be effective (Gómez-Penedo et al., 2023; Türkçapar, 2019; Butler et al., 2006). At the core of these preconditions is the presence of a specific problem or characteristic that the individual observes in their inner world and social relationships and that causes discomfort or that they wish to change at the cognitive, emotional, behavioral, or relational level. This awareness alone is not sufficient; acceptance that the change sought by therapy is achievable, that is, the person's belief that "this goal can be achieved with the methods proposed by the cognitive-behavioral approach and with the therapist's support," is also necessary. This acceptance forms the basis of motivation and commitment to treatment (Joaquim et al., 2023; Bieling et al., 2022; Beck, 2020).

Another situation that is often overlooked in psychotherapy and therefore negatively affects therapy outcomes is the assumption that simply being aware of the problem or wanting to change is sufficient for therapy. In reality, change is a multilayered process that involves acquiring knowledge, learning new ways of thinking and behaving, trying them out in safe environments, learning from mistakes, and integrating what has been learned into daily life (Gómez-Penedo et al., 2023; Türkçapar, 2019). During this process, the client may frequently

Experience ambivalence, withdrawal, fluctuations in motivation, or difficulties in implementation; these are natural and expected stages, but if not handled appropriately, they can interrupt the progress of therapy (Bieling et al., 2022; Beck, 2020; Türkçapar, 2019).

If we need to address the prerequisites for successful therapy more concretely: the client's goal for change must be clear; they must have realistic expectations regarding the therapy method and therapist; they must be willing to commit time to therapy and complete assignments; they must be capable of establishing an emotionally secure relationship; and their environmental/living conditions must be relatively favorable, not hindering their ability to continue therapy (Dobson & Dozois, 2021). Furthermore, ensuring compatibility between cultural, linguistic, and personal values and the therapeutic approach is also critical, as method-client incompatibility disrupts the client's learning process and the sustainability of therapeutic gains (Dobson & Dozois, 2021; Beck & Dozois, 2011). The therapist's role is also decisive here: In the therapy process, the therapist is not only an expert who applies techniques; they are also a companion who assesses the client's motivation, resolves ambivalence together, identifies learning barriers and intervenes with appropriate teaching strategies, and makes adjustments according to the client's own learning style. Jointly setting therapy goals, strengthening the therapeutic alliance, and progressing in small steps with achievable goals make the "teacher-student" interaction required by the learning analogy more effective (Chand et al., 2023; Nakao et al., 2021).

Ultimately, "change" in psychotherapy requires choice and conscious effort; awareness or good intentions alone are not sufficient for sustainable learning and skill internalization (Dobson & Dozois, 2021). For therapy to be successful, several prerequisites must be met simultaneously, including the client's readiness, motivational state, method-client fit, quality of the therapeutic relationship, and suitability of life circumstances. When these conditions are met, therapy can become a process of acquisition based on repetition, practice, and integration into life, similar to learning a new language; otherwise, learning and lasting change cannot be expected (Bieling et al., 2022; Beck, 2020; Türkçapar, 2019).

2.1. Stages of Change in Cognitive Behavioral Therapy

The question of how human behavior and attitudes change has been intensively researched within the framework of motivational theory, drawing particularly on experiences in the field of addiction. An important starting point in the development of this theory is the observation that individuals who quit substance use on their own have higher long-term success rates compared to those who try to quit with professional treatment support (Beck, 2020; Türkçapar, 2019). This finding demonstrated that change becomes sustainable not only through external interventions but primarily through the individual's internal processes (Türkçapar, 2019; Stevens et al., 2019; Magill et al., 2019).

Motivational theory emphasizes that, especially in areas where strong biological, psychological, and environmental factors are intertwined, such as substance addiction, the individual's internal motivation for change is one of the most critical determinants of the treatment process (Stevens et al., 2019; Magill et al., 2019). This approach posits that factors such as the person's desire for change, understanding why this change is important to them, establishing a connection between their change goals and their values, and being aware of their level of readiness for change are decisive in both initiating and sustaining behavioral change (Bieling et al., 2022; Türkçapar, 2019; Stevens et al., 2019). Furthermore, motivational theory suggests that change is not a linear process; individuals often undergo natural stages, including indecision, resistance, back-and-forth movement, and ambivalence. Therefore, what is important in the change process is for the individual to recognize these stages and be willing to move forward based on their own internal motivations. According to the theory, although external pressures, coercion, or the expectations of others may trigger change in the short term, the factual basis for long-term transformation is the person's own internal desire, self-efficacy perception, and personal beliefs about change (Dobson & Dozois, 2021; Türkçapar, 2019; Stevens et al., 2019).

Therefore, motivational theory approaches change in psychotherapy not as a "technique applied from the outside," but as a journey initiated within the individual and guided by the therapist. In other words, the effectiveness of the methods used in therapy largely depends on how ready the individual is for change, why they want this change, and what kind of transformation they aim for in their life (Dobson & Dozois, 2021; Türkçapar, 2019). This perspective clearly demonstrates the importance of therapeutic interventions focusing on strengthening the individual's internal motivation, exploring ambivalence, and helping the person recognize their own reasons for change (Türkçapar, 2019; Stevens et al., 2019; Magill et al., 2019). For change to be achieved through psychotherapy,

- The individual must be aware of their problem or distress,
- They must believe that this problem or distress can be reduced or eliminated,
- They must believe that the recommended form of assistance can bring about this change.
- The counselor must have the ability to teach the individual the skills necessary to make these changes.
- The stage an individual is at in terms of readiness for change is critical (Türkçapar, 2019; Özdel, 2015; Gençtan, 1993).

Motivational theory classifies the stages individuals go through in terms of change into four phases: (Türkçapar, 2019; Gençtan, 1993)

1. <u>First stage: Precontemplation stage:</u>

The pre-contemplation stage is the phase in which the individual has not yet recognized that they have a problem, has not accepted it, or is not ready to evaluate the consequences of their problematic behavior in terms of its impact on their own life. During this period, the person generally does not see the need for change, does not perceive their current situation as threatening or problematic, and therefore lacks internal motivation for behavioral change (Dobson & Dozois, 2021; İlgar & İlgar, 2019; Beck & Dozois, 2011). If the person has entered psychotherapy, it is often not of their own volition; it has been driven by family pressure, workplace demands, legal obligations, or other external factors. Therefore, the client may come to the therapy setting with a reluctant, distant, or resistant attitude (Dobson & Dozois, 2021; Türkçapar, 2019).

At this stage, it is not yet appropriate to initiate the structured interventions of standard cognitive-behavioral therapy with the client, as these techniques require the client's active participation, acceptance of the need for change, and a willingness to work toward specific goals. Since individuals in the pre-contemplation stage do not yet have an internal conviction that "something needs to change," direct technical applications are often ineffective and may lead to resistance from the client (Dobson & Dozois, 2021; Türkçapar, 2019; Beck & Dozois, 2011). Therefore, the fundamental intervention during this phase is to facilitate the individual's awareness. The therapist's goal is to help the person discover the gap between their current situation and their desired ideal lifestyle, values, or goals (Türkçapar, 2019; Beck & Dozois, 2011). In this process, the therapist:

- Addresses important areas of the client's life (health, relationships, work, academic life, daily functioning, etc.) to make the effects of the problem in these areas visible.
- Creates a safe space for conversation by approaching the client with a non-judgmental attitude.
- Helps the client identify their values and goals in their own words (Türkçapar, 2019).
- Helps the client gently question how their current behavior is preventing them from achieving these goals.
- Supports the client in discovering the potential personal benefits of change to foster their internal motivation (Dobson & Dozois, 2021; Türkçapar, 2019; Beck & Dozois, 2011).

This approach aims to help the individual develop an internal "why" rather than forcing or persuading them. This is because when individuals realize that change is consistent with their values and that their current situation is detrimental to them in the long term, they become more willing to move from the pre-contemplation stage to the next stage, the contemplation stage (Nakao, 2021; Türkçapar, 2019).

In summary, the pre-contemplation stage is a preparatory phase where the awareness necessary for change to begin has not yet formed, but where this awareness can be gradually developed through therapeutic relationships and discovery-based interventions (Nakao, 2021; Dobson & Dozois, 2021; Türkçapar, 2019; Beck & Dozois, 2011).

2. <u>Second stage: The planning (thinking/indecision) stage:</u>

At this stage, the individual is now aware that their situation is a "problem" and has begun to desire change genuinely. However, this desire does not yet translate into decisive action because the client experiences profound ambivalence about whether change is possible. Therefore, the person both wants to change and fears change (Nakao, 2021). The therapist's primary task at this stage is to bring the client's mental ambivalence to light and address it with an attitude of exploration, without judgment. An important technique is to help the client consider the pros and cons of change, i.e., the questions "How will change benefit me?" and "What will happen if I do not change?" In this way, the person touches their own internal motivation and begins to express the personal reasons necessary for change more consciously (Chand, 2023; Nakao, 2021; Türkçapar, 2019).

For example, a client with obsessive-compulsive disorder may acknowledge their problem but believe it cannot be changed. Thoughts such as "I am so used to being this way," "I will feel terrible if I do not do it," or "I will lose control if I break my routines" simultaneously generate both desire and fear regarding change (Türkçapar, 2019). In this case, all of the client's assumptions are listened to with therapeutic curiosity, and then examined together to determine whether they are absolute truths. The therapist can plan safe and small-scale behavioral experiments so that the individual can see that change is possible (Türkçapar, 2019; Beck & Dozois, 2011). For example:

- The client tries to reduce handwashing time by just 10 seconds; thus, they can experience that the things they perceive as "catastrophic" do not occur.
- Someone with a need for symmetry may try leaving an object on the table "out of place" for a short time.
- Someone experiencing a compulsion to check things may try checking the stove only once when leaving home and observing the results (Van Dis et al., 2021; Hirsch et al., 2019; Türkçapar, 2019).

These types of micro-experiments allow the client to question their belief that "change is not possible" and boost their self-confidence. In addition, by discussing the client's possible obstacles, fears, and sources of motivation in detail, both the psychological and behavioral foundations of the change process are strengthened (Van Dis et al., 2020; Hirsch et al., 2019). Thus, the client becomes more prepared to move on to the next stage, the "action" phase. To show a patient in this phase that change is difficult but possible, several simple behavioral experiments can be conducted with the client (Hirsch et al., 2019; Türkçapar, 2019):

After asking an intriguing question such as, "*If you could change something you have been doing your entire life within a week, would you believe that change is possible in this area too?*", the patient can be asked, "*Which hand do you use to hold your toothbrush when brushing your teeth?*" In this case: "*For your entire life, for about 25 years, you have brushed your teeth holding the toothbrush in your right hand. Let us say you wanted to change this, that is, if you held your toothbrush with your left hand next week, what would you need to do to make this change?*" (Türkçapar, 2019). In summary, motivational interviewing should be prioritized with clients in the pre-contemplation and contemplation stages. Applying cognitive behavioral therapy during these stages would not be an appropriate approach. The fundamental principle of motivational interviewing is that the motivation to change must come from the individual themselves and cannot be imposed from outside (Dobson & Dozois, 2021; Türkçapar, 2019; Beck & Dozois, 2011; Butler et al., 2006).

3. Third stage: The preparation stage:

This stage is a critical phase in which the client begins to both want and plan for change. The person now realizes that change is necessary and has a much clearer idea, in this stage, than in previous ones, that "I must do something to solve this problem." At this stage, the individual has begun to set concrete and achievable goals, moving beyond a general desire for improvement (Türkçapar, 2019; Beck & Dozois, 2011). For example, an ambiguous statement such as "*I need to reduce my anxiety*" is replaced by measurable goals such as "*I will reduce my daily checking behavior by half*" (Dobson & Dozois, 2021; Türkçapar, 2019).

A key characteristic of clients in the preparation stage is that they have mentally prepared the necessary conditions for change. At this stage, the client can more realistically assess their confidence in the change, their available resources, and potential obstacles. It is common for clients to seek psychotherapy on their own accord during this period because their motivation for change has shifted from external to internal resolve (Nicoară et al., 2023; Dobson & Dozois, 2021; Türkçapar, 2019). The therapist's primary task at this stage is to help the client structure their goals in a realistic, small, measurable, and achievable way. As Türkçapar (2019) also points out, setting significant and difficult-to-achieve goals during the preparation period can undermine the client's motivation; therefore, the treatment process should be structured around small steps. For example:

- For a client with panic disorder, a small exposure goal such as "*going outside for short periods twice a week*" can be set.
- For a client with depression, behavioral activation steps such as "*a 10-minute walk every day*" can be planned.

For individuals with obsessive-compulsive disorder (OCD), a simple but effective behavioral exercise such as "*delaying the ritual for 5 minutes*" can be recommended (Dobson & Dozois, 2021; Türkçapar, 2019).

During the preparation phase, the support mechanisms the client will need during the change process (family, friends, daily routine adjustments, time management) are also evaluated. Potential relapse points are discussed, and strategies for coping with them are developed. These preparations enable the client to transition to the next phase, the "action" phase, more strongly and securely (Türkçapar, 2019; Beck & Dozois, 2011). Following this integrated preparation, cognitive behavioral therapy can be sustained in a structured manner, as the client now has the internal motivation to engage in both cognitive restructuring and behavioral interventions (Türkçapar, 2019).

4. Fourth phase: Action phase:

This phase is the stage where the change process is actively implemented, and the client begins to apply what they have learned in therapy to their behavior, thoughts, and daily life. The action phase is the stage where the core interventions of cognitive behavioral therapy are used most intensively. The client now not only knows that change is possible but also takes concrete steps to achieve it (Dobson & Dozois, 2021; Türkçapar, 2019).

At this stage, therapy assumes a more structured and technically focused approach. The therapist systematically applies the necessary cognitive and behavioral interventions to help the client achieve their goals. As Türkçapar (2019) emphasizes, in order for this to be carried out correctly, careful consideration must be given to whether the client has entered the action phase, because cognitive techniques are only effective when the person is truly ready for change (Türkçapar, 2019; Beck & Dozois, 2011). Some basic applications used in the action phase are as follows:

- ✓ Cognitive Restructuring: The client is helped to recognize their automatic thoughts, question them, and develop more functional alternative thoughts.
- ✓ Exploring the emotion–thought–behavior connection: The client gains a clearer understanding of which emotion a particular thought triggers and how this translates into behavior (Gumport et al., 2015).

- ✓ Behavioral Experiments: The client is encouraged to have small but planned encounters with behaviors they fear or avoid. These experiments both test cognitive assumptions and expand the client's functional behavior repertoire (Dobson & Dozois, 2021; Türkçapar, 2019).
- ✓ Exposure: Particularly in cases of anxiety, OCD, or post-traumatic issues, the client systematically confronts situations they physically or mentally avoid.
- ✓ Behavioral Activation: Activities that evoke feelings of pleasure, interest, and success are structured for individuals with depression, aiming to elevate their mood.
- ✓ Skill training: The client is taught new skills, including emotion regulation, problem-solving, and coping with stress (Dobson & Dozois, 2021; Türkçapar, 2019; Gumport et al., 2015).

A key feature of the action phase is that the client becomes an active participant in the therapy process. The person makes an effort to apply what they have learned not only during the session but also outside of it. Therefore, homework assignments, behavior

Monitoring forms, emotion logs, and behavior trials play a critical role during this phase (Türkçapar, 2019). Additionally, maintaining the client's motivation is crucial during the action phase of therapy. The therapist makes the small successes the client experiences during the process visible and reinforces them (İlgar & İlgar, 2019). When obstacles or setbacks occur, they are treated not as "failures" but as natural parts of the change process (Dobson & Dozois, 2021; Türkçapar, 2019; Gumport et al., 2015). At the end of this phase, the client has achieved many of the changes they aimed for. The individual's meaningful progress at both the cognitive and behavioral levels forms the basis for transitioning to the next phase, the maintenance phase (Türkçapar, 2019; Beck & Dozois, 2011).

5. Fifth phase: Maintenance and Relapse Prevention Phase

The maintenance phase aims to sustain the skills and changes gained by the client during therapy in the long term. The primary goal in this phase is for the client to transition from being an active client to becoming an individual who can independently sustain their own change in daily life (Dobson & Dozois, 2021; Türkçapar, 2019). The cognitive and behavioral skills learned during the action phase have now become more automatic and a natural part of the client's life (Türkçapar, 2019).

One of the most important features of the maintenance phase is the focus on **recognizing, preventing, and managing** possible **relapses**, along with "continuing" the change. This is because clinical observations and research show that relapses that may occur after therapy are a natural part of the process, but when the client can recognize these relapses early and apply appropriate coping strategies, they can be prevented from turning into a permanent relapse (Ak et al., 2020; İlgar & İlgar, 2019; Türkçapar, 2019).

During this period, the work between the therapist and the client generally focuses on the following topics:

- **Identifying early warning signs:** Together with the client, thoughts, feelings, and behaviors that increase the risk of relapse are identified. For example, increased avoidance for someone with an anxiety disorder, social withdrawal, or loss of energy for someone experiencing depression are considered early signals (Ak et al., 2020; İlgar & İlgar, 2019; Türkçapar, 2019).
- **Creating coping plans:** The client is helped to create a ready action plan to cope with risky situations. This plan includes both cognitive skills (e.g., questioning automatic thoughts) Moreover, behavioral skills (e.g., planning regular activities, maintaining exposure strategies) (Dobson & Dozois, 2021; Türkçapar, 2019; Gumport et al., 2015).
- **Reinforcing gains:** The client's progress made during therapy is reviewed, and the importance of this progress is emphasized. Reinforcing successes helps maintain motivation to sustain change (Ak et al., 2020; İlgar & İlgar, 2019).
- **Strengthening self-efficacy:** The client begins to develop a stronger belief that they can now cope with their problems. The therapist supports the client in recognizing their own skills and trusting them (Özdel & Türkçapar, 2021).
- **Monitoring sessions:** In this phase, the frequency of sessions is reduced (e.g., to once every two weeks or once a month). This practice enables the client to become more independent and discover opportunities to apply what they have learned independently (Ak et al., 2020; İlgar & İlgar, 2019).
- **Building resilience for the future:** The therapist and client plan in advance for potential future life stressors (e.g., job changes, relationship issues, losses) and develop strategies to cope with them. This reduces the risk of relapse during potentially difficult periods (Sakarya & Karaaziz, 2025; Özdel & Türkçapar, 2021).

The maintenance phase is the stage at which the client internalizes the changes provided by the therapeutic process. At the end of this phase, the client not only has reduced their problems but also becomes a more flexible, resilient, and functional individual with coping skills to face future challenges (Dobson & Dozois, 2021; Türkçapar, 2019).

3. FORMULATION IN COGNITIVE BEHAVIORAL THERAPY

One of the most important features that distinguishes cognitive behavioral therapy from other therapies is that the therapy process is conducted clearly and straightforwardly for both the patient and the therapist. Cognitive conceptualization provides the framework that helps the therapist and patient understand the problem. Conceptualization provides as traightforward and understandable roadmap, with the flexibility to be updated in response to new information and shifting goals (Mercin, 2005). Cognitive behavioral formulation can be conducted at three levels: case, syndrome/problem, and situation levels.

1. Formulation at the case level is an attempt to understand the case as a whole, focusing on the relationship between the patient's problems and the underlying cognitive mechanisms (Türkçapar, 2019).
2. Cognitive formulation at the syndrome or problem level is the general cognitive model of a general problem or psychiatric diagnosis, such as depression or social anxiety. For example, the formulation of panic disorder is the experience of anxiety and avoidance responses as a result of the individual catastrophizing innocent physical and mental symptoms (Dobson & Dozois, 2021; Türkçapar, 2019; Gumport et al., 2015
3. Situation-level formulation, on the other hand, is a cognitive explanation of the patient's emotional and behavioral response in a given situation, recorded as negative thoughts in accordance with the A-B-C model, which is done in almost every session (Türkçapar, 2019; Özdel, 2015).

Example:

- Patient's statement: *"I thought they would get angry at me because I am stupid."*

  Expectation: They will get angry at me.
  Attribution: They will get angry because I am stupid.
  Self-belief: I am stupid, so I cannot do things that require intelligence.
  Concern: I do not want them to get angry at me.

The focus of cognitive conceptualization is the client's cognitive response to the problem situation: What was the cognitive picture at the moment the symptoms appeared or intensified? Formulation is the expression of the cognitive mechanism underlying the observed problems. Evidence-based case conceptualization is fundamental in cognitive behavioral therapy. In other words, the formulations presented are based on information obtained from the patient and observations made (Aslan, 2025; Ak et al., 2020).

3.1. How is Formulation Done?

Formulation begins with observations related to emotions, behaviors, and thoughts. In other words, the information obtained and observations made during the interview with the patient can be likened to the data collection stage, which is the first step in forming a scientific hypothesis. These collected data and observations are evaluated in accordance with cognitive theory (Ak et al., 2020). The person's problems are listed, and possible mechanisms based on the underlying core beliefs are considered. The themes that emerge in many cases in the data obtained provide general schemas (Ak et al., 2020; Türkçapar, 2019; Özdel, 2015).

- ✓ What is the common aspect of the person's problems?
- ✓ What kind of belief might someone who behaves this way have?
- ✓ What are the antecedents and consequences of the behaviors?
- ✓ What underlying mechanisms might be causing the problems?
- ✓ What are the preparatory factors for the current problems?
- ✓ Is the underlying mechanism being considered consistent with the preparatory factors of the current problem?
- ✓ What early experiences did the client have that taught them these things?
- ✓ The answers to all these questions help us formulate the cognitive fact (Ak et al., 2020; Türkçapar, 2019).

3.2. Content of Cognitive Fact Formulation

The content of the cognitive formulation consists of a list of the client's problems, core beliefs, and their associated early developmental history that laid the groundwork for their formation, as well as intermediate beliefs and coping strategies caused by core beliefs. Additionally, it includes therapy assumptions and treatment plans that summarize the problems (Yüksel, 2024). In summary, a case formulation is a summary of information about the patient's diagnosis, problems, how these problems developed and persisted, the thoughts and beliefs that accompanied and prepared for these problems and how they developed, the accompanying reactions, and how the patient's psychological disorder emerged based on this information (Yüksel, 2024; Ak et al., 2020).

3.3. Components of Formulation

Early life experiences and core beliefs (schemas): The client's relational experiences during childhood, caregiver attitudes, traumatic events, or experiences such as neglect form the person's core beliefs about themselves, others, and the world. These schemas are usually deep-rooted cognitive structures, such as "I am inadequate," "People are untrustworthy," and "The world is a dangerous place" (Özcan & Çelik, 2017).

Intermediate beliefs (rules, assumptions): Intermediate rules, which are more superficial than core beliefs and operate in the form of "If ... then ...", guide the person's daily behavior. For example: "*If I am not perfect, I will not be valued.*" "*If I show weakness, people will abandon me.*" Intermediate beliefs show how core beliefs are reflected in behaviors and are critical to understanding the client's internal conflicts (Yüksel, 2024; Ak et al., 2020; Özcan & Çelik, 2017).

Triggering situations: Events that activate the client's schemas or intermediate beliefs are important components of the formulation. These situations often involve interpersonal relationships.

Stressors, performance-demanding environments, and sensitive moments such as loss and rejection (Özcan & Çelik, 2017).

Automatic thoughts and emotional responses: Automatic thoughts that arise instantly in response to triggers determine a person's emotional and physiological responses. For example, the thought "*I am not good enough*" can lead to feelings such as anxiety, sadness, or shame, and behaviors such as avoidance (Ak et al., 2020; Özcan & Çelik, 2017).

Behavioral responses and perpetuating cycles: The coping styles developed by the client, such as avoidance, safety-seeking behaviors, aggression, and withdrawal, are often comforting in the short term; however, they contribute to the persistence of problems in the long term. Thus, a mechanism called a vicious cycle develops (Yüksel, 2024; Ak et al., 2020; Özcan & Çelik, 2017).

Fundamentally, the first stage of formulation includes identity information and demographic characteristics. For clients, a

Problem list: This consists of a list of the patient's problems and difficulties expressed in concrete terms in emotional, behavioral, or physiological terms. The patient's psychiatric symptoms or life problems may be included (Bengisoy et al., 2019). Each item on the problem list consists of a few words describing the problem. After defining the problem or leading symptom, a brief description of the accompanying factors in other areas is added (Ak et al., 2020; Bengisoy et al., 2019; Özcan & Çelik, 2017).

Diagnosis: Here, if the client does not have a diagnosis-level condition, only their psychological reactions are noted, or if they have a diagnosis-level problem, the relevant diagnosis or diagnoses are recorded (Bengisoy et al., 2019; Türkçapar, 2019).

Cognitive assumptions: This is the most important part of the formulation. To achieve this, it is advisable to begin with formulations at the problem/situation level; this is the cognitive explanation of the patient's emotional and behavioral response in a given situation, in accordance with the A-B-C model (Türkçapar, 2019).

Case Formulation Plan:

1. Descriptive information
2. Problem list
3. Diagnosis
4. Cognitive assumptions
   a. Situations where problems occur and their formulation
   b. Situation: Emotion, behavior, thought, outcome
   c. Early experiences
   d. Core beliefs
   e. Conditional beliefs and rules
   f. Triggering factors
   g. Problematic situations
   h. Situations that increase the problem
   i. Situations that reduce the problem
   j. Sustaining factors
5. Summary of cognitive assumptions
6. Situations that may positively affect treatment
7. Situations that may negatively affect treatment

4. INTEGRATION OF COGNITIVE BEHAVIORAL TECHNIQUES INTO PATIENT CARE IN PSYCHIATRIC NURSING

Cognitive Behavioral Therapy is a scientifically based and structured psychotherapy approach that focuses on the reciprocal interaction between thoughts, emotions, and behaviors. This approach is now effectively utilized not only in psychotherapy settings but also in clinical nursing, chronic disease management, psychosocial care, rehabilitation, and primary healthcare (Moran & Yılmaz, 2024). The integration of CBT techniques into healthcare improves the quality of care. It enhances patient satisfaction and well-being in the management of patients' psychosocial difficulties, treatment compliance issues, and anxiety and depression symptoms (Ata & Doğan, 2018).

Within the development process of the nursing profession, some principles and techniques of cognitive-behavioral therapy have become fundamental to nursing care and have been integrated into practice. The scope of psychiatric nursing practice is also constantly expanding due to the spread of holistic care and nursing knowledge; nursing practices vary according to the educational background of the nurse, which determines their level of practice (Moran & Yılmaz, 2024; Ata & Doğan, 2018). Psychiatric Nursing standards state that "Nurses provide individual, group, and/or family therapy within an evidence-based, psychotherapeutic framework, within interpersonal relationships and the therapeutic relationship between patient and nurse." The functions of an advanced practice psychiatric mental health nurse include health promotion and protection, as well as long- and short-term therapies, individual, group, couple/marital therapy, family therapy, insight-focused, behavioral, cognitive therapies, and interpersonal therapies (Moran & Yılmaz, 2024; Ata & Doğan, 2018; Demiralp & Oflaz, 2007). The integration of CBT techniques into patient care enhances the communication established between nurses and other healthcare professionals and the patient, increases the patient's motivation for behavioral change, and improves health outcomes.

4.1. The Role and Importance of CBT in Patient Care in Psychiatric Nursing

Psychiatric nurses, due to their counseling roles, undertake important tasks in teaching and developing coping skills, minimizing disability, and protecting and promoting mental health. Additionally, psychiatric nurses can become certified specialists in their field. Certified specialized psychiatric nurses can apply psychotherapy to individuals, families, and groups using the role of psychotherapist in protecting and improving mental health, preventing mental illness and disability, and restoring the individual's functionality and functional impairment to their pre-illness state (Wheeler, 2020; Keser-Özcan, 2020; Duru & Yılmaz, 2023). Considering the increasing evidence of CBT in physical health settings, nurses will be able to meet growing expectations in the future by providing evidence-based treatment, promoting quality improvement, and enhancing efficiency through CBT (Keser-Özcan, 2020). Given the increasing evidence for CBT in physical health settings, nurses will be able to utilize CBT to provide evidence-based treatment, promote quality improvement, and enhance efficiency, thereby meeting growing expectations in the future (Currid et al., 2011).

The experience of illness is not solely a biological process; an individual's past experiences, cognitive schemas, coping styles, and current emotional state directly influence the treatment process. Chronic illnesses, surgical procedures, intensive care processes, or life-threatening health conditions, in particular, can cause patients to develop patterns of behavior based on anxiety, hopelessness, helplessness, and misconceptions (Wheeler, 2020; Keser- Özcan, 2020).

The literature clearly states that psychiatric nurses with appropriate academic and professional training can enter psychotherapy training programs and be certified as psychotherapists when they are qualified to practice CBT (Keser-Özcan, 2020). Regarding the certification of psychiatric nurses, the document published by Horatio European Psychiatric Nurses includes the following recommendations:

- For a country to provide various treatments, access to psychotherapy training should be open to all liberal disciplines, including psychiatric nursing.
- The starting point should be at the basic licensure level (Bachelor's degree or Psychiatric and Mental Health Nurse).
- Psychotherapy certification courses must meet the criteria established by the European Association for Psychotherapy and the World Council for Psychotherapy.
- Countries should not limit the practice of psychotherapy to a single discipline, given both its clinical effectiveness and cost advantages.
- Properly trained psychiatric nurse therapists should be included in mental health services, especially in cases of significant and complex mental illnesses requiring combined psychotherapeutic and psychopharmacological support.
- Nurses who do not provide psychotherapy but care for patients receiving psychotherapy should be trained on how to support the therapist's work (Duru & Yılmaz, 2023; Horatio: European Psychiatric Nurses, 2012).

While psychiatrists and clinical psychologists can assess mental health status in relation to psychiatric disorders, psychiatric nurses should be familiar with care management activities, care planning, and clinical intervention. Thanks to the advantages of their prior education, training, and practical experience, psychiatric nurses appear to be more suited than other professional groups to provide psychotherapy to individuals diagnosed with psychiatric disorders (Duru & Yılmaz, 2023). According to a report published by Horatio European Psychiatric Nurses, 90% of CBT therapists in the United Kingdom have a background in psychiatric nursing. In the United States, psychotherapy is practiced by nurses holding a master's degree or higher. In Australia and Canada, the practice of psychotherapy is similar, although it varies by region and state (Duru & Yılmaz, 2023; Horatio: European Psychiatric Nurses, 2012).

One of the psychotherapeutic areas where psychiatric nurses can be involved is CBT. Some of the fundamentals of CBT are similar to those in nursing, including empathy, establishing relationships with patients, and therapeutic communication. Basic CBT approaches can be utilized by nurses in various settings who aim to bridge the psychological/physiological gap (Wheeler, 2020; Keser-Özcan, 2020). When applying CBT, psychiatric nurses aim to inform the patient, increase their compliance with treatment, and teach them how to cope with stress. Similar to the nursing process, CBT is patient-centered and requires strong.

Collaboration between the therapist and the patient. Another commonality is that both CBT and nursing use an approach based on measurement tools and research evidence (Duru & Yılmaz, 2023). With these characteristics, CBT can be applied by certified psychiatric nurses in any healthcare setting to increase the therapeutic effectiveness of nursing care and the individual's healthy coping behaviors (Duru & Yılmaz, 2023; Stuart, 2014).

4.2. Applications of Integrating CBT Techniques into Patient Care in Psychiatric Nursing

4.2.1. Psychoeducation

One of the most important components of CBT is teaching patients about their illness, its symptoms, and the treatment process clearly and understandably. Information such as how the illness developed, which symptoms are typical, and the impact of stress on the process helps reduce the patient's anxiety. Answering the patient's question, "Why do I feel this way?" increases their confidence in the treatment (Keser-Özcan, 2020). Psychiatric nurses can provide this education in brief interviews and help patients correct their misconceptions (Duru & Yılmaz, 2023; Keser-Özcan, 2020).

4.2.2. Identifying Automatic Thoughts

Patients often find it challenging to identify the thoughts underlying their emotional distress. Psychiatric nurses can identify these thoughts by asking the following questions (Duru & Yılmaz, 2023; Türkçapar, 2019):

- *"What was the first thought that came to your mind in this situation?"*
- *"What emotion did this thought evoke in you?"*
- *"What evidence supports or contradicts this thought?"*

For example, if a patient about to undergo surgery has a catastrophic thought such as "*Something is definitely going to go wrong*," the nurse can guide the patient to question the validity of this thought (Türkçapar, 2019).

4.2.3. Cognitive Restructuring

The identified automatic thoughts are addressed realistically, and more functional alternatives are developed. Psychiatric nurse:

- Helps the patient discuss the accuracy of their thoughts.
- Guides the patient in developing a more balanced perspective.
- Provides examples, analogies, or evidence when necessary.

This technique enhances treatment compliance, particularly in individuals with mental health issues, as well as in areas such as chronic pain, diabetes, heart disease, and oncology (Duru & Yılmaz, 2023; Türkçapar, 2019).

4.2.4. Behavioral Activation

Loss of motivation in managing depression or chronic illness can cause the patient to lead a more passive life. Nurses can use this technique to help the patient reorganize their daily routines. With the behavioral activation principle of CBT (Duru & Yılmaz, 2023; Keser- Özcan, 2020):

- Small and achievable daily activities are planned for the patient.
- As energy levels increase, the activity level is gradually raised.
- The passivity-feeling-destructive cycle is broken.

4.2.5. Adaptation of Exposure Techniques

Avoidant behavior is common in patients with anxiety disorders or phobias. This can hinder treatment compliance. Psychiatric nurses can use simple controlled exposure strategies to:

- Help the patient experience the avoided situation in small steps,
- Help the patient notice that anxiety decreases over time,
- Support the patient in strengthening their coping skills.

For example, a patient who experiences excessive anxiety about medical procedures can be exposed to the pre-procedure stages slowly and in a controlled manner (Duru & Yılmaz, 2023; Türkçapar, 2019).

4.2.6. Supporting Problem-Solving Skills

The BDT problem-solving approach guides the patient in: identifying the problem, generating solution options, planning for the most appropriate option, and taking steps to implement and evaluate the solution. Psychiatric nurses can effectively use this approach, particularly in chronic disease management, rehabilitation, and home care processes (Türkçapar, 2019; Özcan & Çelik, 2017).

5. APPLIED CASE EXAMPLES

5.1. Example Case Formulation-1

Descriptive information: Ms. K., 23 years old, female, student
Problem list-1:

- Anxiety in social settings: She stated that she has experienced anxiety and excitement in social settings such as meeting new people, talking, addressing the class, talking to teachers, attending friend gatherings, etc., which began in elementary school and intensified in high school.
- Thoughts: Thoughts such as “I am embarrassed,” “I will not be able to talk,” “My voice is shaking,” “People will notice my hands are shaking,” “This will never change,” and “I will not have any friends.”
- Behaviors: Avoidance of social groups, trying to stay in the background when with people, talking little, being quiet, and moving little.
- Depressive mood: Hopelessness and pessimism secondary to social anxiety experienced for many years.

Issue list-2:

- Suicidal thoughts: Suicidal thoughts arise due to the continuation of social anxiety and the resulting hopelessness caused by its impact on their social life at school.
- Panic attacks: 3-4 episodes of nighttime distress accompanied by fear of death.
- Thoughts: “I am dying,” “I am going crazy,” “I am going to lose myself.”

- Behaviors: Seeking medical help, undergoing medical examination
- Possible Medical Diagnosis: Social anxiety disorder

Cognitive assumptions:
Situations where the problem occurs and its formulation

Situation 1: Playing backgammon with friends
- ✓ Emotion: Anxiety, excitement
- ✓ Behavior: Hiding hands, playing quickly
- ✓ Thought: "They will notice my hands are shaking."
- ✓ Result: "I will be embarrassed, they will make fun of me."

Situation 2: Playing the guitar
- ✓ Emotion: Excitement
- ✓ Behavior: Trying to look relaxed
- ✓ Thought: "They will realize I am excited."
- ✓ Result: "I will be seen as deficient (sick)."

Early experiences: Dental treatment before elementary school; a critical, distant, and cold father; being teased by classmates due to a skin condition in elementary school

Core beliefs:

Self: "I am different (due to negative traits)," "I am inadequate," "I am flawed," "I am unwanted."

Others: Mocking, critical, exclusionary

Conditional beliefs and rules:
- "I must not make mistakes."
- "If I do not make mistakes, I will be seen as normal."
- "If I succeed and appear calm, my differences and inadequacies will not be exposed."

Triggering factor:
- The problem intensified after changing classes in high school

Situations where the problem occurs:
- Being around other people; situations that require talking to people, eating, one-on-one conversations; having photos taken

Situations that exacerbate the problem:
- Joining a group after it has already formed, being caught unprepared, talking to the opposite sex, and people who are perceived as sarcastic

Situations that reduce the problem:
- Being well-prepared, supportive people

Sustaining factors:

- Avoiding social settings and gatherings, speaking little in social settings, holding something in one's hand, feeling that one's performance was poor after unavoidable social events, and reflecting on this, which negatively affects one's mood

Summary of cognitive assumptions:

- K. Beliefs of inadequacy and not being wanted become active when he is with other people or when performing any activity in environments where they are present. His father's critical and cold attitude, orthopedic problems when he started walking, and his elementary school friends teasing him taught him that he was flawed, inadequate, and different, and that other people were critical and mocking.

These schemas became active with the transition to high school classes. When entering social environments, negative automatic thoughts associated with his schemas, such as "*I got excited, people noticed, I was humiliated*," become active, causing him to feel fear and excitement, and consequently avoid social interactions. As he experiences anxiety symptoms after unavoidable social interactions, his belief solidifies, and he becomes hopeless. This hopelessness sometimes leads to suicidal thoughts.

Factors that can positively influence treatment:

- High motivation, supportive family attitude, above-average intelligence level

Factors that may negatively affect treatment:

- The problem has persisted for years, and the ability to alleviate the problem through avoidance

In summary, with case formulation, assumptions are made about the factors that prepare, cause, maintain, exacerbate, and alleviate the individual's distress, and treatment is carried out accordingly.

5.2. Example Case Formulation-2

Descriptive Information:

Patient: 32 years old, female, single. Diagnosis: Major Depressive Disorder

Reason for Referral: Persistent low mood, lack of motivation, inability to cope with workload, intense feelings of guilt, difficulty getting out of bed in the morning, decreased self-care. Setting: Psychiatric ward; short-term hospitalization.

List of Problems:

Issues highlighted in the nursing assessment:

- Mood: Sadness, hopelessness, guilt.
- Cognitive level: Negative automatic thoughts ("I am a failure," "Nobody loves me," "I will never get better").
- Behavioral level: Decreased activity, social withdrawal, decreased personal care.
- Physiological symptoms: Sleep disturbance, decreased appetite, fatigue.
- Functionality: Difficulty going to work, procrastination.

Summary of the Formulation (with CBT Model):

Triggering Situation:
- Receiving feedback on "areas for improvement" during a performance review at work.

Automatic Thoughts:
- "So I am inadequate."
- "I will not be able to keep this job."
- "No one is satisfied with me anyway." Emotions:
- Sadness (8/10)
- Anxiety (6/10)
- Guilt (7/10)
- Hopelessness (8/10)

Physical/Bodily Reactions:
- Fatigue
- Loss of appetite
- Headache
- Desire to cry

Behaviors:
- Spending more time in bed
- Putting off going to work
- Canceling social activities
- Reduced self-care

This cycle **reinforces depressive symptoms**, reduces functionality, and strengthens negative thoughts.

Underlying Cognitive Structures:

Intermediate Beliefs

- “Making mistakes is unacceptable.”
- “If something is flawed, I am completely worthless.”
- “Being criticized means being abandoned.”

Core Beliefs (Core Schemas):

- **Inadequacy schema:** “I am not a valuable person.”
- **Inadequacy schema:** “I am a failure.” These schemas perpetuate the depressive cycle.

Application of CBT Interventions and Techniques in Nursing:

- The following techniques have been adapted for use by psychiatric nurses in their daily care process.

1. Psychoeducation and Modeling:

o The nurse explains the thought-feeling-behavior relationship to the patient in simple terms:

Example explanation:

- “When a negative thought arises in your mind, it affects your feelings and behaviors.

When we explore these relationships together, change becomes easier.” Objective: awareness, motivation, treatment compliance.

2. Emotion Tracking Form:

- The nurse gives the patient a short form to track their emotions daily.
- Emotion (sadness, anxiety, guilt, etc.)
- Intensity (0–10)
- Thoughts at that moment

This application helps patients develop emotional regulation skills in collaboration with the nurse.

3. Identifying Automatic Thoughts (Using Socratic Questioning):

The nurse asks the patient:

- “What evidence supports this thought?”
- “Is there any evidence to the contrary?”
- “If a friend were going through this, what would you tell them?” The nurse asks questions such as these.

Purpose: To soften rigid, distorted thoughts.

Example:
Patient: "I am a failure."
Nurse: "Is there only one incident that supports this? Can we recall situations where you were successful?"

4. Developing Alternative Thoughts:

For each identified negative thought, a new alternative thought is written down.
Example:
Automatic thought: "I will never get better."
Alternative thought: "I have gotten through difficult times before, and I can approach this process step by step."

5. Activity Schedule and Behavioral Activation:

- The nurse plans small daily activities with the patient:
o 10-minute walk
o Taking a shower
o Short visit with a friend
o Tidying up the room
o A short breathing exercise
Goal: Break the cycle of depression through behavioral activation.

6. Strengths List (Collaborative Work with the Nurse):

With the patient:
- Skills
- past successes
- Positive personality traits
- Support resources are listed.
Goal: to increase self-efficacy and weaken negative schemas.

7. Problem-Solving Training:

The nurse teaches the patient a 6-step problem-solving process for a current concern or problem:
- Defining the problem
- Setting goals
- Generate possible solutions
- Selecting the most appropriate solution

- Taking action
- Evaluating the outcome

8. Coping Cards:

The nurse prepares short coping phrases that the patient can use during a crisis:
- "This feeling is temporary."
- "My thoughts are not the reality itself."
- "I can calm my body by focusing on my breathing right now." These cards can be carried in the patient's pocket or notebook.

9. Behavioral Experiments (with a Nurse):

Small steps are planned to test the patient's negative assumption.
Example:
To a patient who says, "No one talks to me,"
- A short greeting experiment with one person in the dining room can be conducted with the nurse.
Objective: *To demonstrate that negative beliefs are not realistic.*

10. Trust Relationship, Empathy, and Collaborative Experimentation

The nurse-patient relationship is central to CBT. The nurse:
- listens without judgment,
- reflects feelings,
- frames change as "difficult but possible,"
- guides the patient to find their own solutions.

This is the nursing equivalent of the collaborative experimentation principle of CBT. Reflections on the Outcome and Care Plan:

This case formulation and techniques help the nurse:
- Understand the root causes of the patient's problems,
- structure the daily care plan,
- increase motivation,
- set cognitive and behavioral goals,
- monitoring and reducing symptoms.

Thus, a cognitive-behavioral framework is incorporated into psychiatric nursing care.

REFERENCES

Ak, M., Kırpınar, İ., Atmaca, M., Erkan, A., Güler, Ö., Kesici, Ş., & Kumsar, N. A. (2020). *Cognitive behavioral therapy in clinical practice-2*. Nobel Academic Publishing.

Aslan, B. (2025). Cognitive-Behavioral Case Formulation of Panic Disorder. *Turkish Journal of Integrative Psychotherapy*, *8*(15), 89–102.

Ata, E. E., & Doğan, S. (2018). The effect of a brief cognitive behavioral stress management program on mental status, coping with stress attitude, and caregiver burden while caring for schizophrenic patients. *Archives of Psychiatric Nursing*, *32*(1), 112–119. PMID: 29413060

Beck, A. T., & Dozois, D. J. (2011). Cognitive Therapy: Current Status and Future Directions. *Annual Review of Medicine*, *62*(1), 397–409. PMID: 20690827

Beck, J. S. (2020). *Cognitive behavior therapy: Basics and beyond.* Guilford Publications.

Bengisoy, A., Özdemir, M. B., Erkıvanç, F., Şahin, S., & İskifoğlu, T. Ç. (2019). Content analysis of research articles using cognitive behavioral therapy 1997-2018. *Turkish Psychological Counseling and Guidance Journal*, *9*(54), 745–793.

Bieling, P. J., McCabe, R. E., & Antony, M. M. (2022). *Cognitive-behavioral therapy in groups*. Guilford publications.

Bieling, P. J., McCabe, R. E., & Antony, M. M. (2022). *Cognitive-behavioral therapy in groups*. Guilford publications.

Butler, A. C., Chapman, J. E., Forman, E. M., & Beck, A. T. (2006). The Empirical Status of Cognitive-Behavioral Therapy: A Review of Meta-analyses. *Clinical Psychology Review*, *26*(1), 17–31. PMID: 16199119

Chand, S. P., Kuckel, D. P., & Huecker, M. R. (2023). Cognitive behavior therapy. In *StatPearls* [Internet]. StatPearls Publishing.

Currid, T. J., Nikčević, A. V., & Spada, M. M. (2011). Cognitive behavioral therapy and its relevance to nursing. *British Journal of Nursing (Mark Allen Publishing)*, *20*(22), 1443–1447. PMID: 22241494

Demiralp, M., & Oflaz, F. (2007). Cognitive-behavioral therapy techniques and psychiatric nursing practice. *Anadolu Journal of Psychiatry*, *8*(2), 132–139.

Dobson, K. S., & Dozois, D. J. (Eds.). (2021). *Handbook of cognitive-behavioral therapies*. Guilford Publications.

Duru, H. A., & Yılmaz, M. (2023). The role of the psychiatric nurse in cognitive behavioral therapy applied to patients diagnosed with depression: A literature review. *Mersin Üniversitesi Saglik Bilimleri Dergisi*, *16*(1), 131–146.

Gençtan, E. (1993). *Psychoanalysis and Beyond* (5th ed.). Remzi Kitabevi.

Gómez-Penedo, J. M., Babl, A., Dyresen, A., Fernández-Álvarez, J., & Flückiger, C., & grosse Holtforth, M. (2023). Problem mastery and motivational clarification as mechanisms of change in cognitive-behavioral therapy for depression: Secondary analysis of a randomized controlled trial. *Behaviour Research and Therapy*, *167*, 104343. PMID: 37307656

Gumport, N. B., Williams, J. J., & Harvey, A. G. (2015). Learning cognitive behavior therapy. *Journal of Behavior Therapy and Experimental Psychiatry*, *48*, 164–169. PMID: 25898288

Hirsch, C. R., Beale, S., Grey, N., & Liness, S. (2019). Approaching cognitive behavior therapy for generalized anxiety disorder from a cognitive process perspective. *Frontiers in Psychiatry*, *10*, 796. PMID: 31780964

Horatio: European Psychiatric Nurses. (2012, July). Psychiatric/mental health nurses and psychotherapy: Position document. http://www.horatioweb.eu/downloads/Psychotherapy_position_paper.pdf. Retrieved December 10, 2025.

İlgar, M. Z., & İlgar, S. C. (2019). Cognitive behavioral change and motivational interviewing. *Theory and Practice in Education*, *15*(1), 47–73.

Joaquim, S. B., Simões de Almeida, R., & Marques, A. J. (2023). Transdiagnostic cognitive behavioral group interventions: A systematic review. *Cognitive Therapy and Research*, *47*(3), 303–326.

Keser Özcan, N. (2020). Depressive disorder. In F. Oflaz & N. Yıldırım (Eds.), *Psychiatric nursing certification topics* (pp. 417–431). Psychiatric Nursing Association Publications No:1, Akademisyen Nobel Medical Bookstores.

Magill, M., Ray, L., Kiluk, B., Hoadley, A., Bernstein, M., Tonigan, J. S., & Carroll, K. (2019). A meta-analysis of cognitive-behavioral therapy for alcohol or other drug use disorders: Treatment efficacy by contrast condition. *Journal of Consulting and Clinical Psychology*, *87*(12), 1093. PMID: 31599606

Mercin, L. (2005). Comparison of the Characteristics of Piaget and Kohlberg's Theories of Moral Development. *Dicle University Journal of Education*, *5*, 73–86.

Moran, M., & Yılmaz, S. (2024). The use of cognitive behavioral therapy in psychiatric nursing studies. *YOBÜ Health Sciences Faculty Journal*, *5*(1), 91–100.

Nakao, M., Shirotsuki, K., & Sugaya, N. (2021). Cognitive–behavioral therapy for management of mental health and stress-related disorders: Recent advances in techniques and technologies. *BioPsychoSocial Medicine*, *15*(1), 16. PMID: 34602086

. Nicoară, N. D., Marian, P., Petri , A. O., Delcea, C., & Manole, F. (2023). A review of the role of cognitive-behavioral therapy on anxiety disorders of children and adolescents. *Pharmacophore, 14*(4-2023), 35-39.

Özcan, Ö., & Çelik, G. G. (2017). Cognitive behavioral therapy. *Turkey Clinics*, *3*(2), 115–120.

Özdel, K. (2015). Cognitive Behavioral Therapies from Past to Present: Theory and Practice. *Türkiye Klinikleri*, *8*(2), 10–20.

. Özdel, K., Kart, A., & Türkçapar, M. H. (2021). Cognitive Behavioral Therapy in the Treatment of Bipolar Disorder. *Archives of Neuropsychiatry/Nöropsikiyatri Arşivi, 58.*

Sakarya, G., & Karaaziz, M. (2025). A Review of Social Anxiety Disorder and Cognitive Behavioral Therapy. *Journal* of *Social. Human, and Administrative Sciences*, *8*(8), 638–656.

Stevens, M. W., King, D. L., Dorstyn, D., & Delfabbro, P. H. (2019). Cognitive–behavioral therapy for Internet gaming disorder: A systematic review and meta-analysis. *Clinical Psychology & Psychotherapy*, *26*(2), 191–203. PMID: 30341981

Stuart, G. W. (2014). *Principles and practice of psychiatric nursing* [E-book]. Elsevier Health Sciences.

Türkçapar, H. (2019). Cognitive Behavioral Therapy: Basic Principles and Application. Epsilon Publications, 13th Edition, Istanbul.

Tzur Bitan, D., Shalev, S., & Abayed, S. (2022). Therapists' views of mechanisms of change in psychotherapy: A mixed-method approach. *Frontiers in Psychology*, *13*, 565800. PMID: 35496206

Van Dis, E. A., Van Veen, S. C., Hagenaars, M. A., Batelaan, N. M., Bockting, C. L., Van Den Heuvel, R. M., & Engelhard, I. M. (2020). Long-term outcomes of cognitive behavioral therapy for anxiety-related disorders: A systematic review and meta-analysis. *JAMA Psychiatry*, *77*(3), 265–273. PMID: 31758858

Wheeler, K. (2020). Advanced psychiatric nursing practices: Evidence-based practice guide (A. Atlı Özbaş & N. Gürhan, Trans. Eds.; 2nd ed.). Ankara Nobel Medical Publishers.

Yüksel, A. (2024). Cognitive Behavioral Therapy Case Formulation for Social Phobia. *Turkey Journal of Integrative Psychotherapy*, *7*(14), 65–71.

Chapter 4
Mindfulness and Acceptance-Based Approaches

Ercan Tunç
https://orcid.org/0000-0002-3485-953X
Ondokuz Mayıs University, Turkey

ABSTRACT

This chapter examines the theoretical foundations and clinical applications of mindfulness- and acceptance-based approaches within contemporary psychosocial intervention frameworks. Core processes such as present-moment awareness, acceptance, cognitive defusion, self-as-context, values, and committed action are outlined to demonstrate how these mechanisms enhance psychological flexibility. Evidence supporting Mindfulness-Based Stress Reduction and Acceptance and Commitment Therapy is reviewed, with emphasis on their relevance to emotional regulation, chronic illness management, and holistic nursing practice.

INTRODUCTION

Psychosocial interventions constitute a diverse and expanding set of structured, theory-driven, and empirically validated approaches designed to address individuals' psychological, emotional, behavioral, and social difficulties. These interventions are grounded in the understanding that human functioning cannot be separated from the interpersonal, cultural, and environmental contexts in which individuals live. Accordingly, psychosocial interventions emphasize the interconnected nature of cognition, emotion, behavior, and social interaction, with the ultimate goal of

DOI: 10.4018/979-8-3373-6526-8.ch004

improving individuals' quality of life, strengthening adaptive functioning, and promoting long-term well-being (King & Ollendick, 2008).

For an intervention to be classified as psychosocial, several foundational criteria must be met. First, the intervention must be based on a clear theoretical framework that defines its mechanisms of action, clinical targets, and hypothesized outcomes (Yule, 2006). This theoretical grounding distinguishes structured psychosocial programs from ad hoc or purely intuitive helping strategies. Second, psychosocial interventions require a well-defined problem area and a clearly described target population. For instance, interventions aimed at women under the age of 30 who experience chronic interpersonal conflict or domestic stress in specific cultural contexts (e.g., Turkey) must consider both individual and sociocultural determinants of distress (Arranz et al., 2016). The precision with which the target population is described influences not only the intervention's applicability but also its capacity to produce replicable and meaningful outcomes.

A third essential criterion is empirical support. A psychosocial intervention must demonstrate its effectiveness through rigorous scientific methods, including randomized controlled trials, quasi-experimental studies, longitudinal follow-ups, and clinically meaningful effect size analyses (David & Montgomery, 2011). Effectiveness is evaluated both statistically and clinically, meaning that an intervention should not only produce significant quantitative improvements but should also yield observable, meaningful changes in individuals' daily functioning, social relationships, and subjective well-being. This dual emphasis on statistical significance and clinical relevance is central to contemporary evidence-based practice.

Within this broad framework, psychosocial interventions encompass a wide range of modalities, including but not limited to cognitive-behavioral therapies, interpersonal and family-based approaches, community-centered interventions, trauma-informed programs, expressive and creative therapies, and technology-assisted models such as telehealth and internet-based psychological support systems (Feather et al., 2016; Jacobsen & Jim, 2008). These approaches, while diverse, share a commitment to structured assessment, theoretically grounded techniques, culturally sensitive practice, and outcome-driven evaluation.

Among these modalities, mindfulness- and acceptance-based approaches have gained significant prominence over the past thirty years, marking one of the most substantial paradigm shifts in both clinical psychology and psychiatric nursing. Rooted in ancient contemplative traditions yet adapted through modern behavioral science, mindfulness and acceptance-based interventions emphasize present-moment awareness, nonjudgmental observation of experience, psychological flexibility, and the cultivation of adaptive coping strategies (Dryden & Still, 2006). Their rapid integration into nursing theory and practice reflects a broader movement toward holistic models that address the psychological and emotional dimensions of patient care in parallel with physical health needs (Guillaumie et al., 2017; White, 2014).

As the evidence base continues to expand, mindfulness and acceptance based interventions are increasingly recognized not merely as complementary practices but as essential components of comprehensive psychosocial care. Their incorporation into health care settings reflects an interdisciplinary movement that bridges psychological science, behavioral medicine, and nursing practice, offering a robust framework for addressing the complex interplay between mind, body, and environment. This book chapter therefore aims to explore these approaches in depth, examining their theoretical foundations, empirical support, mechanisms of change, and practical applications within nursing. By situating mindfulness and acceptance-based interventions within the broader context of psychosocial practice, the chapter seeks to provide a comprehensive and evidence-based perspective that can guide both clinical application and future research.

1. CORE CONCEPTS: MINDFULNESS AND ACCEPTANCE

Mindfulness and acceptance-based approaches represent a group of psychological interventions that emphasize the cultivation of conscious, intentional, and non-judgmental awareness of present-moment experiences. These approaches aim to help individuals relate to their internal states with openness, curiosity, and compassion, rather than through rigid, habitual, or reactive coping strategies such as emotional suppression, avoidance, rumination, or experiential denial. As such, mindfulness and acceptance-based models align conceptually with the broader movement known as the "third wave" of cognitive-behavioral therapies, a development that expanded the traditional focus on symptom reduction to include holistic mechanisms of psychological flexibility, value-driven behavior, and enhanced life satisfaction (Cavanagh et al., 2014; Hofmann & Asmundson, 2008).

Mindfulness is fundamentally defined as the deliberate orientation of attention to the present moment with an attitude of openness and receptivity. This includes observing ongoing thoughts, bodily sensations, emotional responses, urges, and environmental stimuli as they arise, without attempting to judge, suppress, or alter them (Black, 2011). A core component of mindfulness practice is the recognition of attentional drift; individuals learn to notice when the mind has wandered and to gently redirect attention back to a chosen focal point, such as the breath, bodily sensations, or a daily activity (Kostanski & Hassed, 2008). Through this repeated act of noticing and returning, mindfulness strengthens metacognitive awareness, attentional control, and the ability to consciously shift one's internal stance from reactivity to observation.

Acceptance constitutes another essential element of these approaches. In psychological terms, acceptance refers to willingly making space for internal experiences—including painful emotions, intrusive thoughts, physical discomfort, and urges—especially in situations where avoidance or resistance has proven ineffective or harmful. Importantly, acceptance should not be mistaken for resignation, indifference, or passivity. Instead, it reflects an active, intentional stance of openness toward internal events, combined with a commitment to engage in behaviors that are consistent with one's personally endorsed values (Kostanski & Hassed, 2008; Stewart, 2004). Acceptance thereby encourages individuals to move toward meaningful life directions rather than becoming preoccupied with the futile struggle to eliminate internal distress.

Both mindfulness and acceptance processes act to reduce cognitive fusion, which refers to the tendency to perceive thoughts, images, and internal narratives as literal truths or mandatory directives. Cognitive fusion often leads individuals to behave in ways governed by internal events rather than by context, values, or long-term goals. By contrast, mindfulness and acceptance practices help individuals recognize that thoughts are merely transient mental events—products of the mind rather than objective realities (Blackledge, 2007). This shift enables a more flexible response to internal experiences, allowing individuals to behave in accordance with what the situation requires rather than with what intrusive thoughts demand.

Together, these processes foster a broader construct referred to as psychological flexibility, which is central to acceptance- and mindfulness-based frameworks such as Acceptance and Commitment Therapy (ACT). Psychological flexibility involves:

1. Reduced experiential avoidance, meaning the person is less inclined to escape or suppress internal discomfort;
2. Present-moment contact, enabling individuals to engage fully with what is happening "here and now";
3. Cognitive defusion, decreasing the power and believability of distressing thoughts; and
4. Values-guided action, where behaviors are shaped by deeply held personal values rather than by fear, anxiety, or avoidance.

This integration of present-moment awareness, openness, willingness, and value-consistent behavior serves as a pathway from psychological rigidity to a functional, adaptive, and meaningful life. As Levin and Hayes (2011) describe, interventions grounded in these processes help individuals transform their relationship with their internal experiences, not by removing distress, but by teaching them how to live effectively with it while pursuing actions that align with what matters most to them.

Mindfulness and acceptance-based approaches therefore represent a major conceptual and clinical shift within the cognitive-behavioral tradition, one that aligns closely with contemporary understandings of human suffering, resilience, and well-being. Their emphasis on metacognition, intentional awareness, and value-oriented behavior makes them particularly suitable for diverse populations and settings, including nursing practice, where emotional regulation, chronic illness management, and person-centered care are central clinical priorities. This increasing prominence can be interpreted as a response to the limitations of strictly symptom-focused models in addressing chronic stress, emotional labor, and moral distress in healthcare contexts (Guillaumie et al., 2017; Slatyer et al., 2018). In nursing, where sustained exposure to suffering and high-stakes decision-making is common, approaches that strengthen psychological flexibility offer a clinically relevant framework for both patient care and staff well-being (Halm, 2017; Ramaci et al., 2019).

2. MINDFULNESS-BASED STRESS REDUCTION (MBSR)

The primary objective of Mindfulness-Based Stress Reduction (MBSR) is to systematically train individuals in meditation-based techniques that facilitate the development and deepening of mindfulness. Designed originally by Jon Kabat-Zinn in the late 1970s, MBSR has evolved into one of the most widely studied and empirically supported mindfulness programs in clinical, community, and health care settings. Fundamentally, the program teaches participants to observe their internal experiences—thoughts, emotions, bodily sensations, impulses—with openness, curiosity, and non-judgment, thereby transforming how they relate to stress, discomfort, and psychological challenges (Bishop, 2002). Through repeated practice, individuals begin to recognize that internal experiences do not necessarily reflect objective reality but rather constitute mental events that arise, unfold, and pass within awareness (Praissman, 2008). This shift supports the cultivation of psychological flexibility and emotional regulation, enabling individuals to avoid becoming entangled in stress-induced thoughts or maladaptive reactive patterns (Pan et al., 2024). Consistent with this mechanism-focused rationale, prior evidence indicates that MBSR is associated with reductions in perceived stress and emotional distress, alongside improvements in emotion regulation and attention-related outcomes in healthcare and clinical populations (Grossman et al., 2004; Guillaumie et al., 2017).

2.1. Meditation Practices and Mechanisms of Change

A central meditation practice in MBSR is the sitting meditation. In this practice, the individual adopts an upright, stable posture either on a cushion on the floor or seated in a chair. Attention is gently directed toward the breath, typically focusing on sensations at the nostrils, chest, or abdomen. Inevitably, attention drifts to thoughts, memories, concerns, external noises, or bodily sensations. When this shift occurs, the practitioner is instructed to notice the distraction—recognizing it without criticism or struggle—and then gently returning attention to the breath (Bishop, 2002; Black et al., 2009; Kabat-Zinn, 2016). Rather than viewing mind-wandering as a failure, the practitioner is encouraged to understand it as a natural function of the mind. The act of noticing distraction and returning to the breath is itself a central component of mindfulness training: it strengthens metacognitive awareness, attentional control, and the ability to respond rather than react automatically.

In sitting meditation, emphasis is placed on observing internal experiences with neutrality, without adding judgment, meaning, or narrative (Rodriguez et al., 2018). Thoughts and feelings are treated as transient mental events rather than as commands or truths, helping individuals develop the skill of non-reactivity. Over time, this reduces emotional reactivity and habitual cognitive fusion, allowing individuals to step back from distressing thoughts instead of becoming absorbed by them (Bishop, 2002; Black et al., 2009; Haberlin, 2024; Kabat-Zinn, 2016; Rodriguez et al., 2018).

2.2. Structure and Components of the MBSR Program

MBSR is typically delivered in eight- to ten-week group-based formats, with weekly sessions lasting approximately 2 to 2.5 hours (Bazzano et al., 2015). Many programs also include a full-day silent retreat around the sixth week. Sessions are highly experiential, combining meditation practice, psychoeducation, group discussions, and reflective exercises. The structure is intentionally designed to develop mindfulness skills in a gradual, cumulative manner.

Across sessions, a variety of mindfulness practices are introduced, including:

- Body scan meditation, which cultivates awareness of bodily sensations from head to toe.
- Mindful breathing, emphasizing present-moment focus via breath awareness.
- Gentle hatha yoga, integrating mindful movement and body awareness.
- Sitting meditation, emphasizing observation of thoughts, emotions, and sensory experiences.
- Walking meditation, developing mindfulness during movement.
- Loving-kindness (metta) practices, in some extended MBSR variations, to promote compassion.

The program also includes psychoeducational components, in which participants receive information about the physiological and psychological mechanisms of stress, the role of automatic thoughts, and the impact of emotional avoidance on health and well-being (Grossman et al., 2004; Imel et al., 2008). This educational foundation enhances participants' understanding of how mindfulness can interrupt maladaptive stress cycles and promote more adaptive emotional responses.

2.3. Homework, Daily Practice, and Skill Transfer

A central aspect of MBSR is the emphasis on daily formal and informal practice between sessions. Homework is not supplementary but foundational, intended to help participants generalize mindfulness skills to everyday life. Formal practices typically involve 30–45 minutes of meditation per day, guided by audio recordings. Informal practices encourage the application of mindfulness to routine activities such as eating, walking, showering, interpersonal communication, and moments of stress (Kabat-Zinn, 2016). Through consistent daily practice, individuals strengthen the neural and psychological pathways associated with attentional regulation, emotional awareness, and non-reactivity. This enables participants to respond to stressors with greater clarity and stability, rather than resorting to habitual avoidance or automatic emotional responses (Bishop, 2002). During each session, instructors review participants' experiences, challenges, and observations from the previous week, helping them refine their practice and integrate insights into daily functioning. The curriculum evolves progressively from week to week. Early sessions introduce basic skills such as body awareness and breath-focused meditation. Mid-program sessions incorporate mindful movement and advanced attentional practices. Later sessions help participants identify which practices best support their daily lives and guide them in creating sustainable mindfulness routines (Dobkin et al., 2014).

Figure 1.

Session	Theme	Mindfulness practices/ exercises	Homework
1	"[T]here is more right with you than wrong with you"	Awareness of positive self Moment by moment awareness of eating and breathing Guided body scan meditation	CD—guided body scan meditation Eat one meal mindfully
2	"[H]ow you see things (or don't see them) will determine in large measure how you will respond to them"	Guided body scan meditation Wandering mind—acceptance and refocusing Expanding awareness to identify and solve problems Guided sitting meditation with awareness of breathing	CD—guided body scan meditation Sitting meditation Pleasant events calendar Mindfully engage in routine activities
3	"There is pleasure and power in being present"	Guided mindful yoga Guided sitting meditation with awareness of breathing	CD guided (alternating) body scan meditation and mindful yoga Sitting meditation with awareness on breathing Unpleasant events calendar Capturing present moments Awareness of "automatic pilot" moments
4	"Awareness of being stuck in one's life and how to get unstuck"	Guided sitting meditation with awareness on breathing, sensations, body as a whole Listening and trusting in inner wisdom Awareness of stress and stress reactivity Loving kindness (i.e..	CD guided (alternating) body scan meditation and mindful yoga Sitting meditation with awareness on breathing, sensations, and body as a whole Awareness of stress reactions, feeling stuck, and shutting off
5	"Reacting and responding to stress"	Guided sitting meditation with awareness on thoughts and focus on stillness Mindfulness in problem-focused and emotion-focused coping strategies to stress Mindful pain management Loving kindness meditation	CD guided sitting meditation, alternating with body scan meditation or yoga Difficult communications calendar Awareness of moments of reacting Mindful responses to stress
6	"Maintaining your center in interpersonal relationships"	Guided sitting meditation Optional mountain and/ or lake meditation Guided mindful yoga Loving kindness meditation	CD guided sitting meditation, alternating with body scan meditation or yoga Awareness of consumption
7	"How what we take in (diet in the broadest sense of the term) affects our health and well-being"	Awareness of attachment to place Sitting meditation with choiceless awareness Mindfulness of moving out of self-destructive diet practices Mindful communication Loving kindness meditation	Non-guided formal mindfulness practice Informal practices Awareness of consumption
8	"Keeping up the momentum and discipline"	Body scan Sitting meditation Loving kindness meditation Review	Continuing guided and non-guided formal mindfulness practice Informal practices Short- and long-term health goals

Overall, MBSR is delivered in an 8–10 week group format that combines structured mindfulness practices, psychoeducation about stress, and between-session homework to promote skill transfer into daily life (Grossman et al., 2004; Imel et al., 2008; Dobkin et al., 2014; Del Rosario & Beshai, 2022).

3. ACCEPTANCE AND COMMITMENT THERAPY (ACT)

Acceptance and Commitment Therapy (ACT) is a central model within the "third wave" of cognitive-behavioral therapies, a movement that evolved from earlier behavioral (first wave) and cognitive (second wave) paradigms. While first-wave behavioral therapies emphasized observable behavior and conditioning principles, and second-wave cognitive therapies focused on identifying and modifying dysfunctional beliefs, third-wave approaches broadened the scope of intervention by incorporating mindfulness, experiential acceptance, contextual learning, and values-oriented change processes. ACT is one of the most influential and widely researched models emerging from this evolution (Hayes, 2004).

3.1. Theoretical Foundations of ACT

ACT's primary clinical aim is to cultivate psychological flexibility, defined as the capacity to remain in contact with the present moment while choosing actions aligned with personal values, even in the presence of internal discomfort. Psychological flexibility represents an overarching adaptive process that integrates two major therapeutic pillars:

1. Mindfulness and acceptance processes, which foster openness to internal experiences; and
2. Values and committed action, which guide behavior toward personally meaningful life directions (Larmar et al., 2014).

This dual structure positions ACT as a comprehensive behavioral model that addresses both private events (thoughts, emotions, memories, bodily sensations) and overt behavior in a coherent, context-sensitive way. From a nursing perspective, this focus is particularly relevant because psychological flexibility may buffer the impact of ongoing occupational stressors by supporting adaptive responding in emotionally demanding clinical situations (Zarvijani et al., 2021).

3.2. Functional Contextualism: Philosophical Underpinnings

ACT is grounded in functional contextualism, a modern behavioral philosophy emphasizing that the meaning and function of psychological events are determined by the context in which they occur. From this viewpoint, internal experiences are neither inherently good nor bad; their significance depends on the historical and situational factors surrounding them (Hayes, 2004; Kul & Türk, 2020).

Functional contextualism asserts that:

- Psychological phenomena must be understood within their learning history, including reinforcement patterns, relational learning, and prior coping strategies.
- Present situational variables—antecedents, consequences, environmental cues—shape whether a behavior is adaptive or maladaptive.
- Interventions should aim not at altering the form or frequency of private events but at changing how individuals respond to these events within relevant contexts.

A behavior is considered functional when it effectively serves one's values within a given context. Conversely, a behavior becomes *dysfunctional* when it rigidly persists despite failing to promote valued living (Kul & Türk, 2020). This perspective shifts the therapeutic goal from symptom elimination to transformational change in patterns of behavior.

3.3. Relational Frame Theory (RFT): Language, Cognition, and Human Suffering

Another central theoretical component of ACT is Relational Frame Theory (RFT), a behavioral account of language and cognition. RFT proposes that language is learned through the ability to relate stimuli in arbitrary, symbolic ways—for example, understanding that "A is greater than B" or that "pain means danger," even when the associations are not inherently physical (Belisle & Tarbox, 2024).

According to RFT:

- Relational responding forms the basis for complex cognitive abilities, including reasoning, problem-solving, identity formation, and social behavior.
- Human suffering often arises because language enables individuals to construct negative meanings, global narratives, and catastrophic predictions about their experiences (Terzioğlu & Yavuz, 2023).
- Through language, thoughts acquire functional properties—fearful, avoidant, self-critical—that shape behavior, sometimes in maladaptive ways.

Since language itself is a learned behavior, ACT interventions can modify its influence by altering how individuals relate to their thoughts. This is accomplished not by disputing their content, as in traditional cognitive therapy, but by changing the **context** in which language operates (Belisle & Tarbox, 2024; Terzioğlu & Yavuz, 2023).

3.4. The Six Core Processes of Psychological Flexibility

ACT conceptualizes the development of psychological flexibility through six interconnected processes, which together form the model:

1. Cognitive defusion: Learning to observe thoughts as transient verbal events rather than literal truths. A common defusion exercise involves shifting from "I am inadequate" to "I am having the thought that I am inadequate," thereby weakening the thought's believability.

Cognitive defusion is a core process within acceptance- and mindfulness-based therapeutic models, designed to transform the way individuals relate to their own thoughts. Rather than focusing on the content of thoughts, as in traditional cognitive approaches, defusion emphasizes the function of a thought and the influence it exerts on behavior. The underlying assumption is that when individuals become psychologically "fused" with their thoughts, those thoughts gain excessive authority, shaping emotions and actions in ways that may undermine well-being (Yavuz, 2015).

In states of cognitive fusion, a person tends to treat internal verbal events as literal truths or as mandatory instructions. For instance, a thought such as "I am a failure" can quickly be interpreted as an objective and unchangeable fact. Cognitive defusion works to interrupt this automatic process. It helps individuals create psychological distance, enabling them to perceive a thought as a transient mental event rather than as an accurate reflection of reality. This shift does not aim to dispute or replace the thought but to weaken its dominance over behavior (Assaz et al., 2018).

Techniques used to foster defusion often highlight the linguistic nature of thoughts. Reformulating a statement like "I am a failure" into "My mind is producing the thought that I am a failure right now" allows the person to recognize the thought as something generated by the mind, not as a factual statement about the self. This reframing reduces the emotional impact of the thought and makes space for values-based actions, even in the presence of uncomfortable internal experiences (Assaz et al., 2018; Yavuz, 2015).

The primary contribution of cognitive defusion is not to eliminate distressing thoughts but to loosen their grip. By reducing the degree to which thoughts dictate behavior, defusion enhances psychological flexibility: the ability to act in accordance with one's values rather than in response to fear, anxiety, or habitual patterns. It is particularly beneficial for individuals dealing with anxiety, depressive rumination, intrusive self-critical thoughts, or rigid thinking styles, as it introduces a more adaptive and context-sensitive way of responding to internal events (Doorley et al., 2020).

Overall, cognitive defusion represents a shift from attempting to control the content of thought to changing one's relationship with thought. It helps individuals observe thoughts without becoming entangled in them, thereby carving out the cognitive space required for effective action. Because of these mechanisms, cognitive defusion is regarded as a central therapeutic process within Acceptance and Commitment Therapy (ACT) and related interventions (Assaz et al., 2018; Doorley et al., 2020; Yavuz, 2015). Empirical findings suggest that reductions in cognitive fusion are associated with improvements in psychological functioning, indicating that defusion may operate as a meaningful change process rather than a purely descriptive concept (Berghoff et al., 2018; Ramaci et al., 2019).

2. Acceptance: Willingness to allow unpleasant emotions, bodily sensations, memories, and urges to be present without attempting to suppress, avoid, or replace them. Acceptance enables individuals to remain open to experience even when discomfort arises.

Acceptance refers to a deliberate and mindful willingness to remain in contact with one's internal experiences thoughts, emotions, memories, bodily sensations, and impulses even when these experiences are unpleasant or evoke discomfort. Within acceptance- and mindfulness-based models, acceptance is understood as a functional stance: rather than attempting to control, suppress, or alter internal states, individuals practice allowing them to be present while engaging in meaningful action (Hayes et al., 2006). This orientation emerges from the recognition that efforts to eliminate internal distress -particularly through avoidance, suppression, or resistance- often intensify suffering and restrict behavioral flexibility (Larmar et al., 2014).

From a psychological perspective, acceptance is not synonymous with resignation, passivity, or helplessness. It is an active and intentional process grounded in awareness. Individuals learn to observe their internal states with curiosity and openness, recognizing that these experiences fluctuate naturally and need not dictate behavior. By shifting from control strategies toward acceptance, a person reduces the struggle with internal content and frees cognitive and emotional resources that can be used to pursue personally valued goals (Dahl, 2015).

A central component of acceptance is the willingness to experience discomfort when doing so serves an important purpose. For instance, anxiety may arise before a challenging conversation, yet avoidance of discomfort may prevent the person from acting in accordance with personal values such as honesty or relational integrity (Doorley et al., 2020). Acceptance supports the ability to feel anxiety, acknowledge its presence, and nonetheless proceed with value-consistent behavior. In this way, the focus moves from controlling inner experiences to choosing actions that align with long-term well-being (Ong et al., 2024).

Acceptance also transforms the way individuals interpret their internal events. When distressing thoughts or emotions arise, people often respond as if these events are dangerous or must be immediately neutralized. Acceptance introduces a different relational stance: internal experiences are recognized as transient phenomena that do not require immediate reaction. Anxiety is understood as a bodily activation rather than a threat; intrusive memories are acknowledged as mental content rather than accurate representations of the present; and negative thoughts are seen as products of the mind, not as instructions or facts. This shift helps reduce automatic reactivity and broadens the individual's behavioral repertoire (Yavuz, 2015).

Moreover, acceptance plays a central role in weakening experiential avoidance, a pattern in which individuals attempt to escape or control internal events at the cost of their own functioning. Experiential avoidance is linked to a wide range of psychological difficulties, including chronic worry, depression, trauma-related symptoms, and substance use (Tarbox et al., 2022; Yavuz, 2015). Acceptance serves as a corrective process: by learning to stay with discomfort, individuals gradually develop tolerance for emotional and cognitive states they previously perceived as intolerable. This expanded tolerance forms the basis of psychological flexibility, allowing behavior to be shaped by goals and values rather than by the immediate urge to avoid discomfort (Hayes et al., 2006).

In clinical practice, acceptance is often cultivated through structured exercises such as exposure to internal sensations, mindful observation of emotions, or metaphor-based techniques that illustrate the futility of control strategies. These practices help individuals notice how resisting distress often amplifies it, while allowing discomfort to rise and fall naturally facilitates more adaptive functioning. Over time, acceptance-oriented interventions contribute to improved emotional regulation, reduced reliance on avoidance behaviors, and greater engagement in meaningful life activities (Tarbox et al., 2022; Willi et al., 2024).

In summary, acceptance is a sophisticated psychological process that involves opening up to internal experiences with intention and awareness, reducing the dominance of avoidance strategies, and enabling value-oriented action. Rather than aiming to eliminate emotional pain, acceptance helps individuals build the capacity to live effectively with discomfort, thereby fostering resilience, authenticity, and long-term psychological well-being. However, it should be acknowledged that the effectiveness of acceptance-based strategies may vary depending on contextual factors such as implementation fidelity, cultural norms related to emotional expression, and the availability of supervised training for practitioners.

3. Contact with the present moment: Maintaining flexible, nonjudgmental awareness of ongoing experience. This process contrasts with attentional rigidity, rumination, and dissociation, which contribute to psychological distress.

Contact with the present moment refers to the capacity to attend intentionally to one's ongoing experience as it unfolds, rather than being absorbed in memories, predictions, internal narratives, or habitual patterns of distraction. Within mindfulness- and acceptance-based approaches, this process represents a core mechanism through which individuals enhance awareness, regulate emotion, and respond flexibly to situational demands (Walser & O'Connell, 2021).

At its simplest, contacting the present moment involves noticing what is happening right now: the sensations in the body, the movement of the breath, the tone of an emotion, or the quality of a thought as it arises. However, the concept extends beyond mere observation. It includes the willingness to stay in contact with ongoing experience without judgment, analysis, or attempts to modify it. This orientation enables the person to step out of automatic pilot and engage with life more fully (Blackledge & Barnes-Holmes, 2009).

In daily life, much of human suffering emerges not from current events but from mental elaborations -rumination about the past, worry about the future, or internal stories about what a situation means. When attention becomes absorbed in these cognitive processes, the individual loses access to contextual cues and may react based on assumptions rather than the actual demands of the moment (Blanke et al., 2020). Contact with the present moment serves as an antidote to this drift. By anchoring awareness in present experience, individuals reclaim the ability to perceive events accurately and respond with greater intentionality. This process also supports emotional regulation. Many distressing emotions intensify when individuals resist them or attempt to escape them mentally. Present-moment awareness creates an opportunity to observe emotions as they arise in real time -acknowledging their presence, noticing how they manifest in the body, and allowing them to fluctuate naturally. This experiential contact reduces the urgency to engage in avoidance or suppression and fosters a more balanced and compassionate internal stance (Yavuz, 2015).

Clinically, present-moment contact is cultivated through mindfulness practices such as breath awareness, body scans, mindful walking, and sensory grounding exercises. These practices train attention to return repeatedly to the "here and now," strengthening the individual's ability to maintain awareness even in challenging contexts. Over time, attention becomes more stable, less reactive, and more attuned to meaningful aspects of experience (Valdez et al., 2016). Crucially, present-moment contact is not limited to meditative contexts. It also applies to interpersonal interactions, decision-making, and everyday activities. When individuals attend fully to the present moment, they are better able to recognize subtle emotional cues, identify value-consistent choices, and interrupt automatic behavioral patterns (Stern, 2004). This awareness supports psychological flexibility, allowing behavior to be guided by personal values rather than by habitual reactions or internal distractions.

In therapeutic settings, present-moment contact functions as a foundational process that interacts with acceptance, cognitive defusion, and values-based action. By establishing a clear awareness of current experience, individuals gain the grounding necessary to apply these other processes effectively. When attention is anchored in the present, thoughts and emotions become more observable, values become clearer, and behavior becomes more intentional (Ramaci et al., 2019).

In summary, contact with the present moment is a central mechanism of mindfulness- and acceptance-based interventions. It enhances awareness, reduces reactivity, improves emotional regulation, and strengthens behavioral flexibility. By encouraging individuals to engage with experience as it unfolds -rather than being caught in mental elaborations or avoidance patterns. This process supports a more grounded, meaningful, and psychologically resilient way of living.

4. Self-as-context: Developing a perspective-taking sense of self that observes experiences without being defined by them. This "observing self" is stable and continuous, unlike the fluctuating thoughts and emotions that constitute the "conceptualized self."

Self-as-context refers to a fundamental process within acceptance- and mindfulness-based therapies in which the individual learns to experience the "self" not as a collection of thoughts, emotions, or personal narratives, but as the stable, observing perspective from which all internal events are noticed. Rather than defining the self through cognitive content ("I am inadequate," "I am strong," "I am a failure"), this concept emphasizes the context or container in which these thoughts and feelings arise (Godbee & Kangas, 2020).

In everyday life, people often relate to their internal experiences through what is known as self-as-content, meaning they identify with the specific stories the mind generates. When someone thinks, "I am incompetent," the thought is treated as a literal description of the self. Self-as-context, however, introduces a shift in perspective: the individual notices that "My mind is producing the thought that I am incompetent right now." The self becomes the observer of thought, not the thought itself (Yavuz, 2015). This shift loosens the fusion between internal events and behavior, reducing the power of self-critical or distressing mental content. Importantly, this observing self is not a passive or detached stance. It is an active form of conscious awareness that allows individuals to notice thoughts, emotions, bodily sensations, and memories as experiences occurring within awareness rather than experiences that define who they are. Even when internal events are intense or distressing, the observing self provides a stable vantage point -a sense of continuity that persists despite the fluctuations of the inner world (Gowda & Premanand, 2025).

In emotional contexts, self-as-context helps individuals recognize that they have emotions, but they are not identical to those emotions. For example, a person experiencing anxiety may initially feel consumed by it, reacting as though the anxiety reflects a personal truth or imminent danger. Through self-as-context, the individual can instead observe: "Anxiety is arising in my body," without collapsing into the emotion itself (Lu et al., 2025). This non-identification reduces reactivity and opens space for value-guided choices. A major contribution of self-as-context is its ability to counteract rigid self-narratives. People often carry long-standing stories shaped by past experiences -stories about inadequacy, failure, or unlovability. These narratives can become psychologically constraining, limiting behavior and reinforcing avoidance (Yavuz, 2015). By cultivating the perspective of the observing self, individuals learn that these narratives are events in consciousness, not essential truths. This distinction allows for greater psychological flexibility and encourages engagement in behaviors aligned with one's personal values, even when old narratives persist (Lu et al., 2025; Tarbox et al., 2022).

Clinically, self-as-context is developed through mindfulness practices, experiential exercises, and metaphors. Practices may include noticing thoughts as passing events, shifting attention between different sensory experiences, or exploring the continuity of awareness across changing internal states. Metaphors such as "the sky and the weather" (where the self is the sky and emotions are changing weather patterns) help individuals conceptualize the stability of awareness relative to the impermanence of internal content (Gowda & Premanand, 2025).

Ultimately, self-as-context expands the individual's capacity to observe internal experiences without becoming entangled in them. By fostering a broader, more flexible sense of identity -one that is rooted in awareness rather than cognitive content- it supports resilience, emotional stability, and the ability to act according to deeply held values. For this reason, self-as-context is regarded as a central component of psychological flexibility within Acceptance and Commitment Therapy (ACT) and related approaches.

5. Values: Clarifying what truly matters -relationships, contribution, learning, personal growth, health, spirituality- and identifying life directions that bring meaning and vitality. Values function as an internal compass guiding action.

Values constitute a central process within acceptance- and mindfulness-based interventions, particularly within ACT. In this framework, values refer to personally chosen life directions -deeply held principles that guide long-term patterns of behavior rather than specific, time-limited goals. They function as internal compasses, orienting the individual toward meaningful action irrespective of changing emotional states, situational pressures, or transient thoughts (Berryhill & Lechtenberg, 2015).

Unlike goals, which can be achieved and completed, values are ongoing qualities of living. For example, "being a caring partner," "acting with integrity," or "cultivating curiosity" are not tasks to be checked off; they are directions one returns to repeatedly across the lifespan. This distinction is essential, because ACT conceptualizes values not as outcomes but as ways of behaving that embody what matters most to the individual (Chase et al., 2013).

Values also provide context for acceptance and cognitive defusion. When people lack clarity about what they care about, distressing internal experiences tend to dominate behavior. However, when values are clearly articulated, they offer a stable framework for decision-making even when emotions or thoughts are difficult. In this way, values transform acceptance from a passive tolerance of discomfort into an active willingness to experience discomfort in service of meaningful action (Blackledge, 2007; Rangel et al., 2008).

In clinical work, values clarification involves helping individuals explore what they want their lives to stand for in different domains -relationships, education, health, spirituality, community involvement, or personal growth. This exploration encourages reflection on long-standing patterns of behavior as well as unnoticed or unarticulated motivations (Rahal & Gon, 2020). Many individuals discover that their actions have been shaped more by avoidance, fear, or habit than by conscious choice. Values clarification therefore becomes a process of re-aligning behavior with one's authentic commitments rather than with internal struggles (Hayes et al., 2006). Values also play a corrective role in the presence of rigid self-narratives. When individuals define themselves through unhelpful stories ("I am not capable," "I always fail"), those narratives can limit behavioral possibilities. By contrast, values invite a broader view of identity -one that is oriented toward future-directed qualities rather than past-based labels. For instance, a person who believes "I am socially awkward" may still act in accordance with the value of "connecting with others" despite ongoing discomfort. Values open the possibility of growth even when cognitive content does not immediately change (Yavuz, 2015).

Clinically, values-based interventions often include exercises such as guided reflection, imagery, structured worksheets, and discussion of past experiences that highlight what truly matters to the individual (Vowles et al., 2009). Therapists also help individuals differentiate socially imposed expectations from personally chosen commitments. This distinction is particularly important in cultural contexts where identity and behavior are heavily shaped by external norms; values work supports autonomy and self-directed living even within such constraints (Baer, 2015). The functional role of values becomes most evident when integrated with committed action, which involves translating values into concrete behavioral patterns. Values by themselves do not produce change; they provide direction. When combined with willingness, acceptance, present-moment awareness, and behavioral commitment, they form the motivational foundation for psychological flexibility (Tarbox et al., 2022).

In summary, values represent ongoing, personally chosen life directions that support purposeful living. They guide behavior not through obligation or external pressure but through intrinsic meaning. By clarifying what matters most and orienting actions toward these commitments, values help individuals navigate emotional challenges, counteract avoidance patterns, and build lives that feel coherent, authentic, and aligned with their most deeply held principles. For these reasons, values are considered an essential component of acceptance- and mindfulness-based models and a cornerstone of psychological flexibility.

6. Committed action: Translating values into behavior through concrete, achievable goals and sustained behavioral patterns. This stage involves behavior change strategies reinforced by consistency and self-monitoring (Harris, 2006; Hayes et al., 2006; Kul & Türk, 2020).

Committed action refers to the process of taking consistent, goal-directed steps that reflect personally chosen values, even when such actions evoke discomfort, uncertainty, or internal resistance. Within ACT, committed action represents the behavioral expression of values and serves as the practical mechanism through which psychological flexibility translates into meaningful life change (Masudaa & Lillisa, 2006).

At its core, committed action involves patterned, sustained engagement in behaviors that move the individual toward a valued direction. Unlike impulsive or avoidance-driven behavior, committed action is guided by deliberate choice. It requires clarity about what matters and the willingness to take action despite the presence of difficult thoughts, emotions, or bodily sensations. This distinguishes committed action from short-lived motivation or intention; it is a process that unfolds over time and maintains direction even when obstacles arise (Coutinho et al., 2021). A defining feature of committed action is its emphasis on gradual, context-sensitive, and flexible behavior change. Rather than demanding perfection or dramatic transformation, ACT encourages individuals to set realistic, incremental goals that align with their values. These goals can be adjusted as circumstances evolve, making committed action an adaptive process. This flexibility prevents rigid adherence to plans and helps individuals navigate setbacks without abandoning their broader direction (Powers et al., 2009).

In therapeutic practice, committed action is operationalized through behavioral planning, skill development, and the systematic monitoring of progress. Clients may identify specific actions that reflect their values -for instance, initiating a difficult conversation, engaging in health-promoting behaviors, reconnecting with social supports, or dedicating time to personal growth (Mahdavi et al., 2022). Therapists guide individuals in breaking these actions into manageable steps, anticipating potential barriers, and developing strategies for responding to those barriers with acceptance and awareness rather than avoidance or self-criticism (Luoma & Platt, 2015). Committed action is also deeply intertwined with psychological barriers such as fear, self-doubt, and cognitive fusion. Many individuals find that initial attempts to act in line with their values trigger internal resistance; thoughts like "I can't do this," "It's too hard," or "I'll fail anyway" may emerge (Smith et al., 2020). Through acceptance, cognitive defusion, and present-moment awareness, individuals learn to make space for these internal events while moving forward with chosen behaviors. Thus, committed action functions not as an outcome of emotional clarity but as a way of living that coexists with emotional complexity (Masudaa & Lillisa, 2006).

Importantly, committed action is not synonymous with sheer persistence or endurance. Instead, it emphasizes values-based persistence -continuing to act in a valued direction because the action is meaningful, not because of external pressure or rigid determination (Assaz et al., 2018). This approach promotes long-term well-being by reinforcing behaviors that reflect the person's true priorities rather than avoidance patterns or social expectations. Over time, these value-aligned behaviors accumulate, strengthening a sense of purpose, coherence, and life satisfaction. As a central component of psychological flexibility, committed action enables individuals to build lives that reflect their deeper aspirations. It transforms values from abstract ideals into lived behaviors (Viskovich et al., 2021). When integrated with acceptance, defusion, and the observing self, committed action allows individuals to shift from reactive coping toward intentional, value-guided engagement (Berghoff et al., 2018; Blackledge & Barnes-Holmes, 2009).

In summary, committed action represents the behavioral realization of values within ACT. It involves sustained, flexible, and mindful steps toward personally meaningful directions, taken even in the presence of internal discomfort. Through this process, individuals cultivate resilience, expand their behavioral repertoire, and create lasting changes that reinforce a coherent and purposeful life.

These six processes do not operate in isolation; they interact continuously, shaping an individual's ability to navigate internal experiences while engaging in meaningful action.

3.5. Therapeutic Techniques and Clinical Implementation

ACT interventions include a wide variety of experiential, mindfulness-based, and behavioral strategies, such as:

- Cognitive defusion exercises (e.g., repeating distressing thoughts in a humorous tone, labeling thoughts as mental events).
- Acceptance practices (e.g., allowing physical discomfort to be present without resistance, observing emotions with compassion).
- Mindfulness exercises (brief attention practices, body awareness, sensory grounding).
- Values clarification (exploring life domains, identifying intrinsic motivations, articulating long-term intentions).
- Committed action planning (setting short- and long-term value-based goals, creating implementation plans, problem-solving barriers).

In early stages of therapy, clinicians typically help individuals recognize that their existing coping strategies—most commonly experiential avoidance—are rigid, ineffective, or even harmful. After this insight is established, mindfulness and acceptance practices are introduced to help clients experiment with new response patterns and observe the impact of these changes (Larmar et al., 2014).

ACT's integration of acceptance, mindfulness, and behavior change makes it applicable to a wide range of clinical issues, including anxiety, depression, trauma, chronic pain, medical illness, workplace stress, and relational problems. Its adaptability and emphasis on values-driven action also make it particularly relevant in nursing practice, where holistic care and emotional resilience are foundational.

The general aim of ACT is not to forcibly eliminate symptoms but to enhance psychological flexibility. Symptom reduction is often a by-product of increased psychological flexibility (Kul & Türk, 2020). ACT explains the enhancement of psychological flexibility through six interrelated processes: cognitive defusion (learning to see verbal thoughts as merely thoughts—for instance, saying "I'm having the thought that I'm inadequate"); acceptance (making space for unwanted emotions, bodily sensations, and memories instead of avoiding them); contact with the present moment (bringing attention flexibly to the present); the self as context (recognizing a stable observing perspective separate from changing thoughts and feelings); values (clarifying what matters, such as relationships, contribution, learning -one's life compass); and committed action (setting concrete value-aligned goals and taking small, consistent steps toward them) (Harris, 2006; Hayes et al., 2006; Kul & Türk, 2020).

Figure 2. Commitment and Behavior Change Processes

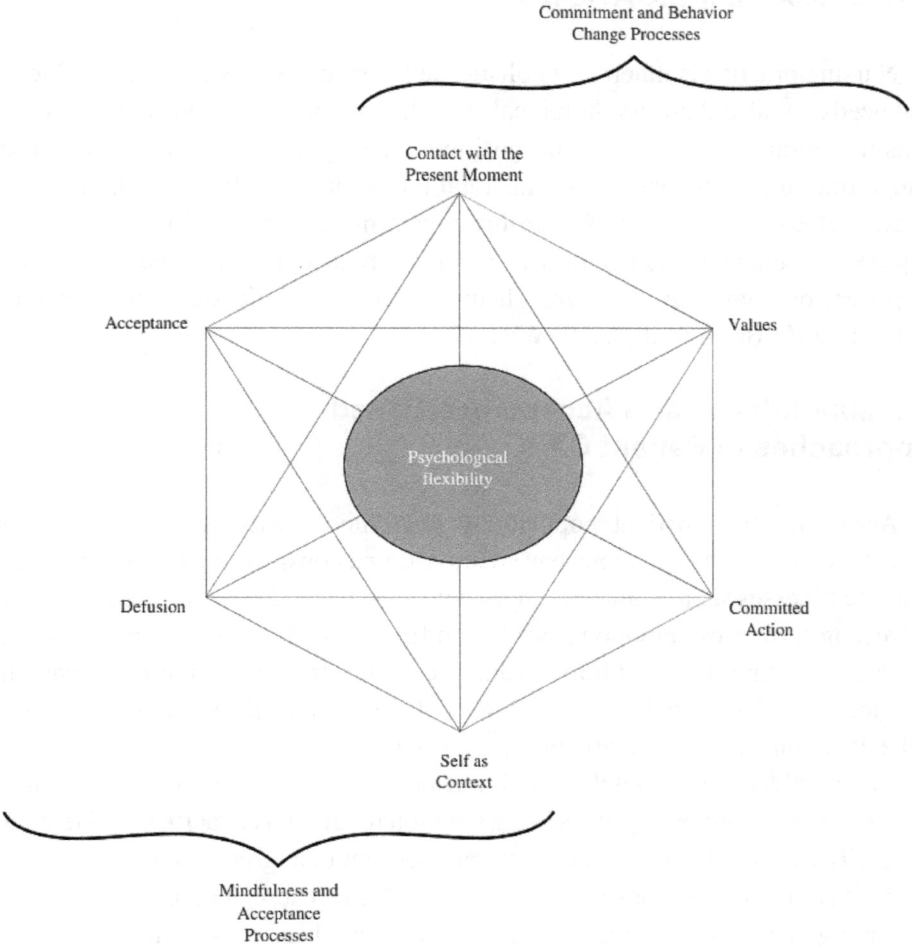

Practical exercises include defusion techniques, acceptance practices that increase openness to inner experience, brief mindfulness tasks, exercises to clarify values, and committed-action planning. The initial therapeutic step is helping individuals realize that their avoidance strategies have not been functional; subsequently, mindfulness and acceptance skills are introduced to help them experiment with alternative response styles (Larmar et al., 2014).

4. APPLICATIONS AND EFFECTS IN NURSING: PRACTICAL IMPLICATIONS

Nursing practice is inherently holistic, addressing not only individuals' biological needs but also their psychological, social, emotional, and spiritual well-being. This multidimensional orientation positions nursing as a discipline in which the integration of psychosocial and behavioral interventions holds substantial clinical relevance (Hoeve et al., 2014). Within this context, mindfulness- and acceptance-based approaches contribute meaningfully to two interrelated domains: the enhancement of patient outcomes and the strengthening of nurses' professional resilience and well-being (O'Brien et al., 2019; White, 2014).

4.1. Mindfulness and Acceptance-Based Approaches in Patient Care

Across multiple patient populations and clinical settings, mindfulness and acceptance-based interventions have demonstrated considerable therapeutic value. Chronic illnesses such as diabetes, hypertension, cancer, and chronic pain often involve long-term stress, emotional burden, and diminished self-management abilities. Research indicates that mindfulness and acceptance training can improve patients' emotional regulation, reduce psychological distress, and enhance their engagement in healthy behaviors and treatment adherence (Gregg, 2013).

Among older adults, mindfulness-based programs have shown efficacy in alleviating depressive symptoms, improving emotion regulation capacities, and reducing sleep difficulties—factors that collectively contribute to greater quality of life and improved functional outcomes (Javadzade et al., 2024). These findings are particularly valuable given the complexity of geriatric care, in which emotional and cognitive vulnerabilities often intersect with chronic medical conditions.

In palliative care environments, where individuals commonly experience existential distress, uncertainty, and emotional turmoil, acceptance-based interventions have been identified as especially beneficial. Studies report reductions in anxiety, depression, and perceived side effects of treatment, as well as improvements in emotional acceptance and coping capacity (O'Hayer et al., 2018). These interventions help patients shift from a struggle-oriented stance toward a more compassionate and adaptive engagement with their remaining life experiences.

More broadly, mindfulness and acceptance-based interventions have demonstrated effectiveness across diverse populations including students, employees in high-stress occupations, and individuals undergoing demanding medical treatments. These approaches consistently reduce stress, improve psychological functioning, and enhance resilience (Keng et al., 2011). Their versatility underscores the clinical potential of integrating such approaches into broader health care frameworks.

4.2. Strengthening Nurses' Professional Well-Being and Resilience

Nursing professionals operate in environments characterized by high emotional demands, heavy workloads, ethical stress, complex patient needs, and exposure to suffering and trauma. These factors contribute to burnout, compassion fatigue, emotional exhaustion, and decreased job satisfaction. As a result, enhancing nurses' psychological resilience has become a significant priority for health care systems.

Mindfulness- and ACT-based programs are increasingly recognized as evidence-based tools for promoting nurses' self-care, emotional stability, and professional competence (Halm, 2017; Slatyer et al., 2018). These programs support nurses in:

- regulating stress responses,
- maintaining focus and attention in high-pressure situations,
- fostering emotional balance during patient care,
- enhancing empathy without sacrificing personal boundaries,
- improving communication and relational skills,
- reducing burnout and compassion fatigue.

An experimental study conducted among psychiatric nurses demonstrated that an ACT-based intervention significantly reduced perceived stress symptoms, suggesting that acceptance and psychological flexibility training can mitigate the negative health effects of occupational demands (Zarvijani et al., 2021). Improvements in stress management directly enhance nurses' overall health, job performance, and ability to engage in compassionate, high-quality care.

4.3. Implications for Nursing Practice

The integration of mindfulness and acceptance-based approaches into nursing practice holds important implications:

1. Enhanced patient-centered care: Nurses trained in mindfulness provide more attuned, empathetic, and present-focused care, improving therapeutic relationships.
2. Greater emotional resilience: Acceptance and mindfulness foster psychological flexibility, allowing nurses to cope with complex emotional encounters.
3. Reduced occupational stress: These approaches offer sustainable self-regulation strategies that can buffer the cumulative effects of workplace stressors.

4. Improved interdisciplinary collaboration: A mindful communication style enhances teamwork and reduces interpersonal conflict.
5. Support for holistic care models: Mindfulness and acceptance align naturally with holistic nursing frameworks that view individuals as biopsychosocial-spiritual beings.

Collectively, these findings indicate that mindfulness- and acceptance-based interventions have the potential to serve as valuable, evidence-based components of both patient care and professional development in nursing. In practice, these implications can be operationalized through brief, structured modules (e.g., short daily mindfulness exercises and values-based reflection) integrated into nursing education and workplace well-being programs, with outcomes monitored using validated indicators such as stress, burnout, and psychological flexibility measures.

Nursing is concerned not only with biological care but also with meeting individuals' psychological, social, and spiritual needs (Hoeve et al., 2014). Therefore, mindfulness and acceptance-based approaches have a twofold value in nursing practice: they support patient well-being and strengthen nurses' professional resilience (O'Brien et al., 2019; White, 2014).

Mindfulness and acceptance-based approaches have been reported to provide considerable support in the treatment processes of chronic illnesses such as diabetes, hypertension, and cancer (Gregg, 2013). Among older adults, mindfulness-based approaches have been found to improve depression, emotion regulation, and sleep problems, enhancing quality of life (Javadzade et al., 2024). In palliative care units, acceptance-based interventions have been effective in reducing patients' anxiety, depression, and treatment side effects (O'Hayer et al., 2018). Acceptance-based applications have been shown to reduce the negative psychological impact of stresses across diverse groups such as students, workers, and cancer patients (Keng et al., 2011).

Research indicates that mindfulness and ACT-based programs are effective in nurses' self-care processes within nursing science (Halm, 2017; Slatyer et al., 2018; Zarvijani et al., 2021). For example, an experimental study on psychiatric nurses reported that an ACT-based intervention significantly reduced perceived stress symptoms. Finding appropriate solutions to cope with these stress symptoms can improve nurses' overall health and work quality (Zarvijani et al., 2021).

CONCLUSION

Mindfulness and acceptance-based approaches—particularly Mindfulness-Based Stress Reduction (MBSR) and Acceptance and Commitment Therapy (ACT)—offer individuals a structured and evidence-based way to respond more flexibly and functionally to difficult thoughts, emotions, and bodily sensations. These approaches strengthen the ability to bring attention to the present moment with openness and non-judgment, to create space for unpleasant internal experiences without resorting to avoidance, and to engage in small yet sustainable actions guided by personal values. In doing so, they aim not merely to reduce symptoms but to enhance daily functioning, deepen self-awareness, and improve overall quality of life.

A substantial body of research demonstrates that mindfulness- and acceptance-based interventions lead to meaningful improvements across diverse clinical populations. In chronic illness, older adulthood, and palliative care settings, such interventions have been linked to reductions in anxiety, depressive symptoms, sleep difficulties, and maladaptive stress responses. These therapeutic gains reflect the broader capacity of mindfulness and acceptance to regulate emotional processes, build resilience, and support adaptive coping.

Within nursing, the relevance of these approaches is twofold. First, they contribute directly to holistic patient care by supporting emotional regulation, treatment engagement, and psychological well-being. Second, they strengthen nurses' own well-being by enhancing self-care, emotional resilience, attentional stability, and professional satisfaction. Studies have consistently shown that mindfulness- and ACT-based programs reduce perceived stress and burnout among nurses, leading to improved mental health and better quality of care.

In practice, brief and regular mindfulness exercises, acceptance and cognitive defusion techniques, and value-aligned goal-setting strategies can be integrated into both clinical interventions and nursing self-care routines. Nevertheless, future research should continue to clarify which components are most effective for specific nursing contexts and populations, and under what implementation conditions these interventions produce sustainable benefits. As evidence grows, mindfulness and acceptance-based models are increasingly recognized as practical, scalable, and beneficial tools not only for improving patient outcomes but also for enhancing the well-being and resilience of nursing professionals.

REFERENCES

Arranz, E. B., Olabarrieta, F., Manzano, A., Martín, J. L., Cruz, N., & Etxaniz, A. (2016). Psychosocial Intervention. *Psychosocial Intervention*, *25*(2), 127–134.

Assaz, D. A., Roche, B., Kanter, J. W., & Oshiro, C. K. (2018). Cognitive defusion in acceptance and commitment therapy: What are the basic processes of change? *The Psychological Record*, *68*(4), 405–418.

Baer, R. (2015). Ethics, values, virtues, and character strengths in mindfulness-based interventions: A psychological science perspective. *Mindfulness*, *6*(4), 956–969.

Bazzano, A., Wolfe, C., Zylowska, L., Wang, S., Schuster, E., Barrett, C., & Lehrer, D. (2015). Mindfulness based stress reduction (MBSR) for parents and caregivers of individuals with developmental disabilities: A community-based approach. *Journal of Child and Family Studies*, *24*(2), 298–308.

Belisle, J., & Tarbox, J. (2024). Relational frame theory and acceptance and commitment therapy. In Roane, H. S., Craig, A. R., Saini, V., & Ringdahl, J. E. (Eds.), *Behavior analysis: Translational perspectives and clinical practice* (pp. 526–547). The Guilford Press.

Berghoff, C. R., Ritzert, T. R., & Forsyth, J. P. (2018). Value-guided action: Within-day and lagged relations of experiential avoidance, mindful awareness, and cognitive fusion in a non-clinical sample. *Journal of Contextual Behavioral Science*, *10*, 19–23.

Berryhill, M. B., & Lechtenberg, M. M. (2015). Acceptance and commitment therapy with adolescents: Identifying and clarifying values. *Journal of Family Psychotherapy*, *26*(1), 25–30.

Bishop, S. R. (2002). What do we really know about mindfulness-based stress reduction? *Biopsychosocial Science and Medicine*, *64*(1), 71–83.

Black, D. S. (2011). A brief definition of mindfulness. *Behavioral Neuroscience*, *7*(2), 109.

Black, D. S., Milam, J., & Sussman, S. (2009). Sitting-meditation interventions among youth: A review of treatment efficacy. *Pediatrics*, *124*(3), e532–e541.

Blackledge, J. T. (2007). Disrupting verbal processes: Cognitive defusion in acceptance and commitment therapy and other mindfulness-based psychotherapies. *The Psychological Record*, *57*(4), 555–576.

Blackledge, J. T., & Barnes-Holmes, D. (2009). Core processes in acceptance and commitment therapy. *Acceptance and commitment therapy: Contemporary theory, research, and practice, 1*, 41-58.

Blanke, E. S., Schmidt, M. J., Riediger, M., & Brose, A. (2020). Thinking mindfully: How mindfulness relates to rumination and reflection in daily life. *Emotion (Washington, D.C.), 20*(8), 1369.

Cavanagh, K., Strauss, C., Forder, L., & Jones, F. (2014). Can mindfulness and acceptance be learnt by self-help?: A systematic review and meta-analysis of mindfulness and acceptance-based self-help interventions. *Clinical Psychology Review, 34*(2), 118–129.

Chase, J. A., Houmanfar, R., Hayes, S. C., Ward, T. A., Vilardaga, J. P., & Follette, V. (2013). Values are not just goals: Online ACT-based values training adds to goal setting in improving undergraduate college student performance. *Journal of Contextual Behavioral Science, 2*(3-4), 79–84.

Coutinho, M., Trindade, I. A., & Ferreira, C. (2021). Experiential avoidance, committed action and quality of life: Differences between college students with and without chronic illness. *Journal of Health Psychology, 26*(7), 1035–1045.

Dahl, J. (2015). Valuing in ACT. *Current Opinion in Psychology, 2*, 43–46.

David, D., & Montgomery, G. H. (2011). The scientific status of psychotherapies: A new evaluative framework for evidence-based psychosocial interventions. *Clinical Psychology : a Publication of the Division of Clinical Psychology of the American Psychological Association, 18*(2), 89–99.

Del Rosario, N., & Beshai, S. (2022). Do you mind? Examining the impact of psychoeducation specificity on perceptions of mindfulness-based programs. *International Journal of Environmental Research and Public Health, 19*(15), 9621.

Dobkin, P. L., Hickman, S., & Monshat, K. (2014). Holding the heart of mindfulness-based stress reduction: Balancing fidelity and imagination when adapting MBSR. *Mindfulness, 5*(6), 710–718.

Doorley, J. D., Goodman, F. R., Kelso, K. C., & Kashdan, T. B. (2020). Psychological flexibility: What we know, what we do not know, and what we think we know. *Social and Personality Psychology Compass, 14*(12), 1–11.

Dryden, W., & Still, A. (2006). Historical aspects of mindfulness and self-acceptance in psychotherapy. *Journal of Rational-Emotive & Cognitive-Behavior Therapy, 24*(1), 3–28.

Feather, J. S., Howson, M., Ritchie, L., Carter, P. D., Parry, D. T., & Koziol-McLain, J. (2016). Evaluation methods for assessing users' psychological experiences of web-based psychosocial interventions: A systematic review. *Journal of Medical Internet Research, 18*(6), e181.

Godbee, M., & Kangas, M. (2020). The relationship between flexible perspective taking and emotional well-being: A systematic review of the "self-as-context" component of acceptance and commitment therapy. *Behavior Therapy, 51*(6), 917–932.

Gowda, P. C., & Premanand, V. (2025). Mindfulness and Differentiation of Self among Adolescents: Mediating Role of Self-as-context. *Indian Journal of Positive Psychology, 16*(1).

Gregg, J. A. (2013). Self-acceptance and chronic illness. In *The strength of self-acceptance: Theory, practice and research* (pp. 247–262). Springer New York.

Grossman, P., Niemann, L., Schmidt, S., & Walach, H. (2004). Mindfulness-based stress reduction and health benefits: A meta-analysis. *Journal of Psychosomatic Research, 57*(1), 35–43.

Guillaumie, L., Boiral, O., & Champagne, J. (2017). A mixed-methods systematic review of the effects of mindfulness on nurses. *Journal of Advanced Nursing, 73*(5), 1017–1034.

Haberlin, S. (2024). Sitting with the data: Experimenting with meditative thematic analysis. *The Qualitative Report, 29*(7), 1969–1980.

Halm, M. (2017). The role of mindfulness in enhancing self-care for nurses. *American Journal of Critical Care, 26*(4), 344–348.

Harris, R. (2006). Embracing your demons: An overview of acceptance and commitment therapy. *Psychotherapy in Australia, 12*(4), 70–76.

Hayes, S. C. (2004). Acceptance and commitment therapy, relational frame theory, and the third wave of behavioral and cognitive therapies. *Behavior Therapy, 35*(4), 639–665.

Hayes, S. C., Luoma, J. B., Bond, F. W., Masuda, A., & Lillis, J. (2006). Acceptance and commitment therapy: Model, processes and outcomes. *Behaviour Research and Therapy, 44*(1), 1–25.

Hoeve, Y. T., Jansen, G., & Roodbol, P. (2014). The nursing profession: Public image, self-concept and professional identity. A discussion paper. *Journal of Advanced Nursing, 70*(2), 295–309.

Hofmann, S. G., & Asmundson, G. J. (2008). Acceptance and mindfulness-based therapy: New wave or old hat? *Clinical Psychology Review*, *28*(1), 1–16.

Imel, Z., Baldwin, S., Bonus, K., & MacCoon, D. (2008). Beyond the individual: Group effects in mindfulness-based stress reduction. *Psychotherapy Research*, *18*(6), 735–742.

Jacobsen, P. B., & Jim, H. S. (2008). Psychosocial interventions for anxiety and depression in adult cancer patients: Achievements and challenges. *CA: a Cancer Journal for Clinicians*, *58*(4), 214–230.

Javadzade, N., Esmaeili, S. V., Omranifard, V., & Zargar, F. (2024). Effect of mindfulness-based stress reduction (MBSR) program on depression, emotion regulation, and sleep problems: A randomized controlled trial study on depressed elderly. *BMC Public Health*, *24*(1), 271.

Kabat-Zinn, J. (2016). Sitting meditations. *Mindfulness*, *7*(6), 1441–1444.

Keng, S. L., Smoski, M. J., & Robins, C. J. (2011). Effects of mindfulness on psychological health: A review of empirical studies. *Clinical Psychology Review*, *31*(6), 1041–1056.

King, N. J., & Ollendick, T. H. (2008). The elegant psychosocial intervention: A heuristic conceptual framework for clinicians and researchers. *Behavioural and Cognitive Psychotherapy*, *36*(3), 253–261.

Kostanski, M., & Hassed, C. (2008). Mindfulness as a concept and a process. *Australian Psychologist*, *43*(1), 15–21.

Kul, A., & Türk, F. (2020). Kabul ve adanmışlık terapisi (ACT) üzerine bir derleme çalışması. *OPUS International Journal of Society Researches, 16*(29 Ekim Özel Sayısı), 3773-3805.

Larmar, S., Wiatrowski, S., & Lewis-Driver, S. (2014). Acceptance & commitment therapy: An overview of techniques and applications. *Journal of Service Science and Management*, *7*, 216–221.

Levin, M., & Hayes, S. C. (2011). Mindfulness and acceptance: The perspective of acceptance and commitment therapy. *Acceptance and mindfulness in cognitive behavior therapy: Understanding and applying the new therapies*, 291-316.

Lu, J., Chen, Y., & Mudathir, D. (2025). Mindfulness and stress among undergraduate students: Examining the mediation roles of self-as-context and cognitive defusion as decentering facets. *Journal of American College Health*, ●●●, 1–8.

Luoma, J. B., & Platt, M. G. (2015). Shame, self-criticism, self-stigma, and compassion in acceptance and commitment therapy. *Current Opinion in Psychology*, *2*, 97–101.

Mahdavi, M., Emadian, S. O., & Hassanzade, R. (2022). Comparıson Of The Effectıveness Of Mındfulness-Based Cognıtıve Therapy And Acceptance And Commıtment Therapy On Health-Promotıng Behavıors In Patıents Wıth Ulceratıve Colıts. *Journal of Positive School Psychology*, *6*(7).

Masudaa, A., & Lillisa, J. (2006). Acceptance and commitment therapy: Model, processes and outcomes. *Behaviour Research and Therapy*, *44*(1), 1–25.

O'Brien, W. H., Singh, R., Horan, K., Moeller, M. T., Wasson, R., & Jex, S. M. (2019). Group-based acceptance and commitment therapy for nurses and nurse aides working in long-term care residential settings. *Journal of Alternative and Complementary Medicine (New York, N.Y.)*, *25*(7), 753–761.

O'Hayer, C. V. F., O'Hayer, K. M., & Sama, A. (2018). Acceptance and commitment therapy with pancreatic cancer: An integrative model of palliative care-a case report. *Journal of Pancreatic Cancer*, *4*(1), 1–3.

Ong, C. W., Barthel, A. L., & Hofmann, S. G. (2024). The relationship between psychological inflexibility and well-being in adults: A meta-analysis of the acceptance and action questionnaire. *Behavior Therapy*, *55*(1), 26–41.

Pan, Y., Li, F., Liang, H., Shen, X., Bing, Z., Cheng, L., & Dong, Y. (2024). Effectiveness of Mindfulness-Based Stress Reduction on Mental Health and Psychological Quality of Life among University Students: A GRADE-Assessed Systematic Review. *Evidence-Based Complementary and Alternative Medicine : eCAM*, *2024*(1), 8872685.

Powers, M. B., Zum Vörde Sive Vörding, M. B., & Emmelkamp, P. M. (2009). Acceptance and commitment therapy: A meta-analytic review. *Psychotherapy and Psychosomatics*, *78*(2), 73–80.

Praissman, S. (2008). Mindfulness-based stress reduction: A literature review and clinician's guide. *Journal of the American Association of Nurse Practitioners*, *20*(4), 212–216.

Rahal, G. M., & Gon, M. C. C. (2020). A systematic review of values interventions in acceptance and commitment therapy. *International Journal of Psychology & Psychological Therapy*, *20*(3), 355–372.

Ramaci, T., Bellini, D., Presti, G., & Santisi, G. (2019). Psychological flexibility and mindfulness as predictors of individual outcomes in hospital health workers. *Frontiers in Psychology, 10*, 1302.

Rangel, A., Camerer, C., & Montague, P. R. (2008). A framework for studying the neurobiology of value-based decision making. *Nature Reviews. Neuroscience, 9*(7), 545–556.

Rodriguez, V. H., Medrano, C. T., & Plaza, I. (2018). Wearable sensors for measuring movement in short sessions of mindfulness sitting meditation: A pilot study. *Journal of Healthcare Engineering, 2018*(1), 7275049.

Slatyer, S., Craigie, M., Heritage, B., Davis, S., & Rees, C. (2018). Evaluating the effectiveness of a brief mindful self-care and resiliency (MSCR) intervention for nurses: A controlled trial. *Mindfulness, 9*(2), 534–546.

Smith, B. M., Smith, G. S., & Dymond, S. (2020). Relapse of anxiety-related fear and avoidance: Conceptual analysis of treatment with acceptance and commitment therapy. *Journal of the Experimental Analysis of Behavior, 113*(1), 87–104.

Stern, D. N. (2004). The present moment as a critical moment. *Negotiation Journal, 20*(2), 365–372.

Stewart, T. M. (2004). Light on body image treatment: Acceptance through mindfulness. *Behavior Modification, 28*(6), 783–811.

Tarbox, J., Szabo, T. G., & Aclan, M. (2022). Acceptance and commitment training within the scope of practice of applied behavior analysis. *Behavior Analysis in Practice, 15*(1), 11–32.

Terzioğlu, M., & Yavuz, K. F. (2023). İlişkisel Çerçeve Kuramı (İÇK): Dil ve Bilişe Ampirik Bir Yaklaşım. *J Cogn Behav Psychother Res*, 188-200.

Valdez, C. E., Sherrill, A. M., & Lilly, M. (2016). Present moment contact and non-judgment: Pilot data on dismantling mindful awareness in trauma-related symptomatology. *Journal of Psychopathology and Behavioral Assessment, 38*(4), 572–581.

Viskovich, S., Pakenham, K. I., & Fowler, J. A. (2021). A mixed-methods evaluation of experiential intervention exercises for values and committed action from an Acceptance and Commitment Therapy (ACT) mental health promotion program for university students. *Journal of Contextual Behavioral Science, 22*, 108–118.

Vowles, K. E., Wetherell, J. L., & Sorrell, J. T. (2009). Targeting acceptance, mindfulness, and values-based action in chronic pain: Findings of two preliminary trials of an outpatient group-based intervention. *Cognitive and Behavioral Practice, 16*(1), 49–58.

Walser, R. D., & O'Connell, M. (2021). Acceptance and commitment therapy and the therapeutic relationship: Rupture and repair. *Journal of Clinical Psychology, 77*(2), 429–440.

White, L. (2014). Mindfulness in nursing: An evolutionary concept analysis. *Journal of Advanced Nursing, 70*(2), 282–294.

Willi, N., Pancoast, A., Drikaki, I., Gu, X., Gillanders, D., & Finucane, A. (2024). Practitioner perspectives on the use of acceptance and commitment therapy for bereavement support: A qualitative study. *BMC Palliative Care, 23*(1), 59.

Yavuz, K. F. (2015). Acceptance and Commitment Therapy (ACT): An Overview. *Turkiye Klinikleri Journal of Psychiatry Special Topics, 8*(2), 21–27.

Yule, W. (2006). Theory, training and timing: Psychosocial interventions in complex emergencies. *International Review of Psychiatry (Abingdon, England), 18*(3), 259–264.

Zarvijani, S. A. H., Moghaddam, L. F., & Parchebafieh, S. (2021). Acceptance and commitment therapy on perceived stress and psychological flexibility of psychiatric nurses: A randomized control trial. *BMC Nursing, 20*(1), 239.

Chapter 5
Positive Psychotherapy and Strengths-Based Interventions

Eda Albayrak Günday
https://orcid.org/0000-0002-0271-2955
Faculty of Health Sciences, Erciyes University, Turkey

ABSTRACT

This study explores the theoretical framework and clinical application of Positive Psychotherapy (PPT) and Strengths-Based Interventions, emphasizing the shift from a pathology-centered to a resource-oriented paradigm in healthcare. Developed by Nossrat Peseschkian, PPT integrates humanistic and psychodynamic elements, defining the "positive" as the total reality (positum) of the individual, which encompasses both symptoms and innate capacities. The approach is grounded in three core principles: Hope, Balance, and Consultation. Central to this framework is the Balance Model, which seeks dynamic equilibrium across four life domains: body, achievement, relationships, and spirituality. The text further delineates the five-stage therapeutic process and the classification of human potential into primary ("to love") and secondary ("to know") capabilities. The study concludes that integrating these transcultural, holistic approaches into nursing practice significantly enhances resilience, professional well-being, and sustainable patient recovery.

INTRODUCTION

Traditional health services have generally approached mental disorders through pathologies, symptoms, and individuals' risk factors. However, with this approach, mental disorders continue to cost the health system billions of dollars annually

DOI: 10.4018/979-8-3373-6526-8.ch005

(Xie, 2013). Current estimates indicate that this economic burden will cost the global economy approximately $2.5 trillion annually by the year 2030 (Günday & Albayrak Günday, 2025). The field of psychotherapy is a dynamic discipline enriched by efforts to understand and improve human mental health, hosting a wide variety of theoretical approaches and clinical applications. Historically, the primary focus of psychotherapy has generally been the elimination of psychopathologies and the alleviation of symptoms. However, in recent years, alternative perspectives aimed at human potentials, strengths, and increasing quality of life have also attracted great interest (Özen & Türkmen, 2023; Açıkgöz & Coşkunsever, 2025).

With the rise of the field of positive psychology, the focus has shifted from how to prevent and reduce lack and suffering to how to achieve happiness, quality of life, and meaning (Seligman & Csikszentmihalyi 2000; Dolev-Amit et al., 2021). Positive psychology interventions aim to increase psychological well-being and support positive emotions, thoughts, and behaviors by developing strengths. These interventions can contribute to longer and sustainable periods between relapses by strengthening recovery (Meyer et al., 2012). One of these approaches is Positive Psychotherapy, developed by Nossrat Peseschkian in Germany in 1968, which incorporates both humanistic and psychodynamic elements (Özen & Türkmen, 2023). Positive Psychotherapy (PPT) is generally a therapy approach born from the positive psychology movement (Walsh et al., 2017). Positive Psychotherapy (PPT) evaluates the individual not only on the basis of symptoms or strengths, but by handling these two dimensions together within a comprehensive framework. This approach aims to systematically develop clients' positive emotions, capacities to find meaning in life, character-specific strengths, supportive relationships, and achievements demonstrated through intrinsic motivation (Rashid, 2015). In Peseschkian's theoretical approach, the concept of "positive" has a deeper and more specific content beyond the meanings of "good" or "favorable" frequently attributed in daily usage. This concept is derived from the words *positum* in Latin, carrying the meanings of "what is given," "what is present," and "what exists as reality" (Marseille, 2025; Sarı, 2015). This etymological foundation constitutes the philosophical basis of Positive Psychotherapy; it is based on handling the individual's strengths, capacities, and potentials alongside difficulties, conflicts, and illnesses in life as "existing realities" without separating them as positive or negative (Marseille, 2025; Sarı, 2015). In the Positive Psychotherapy approach, symptoms are not treated merely as pathological indicators that need to be eliminated; instead, they are evaluated as unique responses developed by the individual against internal and environmental conflicts, coping efforts, and expressions that sometimes assume a specific function in their life (Peseschkian, 1987; Sarı, 2015). This approach transforms the therapeutic process into a holistic process focused on noticing the potential possessed by the individual and creating a more balanced life order, rather than reducing it to merely correcting deficits (Marseille, 2025). In this framework, PPT relies on the assumption that individuals carry certain capacities even in situations where they face difficulties and that making these resources visible is one of the main goals of therapy (Sarı, 2015).

Positive Psychotherapy, developed by Peseschkian, proceeds from the assumption that the human being is essentially a constructive being open to development; and it is grounded upon three basic pillars: the Principle of Hope, the Balance Model, and the Principle of Consultation (Özen & Türkmen, 2023). Among these principles, the Principle of Hope reflects the fundamental belief that even in the face of difficulties, painful experiences, and conflictual life events encountered by the individual, a possibility of change, ways of solution, or a potential not yet revealed is always present (Sarı, 2015). The Balance Model stands out as one of the basic components of Peseschkian's understanding of psychological well-being. This model argues that a healthy and satisfying life depends on handling the four basic areas of human life in a balanced way: body/health, work/achievement, relationships, and future/spirituality (Aypay & Kara, 2018; Peseschkian & Remmers, 2025a; Sarı, 2015). According to the Positive Psychotherapy approach, the way the individual perceives themselves and their environment is closely related to the interest and energy they allocate to these four areas (Aypay & Kara, 2018). In conflictual situations, it is seen that individuals mostly tend excessively towards one of these areas and neglect the others. For example, excessive focus on work and achievement may cause physical health or social relationships to remain in the background over time. The Balance Model aims to support the individual's holistic psychological well-being by targeting the re-establishment of harmony between said areas (Aypay & Kara, 2018; Marseille, 2025). The consultation principle treats the patient as the expert in their own life and consists of five stages. (Marseille, 2025). In Positive Psychotherapy, the therapeutic process is structured over five basic stages. In the observation and distancing stage, the client is listened to with a non-judgmental and neutral attitude; the aim is to understand the current situation and needs. In the inventory and use of information stage, the four areas in the individual's life are evaluated based on the balance model; the coping ways used, existing capacities, and reactions given to problems are addressed. In the situational encouragement stage, the client's strengths and previously useful coping strategies are made visible, and constructive feedback regarding symptoms is presented. In the verbalization stage, the individual's life story and basic conflicts are analyzed within the framework of the balance model. Finally, in the expansion of goals stage, future-oriented goals are determined; the continuity of the therapeutic process is ensured by supporting the client's self-help skills (Gülırmak Güler, 2023; Peseschkian, 2002; Peseschkian, 2005; Peseschkian, 2007; Sarı, 2015).

Positive Psychotherapy offers a unique perspective regarding human nature and assumes that individuals come to the world with two basic capacities: "to love" and "to know" (Sarı, 2015). In this framework, while the capacity to love is defined as "primary capabilities" covering characteristics such as modeling, patience, trust, hope, and faith, the capacity to know is handled under the concept of "secondary capabilities" including behavioral tendencies such as punctuality, cleanliness, order, and obedience (Sarı, 2015). The disruption of the balance between individual development processes and these capabilities is evaluated as a determining factor in understanding the emergence and maintenance of psychopathology (Kiliç & Eryilmaz, 2019).

Positive Psychotherapy, developed by Peseschkian, is an approach standing out with its holistic and integrative structure. This model offers a multifaceted theoretical framework by bringing together the basic principles of humanistic, psychodynamic, cultural, and behavioral psychotherapy schools (Özen & Türkmen, 2023; Peseschkian, 1987). This multidimensional structure allows Positive Psychotherapy not to remain limited to focusing only on symptoms but to handle the individual's life with all its contexts. Besides this, the transcultural aspect of Positive Psychotherapy is one of the distinguishing features of the approach. Peseschkian attributes special importance to understanding the value systems, worldviews, and life practices of clients with different cultural backgrounds and respecting these differences (Marseille, 2025; Peseschkian & Remmers, 2025a). The use of stories, aphorisms, proverbs, and metaphors in the therapeutic process strengthens cultural sensitivity; it supports clients in developing a new sense of confidence and self-efficacy by enabling them to express themselves through indirect and symbolic narratives (Peseschkian, 1987; Marseille, 2025).

Positive Psychotherapy were This approach is not limited to individual therapy; it can also be used in different application forms such as group counseling, family therapy, and family education (Özen & Türkmen, 2023; Sarı, 2015). Studies have revealed that Positive interventions is effective in reducing negative psychological symptoms such as depression and anxiety, as well as increasing positive psychological outcomes such as life satisfaction (Chakhssi et al., 2018; Hendriks et al., 2020; Hoppen & Morina, 2021; Lim & Tierney, 2023). Similarly, various meta-analyses show that Positive Psychology Interventions create significant and positive effects on mental health and subjective well-being in both the general population and clinical samples (Van Agteren et al., 2021; Bolier et al., 2013; Carr et al., 2021).

The strengths-based approach is based on evaluating individuals experiencing mental illness through the strengths they possess and existing resources, rather than defining them through deficits or inadequacies (Xie, 2013; Slade, 2010). It is stated that focusing on strengths and individual resources within the framework of positive psychology and Positive Psychotherapy offers an effective and promising approach in supporting the recovery processes of individuals with mental ailments such as depression, substance use disorders, and psychosis (Schrank et al., 2014). While person-centered nursing practices based on this approach strengthen the process, cooperation established between clients, clinicians, and community-based organizations provides significant contributions to the reduction of difficulties that may be encountered (Xie, 2013). In this context, Positive Psychotherapy and Strengths-Based Interventions stand out in nursing practice, especially mental health nursing, as promising approaches aimed at increasing individuals' mental well-being and resilience by going beyond illness.

THEORETICAL FOUNDATIONS AND DEVELOPMENT OF POSITIVE PSYCHOTHERAPY

Positive Psychotherapy, developed by Nossrat Peseschkian, is a humanistic-psychodynamic and transcultural psychotherapy method whose foundations were laid in Germany (Marseille, 2025; Özen & Türkmen, 2023; Peseschkian & Remmers, 2025b; Peseschkian, 2023). Born and raised in Iran and completing his medical education in Germany, Peseschkian continued his work in this country until his death in 2010. These cultural changes and experiences in Peseschkian's own life led him to create a cross-cultural theory while developing Positive Psychotherapy (Sarı, 2015).

Positive Psychotherapy offers a cross-cultural model for understanding mental health and well-being by bringing together elements from various schools of psychology, including psychodynamic, humanistic, behavioral, medical, and cognitive approaches (Marseille, 2025). Positive Psychotherapy is a conflict-centered and resource-oriented short-term psychotherapy based on cross-cultural observations made in more than 20 cultures. It integrates the humanistic understanding of humans, the psychodynamic theory of disorders, and a culturally sensitive, systematic therapy process in five steps (Peseschkian & Remmers, 2025b).

Positive Psychotherapy relies on a positive understanding of humans that posits every individual possesses innate physical, mental, and spiritual capacities that can be developed. Emphasizing human potential rather than pathology, this approach aims to support individuals' empowerment, self-awareness, and personal development while preserving their connections with their cultural and spiritual identities (Marseille, 2025).

In positive psychotherapy, the concept of "positive" refers to the factual and the actual; symptoms are treated as functional indicators that help the client make sense of the situation they are experiencing (Özen & Türkmen, 2023; Peseschkian & Remmers, 2025b). Symptoms are addressed as coping reactions given by the individual to the conflicts they experience; what is given is not only the problems but also the capacity to be healthy and to cope. This approach offers a holistic view of clinical assessment and treatment by making the function and meaning of symptoms visible (Peseschkian, 2023). Based on a positive perspective on humans, this approach bases itself on the balance model in line with the principles of hope, balance, and consultation, and aims to support individuals in coping with conflicts, increasing their quality of life, and self-actualization (Özen & Türkmen, 2023).

Three Basic Principles of Positive Psychotherapy

There are three important principles of positive psychotherapy. These principles are balance, hope, and consultation (Marseille, 2025). These principles constitute the basic components of a balanced life and support the individual's psychological well-being (Peseschkian, 2002; Sarı, 2015).

The Principle of the Balance Model

Positive Psychotherapy approaches humans from a humanistic perspective and bases itself on the resources possessed by every individual. At the center of this approach lies the importance of balance in the individual's life, and this balance is addressed in both clinical and non-clinical settings through the balance model. The balance model is based on four basic life areas where the individual sustains their life and functions: body/senses, achievement/activities, contact/environment, and fantasy/future. These areas directly affect the individual's life satisfaction, self-worth, and way of coping with conflicts and difficulties (Peseschkian, 2023; Peseschkian 2002). Although these four capacities are potentially present in every individual, some areas may be more developed compared to others depending on factors such as education, environmental conditions, and the social period lived in (Marseille, 2025; Peseschkian 2002).

The individual's life energy, activities, and reactions are shaped within these areas. According to Peseschkian's balance model, individuals cope with conflicts through these four areas of life; however, cultural tendencies can determine which areas are emphasized more. For example, while body and achievement-oriented coping styles are more common in Western cultures, relationship and future-oriented coping mechanisms are more prominent in Eastern cultures. Disruption of the balance between these areas can lead to the emergence of mental problems and negative symptoms (Marseille, 2025; Peseschkian 2002).

- Body/Senses area: Nutrition, affection and intimacy, sexuality, sleep, relaxation, sports, appearance, and clothing.
- Achievement/Activities area: Work, profession, career, money.

- Contact/Relationships area: Spouse/partner, family, friends, acquaintances and strangers, community life.
- Future/Fantasy area: Existential questions, spirituality, religious practices, future plans, and imagination (Peseschkian, 2023; Peseschkian 2002).

One of the main goals of treatment is to help the client recognize their own resources and mobilize these resources in a way that provides a dynamic balance. This goal is based on the balanced distribution of the individual's life energy ideally. According to Positive Psychotherapy, the individual experiences mental problems not because of the overemphasis on one life area, but as a result of the neglect of some areas (Peseschkian, 2023; Peseschkian & Remmers, 2025a).

The Principle of Hope

Hope means that clients are capable individuals in solving their problems and have the belief that problems can be solved (Eryılmaz, 2017). The principle of hope expresses the individual's belief in the existence of solution possibilities despite the problems experienced and their active effort in this direction; in Positive Psychotherapy, hope is not a passive expectation but a dynamic attitude that strengthens participation in the process (Peseschkian, 2002). Hope is based on a positive understanding of the human being and focuses not only on eliminating malfunctions but on understanding the real and functional aspects of these experiences. The therapist supports the individual in approaching symptoms with a new perspective by making their purpose and meaning visible. In this context, symptoms are treated as signals indicating capacities to respond to conflicts and the need to re-establish life balance (Marseille, 2025).

The Principle of Consultation

The Principle of Consultation emphasizes that the individual's problems are not limited only to their inner world, but also stem from their interactions with their environment, and that solutions can also be found in cooperation with this environment. This principle emphasizes the importance of informing individuals with mental disorders and their families about the problems and solutions (Eryılmaz, 2011). From a legal perspective, this informing process is not only a therapeutic requirement but also a fundamental duty of care, as the psychiatrist is obligated to provide comprehensive information to ensure the patient's right to self-determination and valid consent (Günday, 2015). This principle also supports the transcultural dimension of PPT, as cultural and social contexts deeply affect the individual's problems and ways of solution (Peseschkian & Remmers, 2025a).

In Positive Psychotherapy, the therapeutic process consists of five stages: the Observation/distancing stage, the inventory stage, the Situational encouragement stage, the Verbalization stage, and the expansion of goals stage (Sarı, 2015; Eryılmaz, 2017).

In the Observation/Distancing stage, the therapist listens to the client in a non-judgmental and objective manner; trying to understand the problems brought by the client, their needs, and behavior patterns associated with symptoms. In this stage, the current situation, past experiences, and expectations for the future are handled within a developmental integrity.

In the Inventory stage, the client's life experiences in recent years are evaluated over four basic life areas using the balance model. The client's ways of coping with problems, which life areas they use more intensely, and at what level they engage their basic capabilities are examined; in line with this information, the therapist develops preliminary evaluations regarding the client's basic and current conflicts.

In the Situational encouragement stage, the client's strengths and existing coping resources, which they often ignore, are made visible. Positive interpretations regarding symptoms are shared with the client, and the client's perception of self-worth is supported by developing alternative perspectives.

In the Verbalization stage, the client's basic conflicts are worked on more deeply. Under the guidance of the balance model, awareness and solution development processes are supported so that the individual can establish a more functional balance in the four areas of life. This phase is the longest stage of the therapeutic process.

Finally, in the expansion of goals stage, the client's short, medium, and long-term life goals for the future are addressed. Aiming for the client to develop self-help skills, it is targeted to create a sustainable balance and coping capacity after therapy (Gülırmak Güler, 2023; Peseschkian, 2002, Peseschkian, 2005; Peseschkian, 2007; Sarı, 2015).

Capabilities

Peseschkian's Positive Psychotherapy has a unique understanding of human nature; it accepts that individuals are born with two basic capacities: “to love” and “to know” (Eryılmaz, 2011). These basic capacities are comprehensive categories underlying “primary” and “secondary” capabilities (Cope, 2009).

The Capacity to Love is related to primary capabilities that are innate and develop and take shape especially through the emotional bond established with primary caregivers (Sarı, 2015). This capability is more related to the emotional aspect of the human being (Sarı, 2015). Capabilities such as love, patience, time, contact, sexuality/sensuality, hope, trust, and faith fall into the group of primary capabilities and manifest themselves in this way in development in later years (Eryılmaz, 2011; Sarı, 2015).

The Capacity to Know is related to the human need to understand relationships within reality and is associated with secondary capabilities (Sarı, 2015). This capability is more connected with behavioral aspects (Sarı, 2015). Traits such as punctuality, cleanliness, orderliness, and obedience constitute the group of secondary capabilities (Eryılmaz, 2011). Humans are in need of knowing many things, such as questioning why the apple falls to the ground, why the tree grows, and why there are illnesses and sorrows (Sarı, 2015). The development of these two basic capacities (to love and to know) and the primary and secondary capabilities attached to them, and the balance or imbalances between them, play an important role in the individual's psychological development and the understanding of psychopathology (Eryılmaz, 2011; Özen & Türkmen, 2023).

Positive Interpretation

In Positive Psychotherapy, this refers to taking into account the innate capabilities and capacities of the individual alongside conflicts and symptoms. This approach helps the client look at the situation from different angles by reframing symptoms not just as problems but as a reflection of the individual's true capabilities. Thus, symptoms are addressed through their functional meanings, and the individual's view of themselves and the problems they experience transforms, contributing to the reduction of psychological burden (Eryılmaz, 2020; Sarı, 2015).

Micro-traumas

According to the Positive Psychotherapy approach, these have an important place in the individual's life. Traumatic experiences may limit the individual's effective use of the capacities and capabilities they possess. Especially repetitive and small-scale traumas can accumulate over time and negatively affect the individual's functionality. Therefore, it is emphasized that working on the traumatic experiences individuals experience in their lives contributes to increasing functionality and strengthening psychological well-being (Eryılmaz, 2020; Sarı, 2015).

Conflicts

These are among the basic concepts of Positive Psychotherapy. In this approach, conflicts are addressed at three levels: actual conflict, basic conflict, and inner (key) conflict. In Positive Psychotherapy, **actual conflict** refers to current situations arising from the mismatch between expectations and current life conditions, creating emotional stress in the individual. These conflicts often emerge with daily life events and can trigger unresolved emotional experiences from the past. **Basic conflict** operates at a deeper level and is mostly related to beliefs, values, and expectations internalized in childhood. Even if triggered by a current event, it reflects the tension between the individual's primary and secondary capacities. **Inner (key) conflicts** cover unconscious struggles between opposing desires, values, or ideals and are usually experienced in the form of indecision, dilemma, and repetitive dysfunctional behaviors. These types of conflicts can pave the way for the individual to experience emotional distress and for the deterioration of psychological well-being (Marseille, 2025; Eryılmaz, 2020; Gülırmak Güler, 2023).

Conflict Coping Resources and Model Dimensions

In Positive Psychotherapy, coping with conflicts is addressed through four basic resources: body, achievement, relationships, and future/spirituality. These resources show which areas the individual turns to and how they distribute their energy in the face of conflicts. Additionally, model dimensions conceptualize the basic relationships affecting the individual's self-development. These dimensions are defined as “I” (relationship with oneself), “You” (relationship with partner), “We” (relationship with close circle), and “Primary-We” (relationship with meaning and spirituality). These dimensions are shaped through relationships established with parents during childhood and constitute a model for the individual's subsequent relationships (Eryılmaz, 2020; Sarı, 2015).

Stages of Interaction

Positive Psychotherapy is an approach that addresses the development of individuals within a cultural context and attaches importance to understanding the common and different characteristics between people. In this direction, stages of interaction offer a basic model for making sense of the relationships the individual establishes with both their family and other people. According to Positive Psychotherapy, individuals sustain their psychosocial development by passing through the stages of attachment, differentiation, and detachment throughout their lives. These stages are evaluated as important processes shaping the individual's relational patterns and ways of coping with conflicts (Eryılmaz, 2020; Peseschkian, 2002; Sarı, 2015).

Self-Help

In Positive Psychotherapy, self-help is a fundamental principle aiming for the individual to cope more functionally with conflicts and challenging situations encountered in life. While individuals may occasionally turn to ineffective or dysfunctional coping ways in the face of stressful life events, this principle encourages treating problems as a challenge and a development opportunity. The self-help approach supports the individual in moving away from the "sick role" and becoming an active subject, reducing dependence on the counselor, and using the skills learned in therapy sustainably after therapy (Eryılmaz, 2020; Sarı, 2015; Gülırmak Güler, 2023).

Therapeutic Process and Interventions

While the therapeutic process of Positive Psychotherapy attaches great importance to the quality of the relationship between the client and the therapist, it also proceeds through structured interventions and techniques. At the foundation of the therapeutic relationship, the role of the therapist focuses on empathic listening, unconditional acceptance, and empowering the client (Günday, 2015; Scheel et al., 2012). In this process, instead of handling the client's problems solely within a pathological framework, the therapist guides them to recognize their strengths, existing resources, and capacities; this approach strengthens the client's self-confidence and motivation for change (Marseille, 2025).

A critical step in PPT involves understanding the individual's problems within the framework of the balance model (body/health, work/achievement, relationships/contacts, future/spirituality) (Özen & Türkmen, 2023; Peseschkian & Remmers, 2025a). Through conflict analysis, it is determined in which life areas the problems experienced by the client are concentrated and how the imbalance between these areas has emerged (Peseschkian & Remmers, 2025a). As a result of this analysis, the client's goals focus not only on relieving symptoms but also on re-establishing and developing the balance between the four life areas. The goal-setting process is carried out with the client's participation and by determining concrete, achievable goals (Sarı, 2015).

One of the most distinctive and effective interventions of PPT is the use of stories, aphorisms, and metaphors in therapy (Peseschkian, 1987). Nossrat Peseschkian integrated these narrative forms, especially specific to Eastern cultures, into therapy. These techniques help clients reduce their defenses, look at issues from a different angle, and gain insight (Peseschkian, 1987). A message presented through a story or aphorism can be much more effective than direct advice; because it allows the client to connect with their own internal processes, understand the problem indirectly, and discover their own solutions. Stories also help the client place their own experiences in a broader context by conveying universal themes and cultural wisdom (Peseschkian, 1987; Sarı, 2015).

Some Studies Conducted

A bibliometric analysis conducted shows that interest in Positive Psychotherapy (PPT) has increased in nursing research, especially in the context of psychosocial problems such as depression and stress. However, the fact that the number of studies is still limited reveals that more research is needed. The integration of PPT into nursing practices and education can strengthen holistic care approaches and improve mental health outcomes (Gülırmak Güler, 2025).

Positive psychotherapy has been shown to be superior at a comparable level to active treatment methods in reducing major depression symptoms after an acute treatment process (Seshadri et al., 2021). One study shows that a positive psychotherapy program can be widely used as one of the nursing intervention programs for depression patients (Ko & Hyun, 2015). It was found that the "Positive Psychotherapy Based Kindness and Honesty Model" program effectively developed the practical communication skills of nursing students (Gülırmak Güler et al., 2024a). It is shown that a positive psychotherapy-based hope placement program increased life purpose and raised hope levels in patients with multiple sclerosis (Gülırmak Güler et al., 2024b).

It is suggested in a study that positive psychotherapy is effective in alleviating depression and increasing self-efficacy in undergraduate nursing students (Guo et al., 2017). The results of a research study showed that positive psychotherapy was effective in reducing the mental pressure of breast cancer patients and improving their moods (Dowlatabadi et al., 2016). Likewise, it was determined that positive psychotherapy was effective on happiness, strengths, pleasure, commitment, and semantic measures of life in cancer patients (Meibodi et al., 2021). A study shows that the integration of positive psychotherapy into smoking cessation treatment carries significant potential (Kahler et al., 2015).

STRENGTHS-BASED INTERVENTIONS

A strength can be defined as "a natural capacity for behaving, thinking, or feeling in a way that allows for optimal functioning and performance in the pursuit of valued outcomes" (Ghielen et al., 2018). Strengths-based interventions do not ignore problems or suffering; on the contrary, they emphasize conducting interventions based on individuals' positive potentials and achievable goals rather than deficits (Sousa et al., 2006). Strengths-based interventions aim to promote well-being or other positive outcomes by facilitating the identification of strengths, use and/or development of strengths (Ghielen et al., 2018). It is known that interventions aimed at focusing on strengths yield more desirable psychological outcomes compared to interventions focusing on weaknesses or neutral events (Dolev-Amit et al., 2021). In nursing, the strengths-based approach is a care model containing eight core values that guide nursing action and promote empowerment, self-efficacy, and hope (Gottlieb, 2014).

In a systematic literature review showed that all types of strength-based interventions yielded positive results in terms of well-being, work outcomes (e.g., work engagement), personal growth initiative, and group or team outcomes (e.g., class cohesion) (Ghielen et al., 2018). A 5-week strengths-based residential treatment program for substance use disorders in adolescents provided significant reductions in the frequency of alcohol, cannabis, and opioid use. Improvements in progress toward substance use goals and depressive symptoms were observed along with the treatment (Harris et al., 2016). In another study conducted, it was determined that low-threshold and broad-reach mobile health tools using a strengths-focused approach, such as MyStrengths, have the potential to support people living with chronic diseases in realizing self-management and taking control of their lives (Jessen et al., 2021). Another study examined the effect on mood of framing cognitive and mindfulness-based brief interventions to focus on either strengths or weaknesses. Results showed that presenting the intervention as focused on strengths ensured faster improvement in mood without changing treatment expectations (Murphy et al., 2022). Another study emphasizes the importance of motivational interviewing approaches for specific subgroups in strengths-based and culturally grounded family programs in order to reduce barriers to program participation and prevent adverse childhood experiences (Edwards et al., 2025). One study showed that the positive thinking training approach was effective in increasing resilience and life satisfaction in older adults (Taherkhani et al., 2023). Again, it was determined that strengths-based intervention had a positive effect on the well-being of nursing students (Malik & Sinha, 2025). Another study indicates that reflecting on strengths for a period of 5 weeks before exams prevented the emergence of negative emotions and distress and the decrease in well-being due to the upcoming exam period (Dolev-Amit et al., 2021).

REFERENCES

Açıkgöz, S., & Coşkunsever, A. (2025). Bir Yöntem Olarak Pozitif Psikoterapi Yaklaşımının Manevi Danışmanlık ve Rehberlik Uygulamalarında Kullanılabilirliği. *İslami İlimler Dergisi*, (40), 237-253. https://doi.org/.DOI: 10.34082/islamiilimler.1605479

Aypay, A., & Kara, A. (2018). Pozitif Psikoterapi Denge Modeli Bağlamında Dengeli Yaşam Ölçeği ve Dengeli Yaşam Temel Becerileri Ölçeğinin Geliştirilmesi. *Sakarya University Journal of Education*, *8*(3), 63. DOI: 10.19126/suje.408531

Bolier, L., Haverman, M., Westerhof, G. J., Riper, H., Smit, F., & Bohlmeijer, E. (2013). Positive psychology interventions: A meta-analysis of randomized controlled studies. *BMC Public Health*, *13*(1), 119. PMID: 23390882

Carr, A., Cullen, K., Keeney, C., Canning, C., Mooney, O., Chinseallaigh, E., & O'Dowd, A. (2021). Effectiveness of positive psychology interventions: A systematic review and meta-analysis. *The Journal of Positive Psychology*, *16*(6), 749–769.

Chakhssi, F., Kraiss, J. T., Sommers-Spijkerman, M., & Bohlmeijer, E. T. (2018). The effect of positive psychology interventions on well-being and distress in clinical samples with psychiatric or somatic disorders: A systematic review and meta-analysis. *BMC Psychiatry*, *18*(1), 211. PMID: 29945603

Cope, T. A. (2009). Positive Psychotherapy's Theory of the Capacity to Know as Explication of Unconscious Contents. *Journal of Religion and Health*, *48*(1), 79–89. DOI: 10.1007/s10943-008-9225-7 PMID: 19229628

Dolev-Amit, T., Rubin, A., & Zilcha-Mano, S. (2021). Is awareness of strengths intervention sufficient to cultivate wellbeing and other positive outcomes? *Journal of Happiness Studies*, *22*(2), 645–666.

Dowlatabadi, M. M., Ahmadi, S. M., Sorbi, M. H., Beiki, O., Razavi, T. K., & Bidaki, R. (2016). The effectiveness of group positive psychotherapy on depression and happiness in breast cancer patients: A randomized controlled trial. *Electronic Physician*, *8*(3), 2175. PMID: 27123227

Edwards, K. M., Waterman, E. A., Wheeler, L. A., Xu, W., Herrington, R., Trujllo, P., & Hopfauf, S. (2025). Predictors of Child and Caregiver Attendance in a Strengths-Focused, Culturally Grounded, Family-Based Program to Prevent Adverse Childhood Experiences. *Prevention Science*, •••, 1–12. PMID: 40029566

Eryılmaz, A. (2011). Yetişkin öznel iyi oluşu ile pozitif psikoterapi bağlamında birincil ve ikincil yetenekler arasındaki ilişkilerin incelenmesi. *Klinik Psikiyatri, 14*, 17–28.

Eryılmaz, A. (2017). Pozitif psikoterapiler. *Psikiyatride Güncel Yaklasimlar, 9*(3), 346–362. DOI: 10.18863/pgy.288667

Eryılmaz, A. (2020). *Meta teori: Bir gelişim ve psikoterapi kuramı olarak pozitif psikoterapi.* Nobel Akademik Yayıncılık.

Ghielen, S. T. S., van Woerkom, M., & Christina Meyers, M. (2018). Promoting positive outcomes through strengths interventions: A literature review. *The Journal of Positive Psychology, 13*(6), 573–585. DOI: 10.1080/17439760.2017.1365164

Gottlieb, L. N. (2014). CE: Strengths-based nursing. *AJN The American Journal of Nursing, 114*(8), 24–32. DOI: 10.1097/01.NAJ.0000453039.70629.e2 PMID: 25036663

Gülırmak Güler, K. (2023). *Pozitif psikoterapi temelli umut yerleştirme programının multipl skleroz tanılı bireylerde umut ve yaşam amaçları belirleme düzeyine etkisi.* Doktora Tezi, Ondokuz Mayıs Üniversitesi Lisansüstü Eğitim Enstitüsü Hemşirelik Ana Bilim Dalı.

Gülırmak Güler, K. (2025). Hemşirelik Araştırmalarında Pozitif Psikoterapinin Kullanımı: Bibliyometrik Bir Analiz. *Gümüşhane Üniversitesi Sağlık Bilimleri Dergisi, 14*(2), 823–831. DOI: 10.37989/gumussagbil.1611568

Gülırmak Güler, K., Güleç Keskin, S., & Albayrak, E. (2024a). The power of virtual connections: A randomized controlled trial of online positive psychotherapy training on effective communication skills of nursing students. *Nurse Education in Practice, 77*, 103967. PMID: 38615450

Gülırmak Güler, K., Güleç Keskin, S., & Terzi, M. (2024b). Transformative impact of positive psychotherapy-based hope placement program on life goals and hope level of individuals with multiple sclerosis. *Public Health Nursing (Boston, Mass.), 41*(6), 1402–1417. PMID: 39105489

Günday, H. M. (2015). *Psikiyatristin hukukî sorumluluğu.* Yetkin Yayınları.

Günday, H. M., & Albayrak Günday, E. (2025). Artificial intelligence in mental health practices: Legal liability analysis under Turkish, European, and common law frameworks. *Psikiyatride Güncel Yaklasimlar, 17*(4), 806–821. DOI: 10.18863/pgy.1620119

Guo, Y. F., Zhang, X., Plummer, V., Lam, L., Cross, W., & Zhang, J. P. (2017). Positive psychotherapy for depression and self-efficacy in undergraduate nursing students: A randomized, controlled trial. *International Journal of Mental Health Nursing*, *26*(4), 375–383. DOI: 10.1111/inm.12255 PMID: 27633932

Harris, N., Brazeau, J. N., Rawana, E. P., Brownlee, K., & Mazmanian, D. (2016). A Preliminary Examination of a Strengths-Based Treatment for Adolescent Substance Use Issues Examen préliminaire d'un traitement axé sur les forces destiné aux adolescents ayant des troubles liés à la toxicomanie. Vol. 50 No. 2, 145–163

Hendriks, T., Schotanus-Dijkstra, M., Hassankhan, A., De Jong, J., & Bohlmeijer, E. (2020). The efficacy of multi-component positive psychology interventions: A systematic review and meta-analysis of randomized controlled trials. *Journal of Happiness Studies*, *21*(1), 357–390.

Hoppen, T. H., & Morina, N. (2021). Efficacy of positive psychotherapy in reducing negative and enhancing positive psychological outcomes: A meta-analysis of randomised controlled trials. *BMJ Open*, *11*(9), e046017. PMID: 34489269

Jessen, S., Mirkovic, J., Brendmo, E. H., & Nes, L. S. (2021). Evaluating a strengths-based mHealth tool (MyStrengths): Explorative feasibility trial. *JMIR Formative Research*, *5*(11), e30572. DOI: 10.2196/30572 PMID: 34787580

Kahler, C. W., Spillane, N. S., Day, A. M., Cioe, P. A., Parks, A., Leventhal, A. M., & Brown, R. A. (2015). Positive psychotherapy for smoking cessation: A pilot randomized controlled trial. *Nicotine & Tobacco Research: Official Journal of the Society for Research on Nicotine and Tobacco*, *17*(11), 1385–1392. DOI: 10.1093/ntr/ntv011 PMID: 25646352

Kiliç, N., & Eryilmaz, A. (2019). Investigating narcissistic personality traits in the context of positive psychotherapy. *Archives of Neuropsychiatry*, *56*(1), 40–46. PMID: 30911236

Ko, Y. S., & Hyun, M. Y. (2015). Effects of a positive psychotherapy program on depression, self-esteem, and hope in patients with major depressive disorders. *Journal of Korean Academy of Psychiatric and Mental Health Nursing*, *24*(4), 246–256.

Lim, W. L., & Tierney, S. (2023). The effectiveness of positive psychology interventions for promoting well-being of adults experiencing depression compared to other active psychological treatments: A systematic review and meta-analysis. *Journal of Happiness Studies*, *24*(1), 249–273. PMID: 36373089

Malik, A., & Sinha, N. (2025). Integrating positive psychology into nursing education: A strengths-based intervention. *Journal of Applied Research in Higher Education*, •••, 1–21. DOI: 10.1108/JARHE-12-2024-0738

Marseille, A. (2025). Positive Psychotherapy: A Transcultural Approach to Psychotherapy for the Twenty-First Century. In *Psychotherapy in the Third Millennium-Cross-Cutting Themes and Proposals for Reflection*. IntechOpen. DOI: DOI: 10.5772/intechopen.1007778

Meibodi, R. P., Meftagh, S. D., & Shahangian, S. S. (2021). The effect of positive psychotherapy on happiness and character strength in cancer patients. *Journal of Education and Health Promotion*, *10*, 97. DOI: 10.4103/jehp.jehp_595_20 PMID: 34084844

Meyer, P. S., Johnson, D. P., Parks, A., Iwanski, C., & Penn, D. L. (2012). Positive living: A pilot study of group positive psychotherapy for people with schizophrenia. *The Journal of Positive Psychology*, *7*(3), 239–248. DOI: 10.1080/17439760.2012.677467

Murphy, S. T., Cheavens, J. S., & Strunk, D. R. (2022). Framing an intervention as focused on one's strength: Does framing enhance therapeutic benefit? *Journal of Clinical Psychology*, *78*(6), 1046–1057. DOI: 10.1002/jclp.23302 PMID: 34978712

Özen, Y., & Türkmen, İ. (2023). How Positive Is Positive Psychotherapy? (Examination of Positive Psychotherapy). *Innovare Journal Of Social Sciences*, *11*(2), 7–11.

Peseschkian, H. (2023). Positive psychotherapy: Core principles: Emphasizing capacities and balance can give patients a new perspective on their disorder. *Current Psychiatry*, *22*(1), 5–10. DOI: 10.12788/cp.0317

Peseschkian, H., & Remmers, A. (2025a). Life balance with positive psychotherapy. In *Positive Psychiatry, Psychotherapy and Psychology: Clinical Applications for Positive Mental Health* (pp. 91–99). Springer Nature Switzerland.

Peseschkian, H., & Remmers, A. (2025b). Positive psychotherapy: an introduction. In *Positive Psychiatry, Psychotherapy and Psychology: Clinical Applications for Positive Mental Health* (pp. 11–32). Springer Nature Switzerland.

Peseschkian, N. (1987). *Positive Psychotherapy: Theory and Practice of a New Method*. Springer-Verlag.

Peseschkian, N. (2002). *Günlük yaşamın psikoterapisi (Çev. K. Teksöz)*. Beyaz Yayınları.

Peseschkian, N. (2005). *Pozitif aile terapisi (Çev. M. Naim)*. Beyaz Yayınları.

Peseschkian, N. (2007). *Eğer hiç sahip olmadığın bir şeye sahip olmak istiyorsan, o zaman hiç yapmadığın bir Şey yap (Çev. S. Köseoğlu)*. Beyaz Yayınları.

Rashid, T. (2015). Positive psychotherapy: A strength-based approach. *The Journal of Positive Psychology, 10*(1), 25–40. DOI: 10.1080/17439760.2014.920411

Sarı, T. (2015). Pozitif psikoterapi: Gelişimi, temel ilk eve yöntemleri ve Türk kültürüne uygulanabilirliği. *The Journal of Happiness & Well-Being, 3*(2), 182–203.

Scheel, M., Davis, C. K., & Henderson, J. D. (2012). Therapist Use of Client Strengths. *The Counseling Psychologist, 41*(3), 392. DOI: 10.1177/0011000012439427

Schrank, B., Brownell, T., Tylee, A., & Slade, M. (2014). Positive psychology: An approach to supporting recovery in mental illness. *East Asian Archives of Psychiatry, 24*(3), 95–103. PMID: 25316800

Seligman, M. E., & Csikszentmihalyi, M. (2000). Positive psychology. *The American Psychologist, 55*(1), 5–14. PMID: 11392865

Seshadri, A., Orth, S. S., Adaji, A., Singh, B., Clark, M. M., Frye, M. A., & Fuller-Tyszkiewicz, M. (2021). Mindfulness-based cognitive therapy, acceptance and commitment therapy, and positive psychotherapy for major depression. *American Journal of Psychotherapy, 74*(1), 4–12. DOI: 10.1176/appi.psychotherapy.20200006 PMID: 32985916

Slade, M. (2010). Mental illness and well-being: The central importance of positive psychology and recovery approaches. *BMC Health Services Research, 10*(1), 26. PMID: 20102609

Sousa, L., Ribeiro, C., & Rodrigues, S. (2006). Intervention with multi-problem poor clients: Towards a strengths-focused perspective. *Journal of Social Work Practice, 20*(2), 189–204. DOI: 10.1080/02650530600776913

Taherkhani, Z., Kaveh, M. H., Mani, A., Ghahremani, L., & Khademi, K. (2023). The effect of positive thinking on resilience and life satisfaction of older adults: A randomized controlled trial. *Scientific Reports, 13*(1), 3478. PMID: 36859479

Van Agteren, J., Iasiello, M., Lo, L., Bartholomaeus, J., Kopsaftis, Z., Carey, M., & Kyrios, M. (2021). A systematic review and meta-analysis of psychological interventions to improve mental wellbeing. *Nature Human Behaviour, 5*(5), 631–652. PMID: 33875837

Walsh, S., Cassidy, M., & Priebe, S. (2017). The application of positive psychotherapy in mental health care: A systematic review. *Journal of Clinical Psychology, 73*(6), 638–651. DOI: 10.1002/jclp.22368 PMID: 27482845

Xie, H. (2013). Strengths-based approach for mental health recovery. *Iranian Journal of Psychiatry and Behavioral Sciences*, *7*(2), 5. PMID: 24644504

Chapter 6
Supportive and Interpersonal Psychotherapy in Inpatient Units

Kübra Tan
https://orcid.org/0000-0002-7591-8436
Artvin Coruh University, Turkey

ABSTRACT

In inpatient psychiatric units, treatment focuses not only on managing biological symptoms but also on restoring psychosocial functioning, addressing common issues like impaired relationships, low self-esteem, and social withdrawal. Effective care integrates pharmacological and psychotherapeutic methods, with supportive and interpersonal psychotherapy being especially valuable due to their practicality and efficacy. Supportive psychotherapy enhances coping skills, ego integrity, and resilience during acute crises, while interpersonal psychotherapy targets the connection between symptoms and social interactions, helping patients identify conflicts and develop coping strategies. These approaches promote holistic recovery within a safe therapeutic environment, relying on multidisciplinary collaboration, particularly the continuous, trust-based involvement of psychiatric nurses. This integrated model supports emotional well-being and interpersonal skill rebuilding, contributing significantly to patient recovery as supported by scientific evidence.

DOI: 10.4018/979-8-3373-6526-8.ch006

INTRODUCTION

In inpatient units, the treatment process aims not only to control biological symptoms but also to help individuals regain psychosocial functioning. Due to the nature of psychiatric disorders, problems such as interpersonal relationship impairments, reduced self-esteem, and social withdrawal are frequently observed. Therefore, psychiatric care should incorporate pharmacological treatment and psychotherapeutic approaches. Among these, supportive and interpersonal psychotherapy hold an important place in inpatient clinical settings because of their feasibility and effectiveness.

Supportive psychotherapy aims to strengthen individuals' coping skills, preserve ego integrity, and enhance adaptive capacity. Especially during acute psychiatric crises, it increases resilience and facilitates active participation in the treatment. Interpersonal psychotherapy (IPT), on the other hand, is based on the assumption that psychiatric symptoms are closely related to interpersonal relationship patterns, focusing on the patient's social roles and communication styles. This approach helps patients recognize interpersonal conflicts, understand emotional experiences, and develop new coping strategies.

The use of supportive and interpersonal approaches in inpatient units allows for a holistic treatment perspective. Within a safe therapeutic environment, patients receive emotional support and the opportunity to rebuild their interpersonal skills. Collaboration among nurses, psychiatrists, and psychologists is crucial in this process. Particularly, psychiatric nurses play a key role in implementing these therapeutic interventions effectively through the continuous and trust-based relationships they establish with patients.

This section discusses the importance of supportive and interpersonal psychotherapy in inpatient units, their principles of application, the professional roles involved in the therapeutic process, and their contributions to patient recovery, in light of scientific evidence.

1. THE PSYCHOLOGICAL BURDEN OF HOSPITALIZATION

Many hospitalized patients face serious illness. These conditions are characterized by a high mortality risk, impaired functioning, reduced quality of life, and a significant burden on both the individual and their caregivers. Patients hospitalized with serious medical conditions frequently experience significant psychological distress and impairments (Rokach, 2016). Common psychological difficulties in hospitalized patients include anxiety, depression, decreased quality of life, posttraumatic stress disorder (PTSD), and a sense of identity loss (Vlake et al., 2021; De Carlo et al.,

2020; Boeldt et al., 2019). One study reported that hospitalized patients experience feelings of being overwhelmed, illness-related worry, hopelessness/helplessness, and social isolation (Gerges et al., 2023).

Major psychological stressors in inpatient units include:

- **Uncertainty and loss of control:** Uncertainty about disease progression, treatment, and post-discharge conditions increases feelings of losing control.
- **Role and identity changes:** The suspension or redefinition of daily life roles (e.g., inability to work, dependence on others) may affect personal self-perception.
- **Restrictions on social relationships and interpersonal interactions:** Visiting restrictions, social isolation, or altered interpersonal dynamics within the hospital may reduce perceived social support.
- **Physical environment and institutional dynamics:** Stress factors such as ongoing observation, length of stay, and medical procedures can increase the psychological burden.

For example, a systematic review revealed that *"high levels of psychological stress experienced by hospitalized patients are associated with worse patient outcomes."* (Ford et al., 2023). Under such conditions, psychological support and interpersonal communication are particularly important. Addressing the physical, emotional, and social dimensions of patients is essential. Therefore, this section discusses how nursing care in inpatient units can alleviate this burden and how supportive and interpersonal therapy approaches can be integrated into care.

2. THE BIOPSYCHOSOCIAL APPROACH AND PSYCHOTHERAPEUTIC NEEDS

2.1 Theoretical Foundations of the Biopsychosocial Model

The Biopsychosocial (BPS) model highlights the inadequacy of explaining physical illness solely using biological factors. Originally proposed by George L. Engel, the model suggests that psychological and social factors play a central role in disease development (Bolton, 2023; Xiao et al., 2021). Recent literature indicates persistent gaps in the application of the BPS model in healthcare institutions worldwide. One study stated: *"Although the biopsychosocial approach has become widespread, healthcare personnel pay more attention to patients' physical symptoms and less to their psychosocial status."* (Xiao et al., 2021).

Integrating the BPS model into both diagnostic and treatment processes and care environments ensures consideration of not only the physiological but also the emotional and interpersonal dimensions of the patient. Within this framework, care is related not only to biological recovery but also to psychosocial resilience and the active use of social support.

2.2 The Need for Psychosocial Care in Inpatient Units

Inpatient settings present physical and psychosocial stressors. A study highlighted this emotional burden by stating, *"Hospitalization can be a challenging experience for all patients."* (Alzahrani, 2021). Moreover, hospitalization triggers stress, isolation, and loss of control, which hinder coping (Gerges et al. 2023).

Psychosocial care increases patient participation in the recovery process, improves treatment adherence, and enhances post-discharge functioning. For example, a study assessing psychosocial care needs in surgical units emphasized that meeting these needs is essential for patient well-being, recovery, and positive experiences (Ingstad et al., 2023). This finding suggests that inpatient care should not be limited to biomedical goals, and psychosocial dimensions must be addressed systematically.

2.3 Psychotherapeutic Integration in Nursing Practice

Psychiatric nursing involves dynamic care processes that interact with patients' mood, relational state, and social environment. Through therapeutic relationships and active communication, nurses are in a position to identify and intervene in psychosocial needs. Studies supporting the application of the BPS approach indicate that healthcare teams often fail to focus sufficiently on psychosocial dimensions, which limits the quality of care (Xiao et al., 2021).

Systematically integrating psychotherapeutic principles—creating a trusting environment, maintaining open communication, and reflecting on experiences—into nursing practice can prevent feelings of loneliness, facilitate adjustment, and support the recovery process.

2.4 Assessing Psychotherapeutic Needs in Clinical Settings

Psychotherapeutic needs in inpatient units are often remain invisible or overlooked. Major risk factors include prolonged hospitalization, social isolation, uncertainty, and low levels of social support. For example, a meta-analysis reported significant associations between stress experienced during hospitalization and patient outcomes (Ford et al., 2023).

Thus, nursing care must systematically evaluate patients' emotional states, coping strategies, social support networks, and interpersonal relationships. Implementing supportive and interpersonal psychotherapy models based on these needs can improve the quality of care and patient experience.

3. THEORETICAL FRAMEWORK OF SUPPORTIVE PSYCHOTHERAPY

3.1 Historical Development and Theoretical Foundations

Supportive psychotherapy originates from psychoanalytic theory but differs from classical analysis in that it focuses on strengthening the patient's existing coping capacity. Developed in the mid-20th century as an alternative treatment for individuals with severe mental illness or limited ego strength, its goal is to help patients maintain reality orientation, preserve ego integrity, and cope more functionally with daily challenges (Winston & Schaefer, 2023).

3.2 Core Principles: Trust, Reality Orientation, and Ego Strengthening

The core principles include establishing a safe therapeutic relationship, supporting self-esteem, reconstructing reality, and strengthening adaptive defense mechanisms (Winston & Schaefer, 2023). Reality testing is particularly effective in reducing anxiety, loss of control and helplessness. Ego strengthening aims to enhance the psychological resilience. These principles apply not only to psychiatric patients but also to individuals hospitalized for medical conditions (Holmes 1995).

3.3 Clinical Adaptation of Supportive Therapy

Supportive psychotherapy in inpatient settings is typically brief, goal-oriented, and multidisciplinary in nature. Therapeutic conversations focus on coping strategies, emotional regulation and resilience building (Winston & Schaefer, 2023). Evidence indicates that psychosocial support reduces anxiety and depression and improves treatment adherence (Ford et al., 2023).

3.4 Ethical and Practical Considerations

Ethical boundaries—confidentiality, professional distance, and respect for autonomy—are essential, especially when many healthcare professionals are involved (Wheeler, 2013). Interventions must prioritize the patient's immediate needs and avoid unnecessary in-depth analysis during acute crises.

3.5 Clinical Outcomes and Effectiveness

Research has shown that supportive psychotherapy improves symptom control and self-efficacy. Meta-analytic evidence suggests that it significantly enhances patient adherence (Cuijpers et al., 2020). Supportive therapeutic interactions also reduce burnout among nurses and improve their job satisfaction (Osman et al., 2018; Zhou, 2025).

4. THEORETICAL FOUNDATIONS OF INTERPERSONAL PSYCHOTHERAPY

4.1 Origins and Definition

Interpersonal Psychotherapy (IPT) was developed in the 1970s by Gerald L. Klerman and Myrna M. Weissman as a structured, short-term psychotherapy for depression (Weissman, 2006). It emphasizes that symptoms are influenced not only by biological factors but also by interpersonal stressors.

4.2 Theoretical Background

IPT is based on three major theories.

- **Sullivan's Interpersonal Theory:** Mental health is linked to the quality of interpersonal relationships (Ravitz et al., 2019).
- **Bowlby's Attachment Theory:** provides the basis for addressing grief and loss.
- **Social Role Theory:** This theory emphasizes the impact of role transitions, such as becoming a patient (Markowitz, 2015).

4.3 Therapy Process and Focus Areas

IPT typically lasts 12–16 sessions with four main focus areas:

- **Grief**
- **Role transitions**
- **Interpersonal disputes**
- **Interpersonal deficits**

These themes align closely with the challenges experienced by hospitalized individuals.

4.4 Clinical Adaptation of IPT

IPT can be adapted to short inpatient unit sessions. Nurses can integrate IPT principles by using reflective listening, reframing, and communication-enhancing techniques.

4.5 Cultural and Ethical Dimensions

Therapeutic interventions must be adapted to the cultural norms. Confidentiality and respect for patient autonomy are essential in multi-professional inpatient settings.

4.6 Clinical Effectiveness

Multiple randomized controlled trials support IPT's effectiveness of IPT. It improves both symptoms and social functioning, making it a valuable tool in inpatient settings (Cuijpers et al., 2016; Ravitz et al., 2019).

5. APPLICATION OF SUPPORTIVE PSYCHOTHERAPY IN INPATIENT UNITS

5.1 Clinical Context and Core Principles

Supportive psychotherapy in inpatient units is a short-term, relationship-based approach that focuses on strengthening emotional resources and preserving ego integrity (Winston & Schaefer, 2023). Common stressors, such as uncertainty, loss of control, and social isolation, can weaken ego functions, and supportive techniques aim to reorganize and strengthen these functions.

5.2 Establishing the Therapeutic Relationship

The quality of the therapeutic relationship is the cornerstone of supportive psychotherapies. According to Peplau's Interpersonal Relations Theory (1997), the nurse–patient relationship is inherently healing. Trust-based communication reduces stress, anxiety, and loneliness (Haribhai-Thompson et al. 2022).

5.3 Structure and Process of Sessions

Sessions are typically 15–30 min and follow three phases:

- **Initial phase:** identifying current problems
- **Middle phase:** emotional expression, reality orientation, coping enhancement
- **Termination:** summarizing strengths and reinforcing support

5.4 Supportive Intervention Techniques

Supportive psychotherapy includes many microtechniques frequently used in clinical environments, such as (Table 1):

Table 1.

Technique	Description	Clinical Example
Reality orientation	Helping the patient evaluate their thoughts and feelings on the basis of reality.	"This feeling may be a natural reaction to the illness you are currently experiencing."
Empathic listening	Carefully attending to and reflecting the patient's emotions.	"When you feel lonely, I can understand how heavy that feeling is for you."
Positive reinforcement	Noticing and appreciating the patient's small steps and progress.	"Your active participation in the treatment today was very valuable."
Ego strengthening	Enhancing self-esteem and the sense of self-efficacy.	"You have shown your ability to pull yourself together before; you can get through this as well."
Providing support and hope	Increasing emotional safety and reassurance.	"I know this is a difficult period, but you are not alone."

5.5. Team-Based Practice

Supportive psychotherapy should be implemented using a multidisciplinary team approach. Psychiatrists, psychologists, nurses, and social workers should work in a coordinated manner according to the needs of the patient.

Studies have shown that consistency within a team increases patient satisfaction and treatment adherence (Köbler, 2022). In this process, nurses assume the role of "psychotherapeutic observer"; they detect the patient's emotional reactions at an early stage and provide feedback to the team. This feedback makes it possible to individualize treatment plans.

For example, when a psychiatric nurse notices that a patient's depressive symptoms are increasing and reports this to the team, the psychiatrist may review the medication dose, while the psychologist may add brief IPT sessions, thereby providing comprehensive support.

5.6. Clinical Findings and Effectiveness

The effectiveness of supportive psychotherapy in inpatient settings has been demonstrated in many studies. Winston and Schaefer (2023) state that supportive psychotherapy leads to significant reductions in levels of depression and anxiety. In their meta-analysis, Cuijpers et al. (2019) found that supportive therapy, particularly when implemented in nursing-based practices, is as effective as other short-term psychotherapy. Ford et al. (2023) reported that patients receiving psychosocial support showed significantly higher levels of treatment engagement and self-efficence.

These findings indicate that supportive psychotherapy is a feasible, economical, and humane intervention for inpatient units.

5.7. Challenges in Practice and Suggested Solutions

The most important limitations of supportive psychotherapy are time constraints and high nurse-to-patient ratios. In addition, in some institutions, psychotherapeutic approaches are not associated with the nursing role, which may reduce their frequency of use.

The following recommendations are proposed to overcome these barriers.

Organizing short-term psychotherapy trainings for nurses,

Establishing supervision systems,

Developing care protocols based on psychotherapy,

Prioritizing psychosocial care at the management level.

These steps ensure the sustainability of the supportive approach at the institutional level.

Supportive psychotherapy is a patient-centered approach that strengthens the emotional dimension of nursing care in inpatient settings. Based on trust, empathy, and reality orientation, this model contributes to the patient's recovery physically, emotionally, and socially. When nurses adopt this approach in their daily practice, it not only improves the quality of care but also strengthens patients' psychological resilience and engagement in their recovery.

6. THE APPLICATION OF INTERPERSONAL PSYCHOTHERAPY IN INPATIENT UNITS

6.1. Clinical Context and Rationale for Use

Interpersonal Psychotherapy (IPT) is a time-limited therapy that focuses on social roles, relationship networks, and interpersonal stressors experienced during illness (Markowitz & Weissman, 2012). In inpatient units, the importance of IPT stems from the fact that physical illness affects not only biological processes but also social and emotional relationships of the patient.

Hospitalization causes a dramatic change in the individual's roles: the transition from being an independent person to the "patient" role, loss of autonomy, and shifts in family responsibilities, which create psychosocial stress. IPT uses relationship-focused interventions to facilitate adaptation to such changes (Cuijpers et al., 2016).

Example: A patient with chronic renal failure who is dependent on dialysis and no longer able to continue working expresses role loss by saying, "I am no longer useful." In line with IPT principles, the nurse identifies that the patient is experiencing a "role transition" and works with the patient to develop new areas of adaptation (e.g., supportive roles within the family).

6.2. Stages of Implementation

IPT is generally implemented in three stages (Markowitz 2015):

Initial Phase (Assessment and Focus Setting): The patient's interpersonal relationships were mapped. The primary area of stress (grief, role transition, dispute, or deficit) was identified.

Clinical example: When a patient says, "My spouse no longer comes to visit me," the therapist may identify this as an area of "interpersonal dispute."

Middle Phase (Intervention and Reconstruction): Communication skills were taught. Sources of social support were identified. Emotional awareness and meaning-making were addressed.

For example, when a patient with movement restriction after a stroke says, "No one listens to me anymore," the nurse may reflect the emotion by saying, "You feel invisible," and then discuss with the patient how to open communication channels.

Termination Phase (Strengthening and Sustainability): Therapeutic gains are summarized in this phase. New coping strategies are emphasized in this study. Plans are made to preserve interpersonal bonds after discharge.

6.3. Fields and Foci of Application

6.3.1. Grief and Loss

In inpatient settings, the "grief" process is not limited to bereavement but may also concern the loss of bodily functions or a former lifestyle (Altschul 1984).

For example, when a patient who has undergone amputation says, "My leg is gone, so I am gone too," the therapist conceptualizes this as "symbolic grief" and works on reconstructing identity after loss.

6.3.2. Role Transition

Role transition is the most frequently addressed focus in IPT. The hospitalization process leads to a temporary loss of autonomy and self-regulation (Markowitz & Weissman, 2012).

Example: A parent undergoing long-term treatment says, "I can't take care of my children." The nurse responds, "Your roles have changed during this process, but your presence in the family is still important," thus providing emotional re-framing.

6.3.3. Interpersonal Disputes

Illness and hospitalization may create tension in relationships with family or the healthcare team. In IPT, the goal is to identify the source of conflict and find solutions at the communication level.

Example: When a patient who has tension with a nurse during treatment says, "You are not listening to me," the nurse may respond with a reflective intervention such as, "When you feel unheard, you withdraw; how can we change this together?"

6.3.4. Interpersonal Deficits

Loneliness and lack of social support are common during hospitalization. In such cases, the therapist or nurse works with the patient to rebuild social ties.

For example, when an older patient says, "Nobody calls me," the nurse suggests re-establishing communication with family members, for instance, through phone calls, and helps facilitate this connection.

6.4. IPT Practices in Nursing

Psychiatric nurses play a leading role in applying IPT principles to patients. The integration of IPT into nursing practice can occur at three levels (Wheeler 2013):

Micro Level: Empathic reflection and emotional validation in daily communication.

For example, when a patient says, "Nothing is going to change," the nurse replies, "You feel very hopeless right now; but even small changes can affect your process," thus responding therapeutically.

Meso Level: Participation in group IPT sessions or management of group dynamics.

For example, Group IPT for patients experiencing similar role losses in a depression clinic increases feelings of social support (Ravitz et al., 2019).

Macro Level: Integrating the IPT approach into institutional care protocols—for example, adding an "interpersonal focus area" section to psychosocial assessment forms.

6.5. Clinical Effectiveness and Evidence

When randomized controlled trials over the past 20 years were examined, IPT was found to significantly improve both depressive symptoms and social functioning (Cuijpers et al., 2016). In a study by van Hees et al. (2013), patients who received IPT showed a reduction in their symptoms. Short IPT programs conducted in oncology units have increased patients' adjustment and quality of life after discharge (Markowitz 2015). Moreover, nurses who received IPT training showed significant improvements in communication skills and job satisfaction (Zhou, 2025).

6.6. Ethical and Cultural Sensitivities

When implementing IPT in inpatient units, patients' cultural values and family ties should be considered. In some cultures, the family plays a central role in decision-making; therefore, it is important to consider this context when working on "interpersonal disputes" (Ravitz et al., 2019). Confidentiality, informed consent, and preservation of professional boundaries are ethical priorities.

Interpersonal Psychotherapy in inpatient units is a concrete application of the biopsychosocial approach. By targeting role changes, relationship loss, and social isolation experienced during illness, it brings a human dimension to the treatment process.

IPT demonstrates that psychiatric nursing care is based not only on clinical observation but also on relationship-centered, healing-oriented approaches.

7. THE THERAPEUTIC ROLE OF THE PSYCHIATRIC NURSE

Psychiatric nurses are not only caregivers but also therapeutic specialists who support individuals' emotional, cognitive, and social recovery. Modern psychiatric nursing is shaped by Hildegard Peplau's Interpersonal Relations Theory. According to this theory, the nurse–patient relationship is a therapeutic tool that helps patients understand their internal conflicts and develop adaptive skills (Peplau, 1977). In inpatient units, nurses are the professionals with whom patients spend the most time. Therefore, nursing interactions provide opportunities for psychotherapeutic interventions and physical care (Wheeler, 2013).

7.1. Therapeutic Communication and Emotional Awareness

Communication lies at the core of the psychiatric nurse's therapeutic role. A good therapeutic relationship is built on trust, openness, and mutual respect. In an analytic examination of nurse–patient interviews, Wu (2021) found that techniques such as empathic reflection, emotional validation, and effective use of silence, reduced patient stress. For example, when an anxious, restless patient says, "No one understands me," the nurse responds: "When you feel misunderstood, your sense of loneliness may intensify. Shall we explore together what this feeling means right now?" This response includes both reflection and the introduction of an emotional awareness. Empathy and active listening increase not only patient comfort but also nurses' professional satisfaction. In a systematic review by Zhou (2025), nurses with higher levels of empathy had significantly lower burnout rates.

7.2. Nursing Roles in Psychotherapeutic Interventions

Psychiatric nurses assume three basic roles in the implementation of psychotherapeutic care (Forchuk, 2021):

Supportive Role: Enhancing emotional resilience, maintaining reality orientation, and strengthening self-esteem.

Example: When a depressed patient says, "Nothing has any meaning anymore," the nurse responds, "You feel very helpless right now; shall we identify a small step together?"

Educational Role: Providing information about the illness, treatment process, and coping strategies.

For example, educating a patient with panic disorder about the role of breathing exercises in managing anxiety.

Advocacy Role: Protecting patients' rights, safety, and autonomy.

Example: Ensuring that the patient's preferences are considered when making treatment decisions.

These roles make nursing care not only "helping" but also a healing relational process.

7.3. Role Models of the Psychiatric Nurse

7.3.1. Peplau's Interpersonal Roles

According to Peplau, the nurse assumes different roles at different stages.

<u>Stranger:</u> Establishes trust during the first contact.

<u>Resource Person:</u> Provides information.

<u>Teacher:</u> Teaches adaptation and coping skills to the students.

<u>The Leader:</u> Encourages the patient to actively participate in their care.

<u>Counselor:</u> Helps patients explore their emotions.

<u>Surrogate (Change Agent):</u> Temporarily becomes a trusted figure (Peplau 1997).

This model enables nurses to dynamically manage therapeutic relationships.

Example: On the first day of hospitalization, when an anxious patient perceives the nurse as a "familiar figure of safety," the nurse is temporarily in the surrogate role; over time, the nurse guides the patient to discover their coping resources.

7.4. Therapeutic Role in the Multidisciplinary Team

In inpatient units, the psychiatric nurse is the "relationship builder and observer" of the treatment team. While the psychiatrist is responsible for diagnosis and medication management, the nurse continuously observes the patient's emotional response. These observations, communicated back to the team, support the personalization of the treatment plan (Köbler et al., 2022). For example, when a nurse notices emotional fluctuations after a medication change in a patient, they report this to the psychiatrist. Based on this information, the team adjusts the medication and plans brief supportive sessions for the patient.

7.5. Education, Supervision, and Professional Development

To maintain their therapeutic skills, psychiatric nurses require continuous education, supervision, and self-awareness. Wheeler (2013) noted that when experienced nurses receive regular supervision, a marked increase in patient satisfaction is observed.

The following components are recommended for training programs:

- Emotional awareness and self-reflection activities,
- Role play and case-based learning,
- Empathy development exercises,
- Short-term psychotherapy techniques (e.g., supportive and interpersonal).

For example, in a "therapeutic communication laboratory" in a nursing school, students were found to improve their ability to generate empathic responses in hospital scenarios (McCabe, 2004).

7.6. Challenges Encountered in Practice

The therapeutic role of nurses in inpatient units may be limited by several factors.

High workload: Time pressure restricts therapeutic conversations.

Role ambiguity: In some institutions, psychotherapy is perceived as the role of only psychologists or psychiatrists.

Emotional exhaustion: Long-term stress may lead to empathetic fatigue.

Suggestions to overcome these challenges include the following:

Establishing "psychotherapeutic nursing protocols" at the institutional level,
Providing supervision support and reorganizing working hours,
Clearly defining roles within the team (Winston & Schaefer, 2023).

7.7. Clinical Effectiveness and Patient Outcomes

Recent studies have shown that in clinics where nurses have strong therapeutic communication skills, patients' anxiety and depression scores are significantly lower

(Haribhai-Thompson et al., 2022). It has also been demonstrated that patients' trust in nurses increases treatment adherence and satisfaction (Bahari et al., 2024). For example, in a study conducted in emergency departments, a significant positive relationship was found between patients' trust in nurses and their perceived quality of nursing care (Bahari et al., 2024). This indicates that the nurse–patient trust relationship has the potential to improve treatment participation, adherence to educational programs, and care outcomes in patients with diabetes. These findings show that the therapeutic relationship in nursing directly contributes to clinical effectiveness. The therapeutic role of psychiatric nurses lies at the center of the biopsychosocial care model. Professionals who integrate supportive and interpersonal psychotherapy principles into nursing care lead patients to physical and mental recovery. This role is based on trust, empathy, and professional intuition and directly affects patient satisfaction and clinical outcomes.

8. ETHICAL PRINCIPLES AND PROFESSIONAL BOUNDARIES IN PSYCHOTHERAPEUTIC NURSING

Psychotherapeutic nursing practices are based on respect for human dignity, preservation of privacy, honesty and professional responsibility. While supporting both physical and emotional recovery, the nurse enters the most vulnerable areas of the patient's life; thus, ethical sensitivity is as important as clinical competence (Wheeler, 2013). Therapeutic communication, supportive or interpersonal psychotherapy implemented in inpatient units, places the nurse in deep emotional interaction with the patient. In this interaction, adherence to ethical principles and professional boundaries is essential for both patient safety and the nurse's professional integrity (Peplau 1997).

8.1. Fundamental Ethical Principles

8.1.1. Respect for Autonomy

Every individual has the right to make decisions regarding their life and treatment. Nurses should consider the patient's preferences and apply the principle of informed consent (ANA, 2001). For example, in a psychiatric ward, when a patient refuses medication, the nurse listens to the reasons without judgment and then explains the treatment process and possible consequences in simple language. This process reflects respect for the patient's decision-making abilities.

8.1.2. Beneficence and Non-maleficence

Therapeutic interventions should aim to improve the patient's well-being and minimize the risk of harm. In psychotherapeutic processes, misinterpretation, breaches of confidentiality, or excessive emotional closeness can cause indirect harm. For example, when a nurse realizes that they are reacting with excessive emotional empathy while discussing past trauma with a depressed patient, they share this intense interaction with a supervisor to preserve boundaries (Wheeler, 2013).

8.1.3. Justice

All patients have the right to receive equal, fair, and unbiased care. This principle is particularly important in psychiatric units because of the risk of stigmatization. Nurses are obliged to establish the same level of therapeutic relationship regardless of socioeconomic status, gender, or diagnosis (Beauchamp & Childress, 2019).

8.1.4. Confidentiality and Privacy

Confidentiality of personal information shared by patients during psychotherapeutic processes is essential. Such information should only be accessible to the relevant team members. For example, when providing information to the family, the nurse shares only what the patient has consented to; otherwise, the trust relationship may be damaged. Research has shown that trust in confidentiality enhances treatment adherence (Bahari et al., 2024).

8.2. Maintaining Professional Boundaries

Boundaries in the therapeutic relationship are necessary for patient safety and maintaining the nurse's professional identity. Peplau (1997) emphasized that the therapeutic relationship should be regarded as "professional intimacy" and should not turn into personal or social intimacy.

8.2.1. Emotional Boundaries

Nurses should approach the patient's emotional state with empathy while recognizing and managing their own emotional burden.

For example, if a patient's trauma history triggers the nurse's own past experiences, seeking supervision support is an ethical responsibility (Forchuk, 2021).

8.2.2. Physical Boundaries

Although some patients find touch comforting, physical contact should be carefully evaluated. Physical touch without the patient's consent is a boundary violation.

Example: Before using touch as support for a highly anxious patient, the nurse should ask, "Would you like me to hold your hand to help you feel calmer?"

8.2.3. Social Boundaries

The nursing relationship should be maintained within a professional framework. Social media interactions, personal communications, and accepting gifts are not ethically appropriate (ANA, 2001).

8.3. Supervision and Ethical Decision-Making

Ethical dilemmas are common in psychotherapeutic nursing. When nurses experience uncertainty about emotional transference, confidentiality, or conflicts of interest, they should seek supervision (Wheeler, 2013).

The ethical decision-making process generally consists of four steps (Beauchamp & Childress, 2019).

Identifying the ethical issue,
Determining alternative actions,
Evaluating possible consequences,
Implementing the most ethical options.

For example, when a nurse is uncertain whether to keep a patient's disclosure of domestic violence confidential, they consult the ethics committee and team leader and make a decision based on the principle of non-maleficence.

8.4. Cultural Ethical Sensitivity

Cultural values directly affect nurses' ethical decisions. For example, in some cultures, families may prefer that a poor prognosis not be fully disclosed to the patient. In such cases, nurses must balance the principles of "truth-telling" and "non-maleficence" (Ravitz et al., 2019). For example, if a terminal patient is kept unaware of the severity of the illness at the family's request, the nurse coordinates the level of disclosure with the team to protect both the patient's psychological safety and cultural sensitivity.

8.5. Types of Ethical Violations and Prevention

Research shows that the most common ethical problems in psychiatric units are breaches of confidentiality, boundary violations, and restrictions on autonomy (Giannetta et al., 2021).

Recommendations for preventing such violations include the following:

- Making ethical awareness training continuous,
- Conducting case-based incident analyses,
- Activating ethics consultation committees,
- Encouraging open communication among colleagues.

Adherence to ethical principles in psychotherapeutic nursing determines the reliability and quality of the therapeutic relationship with patients. While being empathic and supportive, nurses should maintain professional boundaries and respect the patient's autonomy, privacy, and cultural values. Nurses with high ethical sensitivity strengthen not only individual patient safety but also the overall ethical climate of their institution.

9. SUPERVISION, SELF-AWARENESS, AND PROFESSIONAL RESILIENCE IN PSYCHOTHERAPEUTIC NURSING

Psychotherapeutic nursing is a discipline that requires not only clinical skills but also the constant development of inner awareness, emotional balance, and professional resilience. Nurses who carry patients' intense emotions, such as trauma, loss, guilt, and hopelessness, stand at the center of the therapeutic process while also needing to protect their own psychological boundaries. In this process, the nurse establishes a healing relationship but maintains a professional distance to avoid emotional overload. The key to maintaining emotional balance in psychotherapeutic practice is self-awareness, regular supervision, and resilience development (Wheeler, 2013). These three components enhance nurses' clinical competence and psychological flexibility. Supervision offers the nurse an opportunity to recognize emotional reactions and countertransference processes; self-awareness allows them to manage the boundaries of the relationship ethically; and resilience enables the nurse to maintain professional presence even under high emotional load. In this context, professional development in psychotherapeutic nursing is possible not only through knowledge but also through self-knowledge and emotional self-regulation. This section addresses the place, importance, and clinical examples of supervision, self-awareness, and professional resilience in psychotherapeutic nursing care.

9.1. The Meaning of Supervision and Its Clinical Importance

Supervision is a structured learning process in which nurses review their professional experiences, recognize their emotional reactions, and continue their professional development. Edwards and Burnard (2003) described supervision as a tool that supports nurses' ethical decision-making, self-reflection, and emotional resilience in clinical practice. For example, a psychiatric nurse realizes that they felt intense anger during a session with a trauma survivor. After the session, the nurse shares this reaction in supervision and recognizes that the emotion stems not from the patient but from their past experiences. This awareness helps nurses develop a more balanced approach to patient care. Research shows that nurses who receive regular supervision have higher job satisfaction and lower burnout levels (McDonough et al., 2025). This indicates that supervision is not only an individual necessity but also an institutional one.

9.2. Types of Supervision and Modes of Practice

9.2.1. Individual Supervision

This is a trust-based process between nurses and supervisors. Personal transference, countertransference, and ethical dilemmas are analyzed in this context. For example, a nurse working in an intensive care unit accompanies a patient through the dying process and feels emotionally exhausted. In individual supervision, nurses share their experiences, recognize their attitudes toward death, and regulate their emotional burden.

9.2.2. Group Supervision

Group supervision provides an environment of shared experiences, learning, and support. It strengthens empathy within the team and fosters professional solidarity (Hawkins & Shohet, 2012). Example: Six nurses working in a psychiatric ward discuss their "fear of boundary violations" in a weekly group-supervision meeting. The supervisor guided the participants to explore their own definitions of ethical boundaries.

9.2.3. Peer Supervision

This is a horizontal model in which professionals at the same level provide feedback to each other. This reduces hierarchical pressure and promotes mutual learning. For example, two nurses can conduct brief "reflective review sessions" after weekly shifts to discuss difficult cases and suggest alternative communication approaches to each other.

9.3. Self-Awareness: The Silent Power of the Therapeutic Process

Self-awareness is the capacity of nurses to recognize their own emotions, values, and boundaries (Geller & Greenberg, 2012). In psychotherapeutic relationships, self-awareness allows nurses to manage the emotions projected onto patients. For example, a depressed patient's statement, "I am useless," may trigger in the nurse an urgent desire to "repair" the patient. A nurse with developed self-awareness recognizes this impulse and adopts a stance of "accompanying" rather than "fixing," thereby maintaining balance in the nurse–patient relationship.

The recommended methods for cultivating self-awareness include:

- ✓ Keeping a journal and engaging in self-reflection,
- ✓ Mindfulness exercises,
- ✓ Empathy-based self-care practices,
- ✓ Emotion diary work (Salem et al., 2025).

These methods increase nurses' emotional resilience and enable more balanced participation in the therapeutic process.

9.4. Professional Resilience

Resilience is a nurse's capacity to maintain psychological integrity in the face of high stress, loss, or crisis (Hart et al., 2014). Prolonged exposure to patients in psychiatric and medical units may increase emotional strain, and resilience acts as a buffer mechanism in such situations. Example: A nurse in an oncology unit feels guilty after the death of a patient whose treatment was unsuccessful. Using resilience skills, nurses seek support through supervision, complete the grief process in a healthy way, and restore a sense of meaning in their professional role.

Strategies that support resilience include (Moore, 2025):

- ✓ Social support networks (colleagues, family),
- ✓ Humor and positive reframing,
- ✓ Physical self-care (sleep, exercise, nutrition),
- ✓ Participation in institutional wellness programs.

9.5. Burnout Syndrome: A Silent Threat

Maslach (2018) defines burnout in three dimensions:

- ✓ Emotional exhaustion,
- ✓ Depersonalization,
- ✓ Reduced sense of personal accomplishment.

Psychiatric nurses are more prone to this syndrome because they carry patients' intense emotional burdens. Zhou (2025) found that nurses with higher levels of empathic communication have significantly lower burnout risk. For example, a nurse who is repeatedly exposed to the anger of a patient experiencing frequent crises becomes emotionally worn out. By sharing this experience during supervision, the nurse recognized burnout symptoms and developed a self-care plan that included weekly walks, relaxation exercises, and participation in a support group.

9.6. Institutional Support Mechanisms

Institutional support is one of the strongest determinants of individual resilience (ICN 2021). The following practices are recommended for an effective psychotherapeutic nursing system:

Reflective Practice Meetings: Nurses share their weekly clinical experiences in a safe environment.
Supervision Systems: Regular individual or group supervision sessions.
Psychological Support Line: Access to professional counseling for staff experiencing post-traumatic stress.
Wellness Programs: Mindfulness training, relaxation techniques, yoga, and stress management workshops.

For example, a university hospital launched a "Nurse Wellbeing Day" program. In this event, nurses participated in emotional sharing sessions and reported reduced burnout and increased job satisfaction (Winston & Schaefer, 2023).

9.7. Ethical Dimension: Supervision and Confidentiality

The confidentiality of information shared during supervision is of great ethical importance. For nurses to reflect on their experiences while protecting patient privacy, the supervision setting must be safe (Forchuk 2021). Violations of ethical boundaries can damage therapeutic trust. Therefore, every supervision process should be framed within a confidentiality agreement.

9.8. Alignment in Education and Clinical Practice

Supervision is not only professional support but also a clinical teaching tool. Regular supervision sessions between newly graduated nurses and experienced specialists accelerate the development of self-awareness (Salem et al., 2025). Supervision, self-awareness, and professional resilience form a triad that ensures the sustainability of psychotherapeutic nursing care. These three concepts protect nurses' emotional health and strengthen the quality of the therapeutic relationship. Regular supervision develops self-reflection skills, self-awareness maintains ethical boundaries, and resilience sustains professional presence under challenging clinical conditions. When psychiatric nurses integrate these three core areas, they become not only healthcare workers but also "specialists in healing relationships."

10. FUTURE DIRECTIONS AND PRACTICE RECOMMENDATIONS IN PSYCHOTHERAPEUTIC NURSING

Psychotherapeutic nursing is evolving within constantly changing healthcare systems, increasingly digital care environments, and culturally diverse societies. In the new era, psychotherapeutic approaches focus not only on face-to-face sessions but also on technology-assisted therapeutic interactions, cross-cultural sensitivity, ethical digital communication, and multidisciplinary integration (Markowitz, 2008; Wheeler, 2013). These developments redefine the nurse's role, transforming it from that of a "care provider" to a "therapeutic professional who regulates psychosocial balance."

10.1. Digital Psychotherapy and Telehealth Applications

In the post-COVID-19 period, telehealth and digital therapeutic platforms have become integral to healthcare services. Digital psychotherapy makes mental health support accessible through mobile applications, online counseling and virtual support groups (Shore et al., 2018).

Clinical Example

A psychiatric nurse plans online follow-up sessions with a patient who fears being discharged because of depressive symptoms. Through a mobile "emotion diary" application, nurses can monitor patients' adherence to treatment. Using real-time feedback, nurses can maintain therapeutic continuity.

The roles of nurses in telepsychiatry are developing at three levels:

E-counseling: Online sessions that support treatment participation,
Remote monitoring: Tracking emotional state and medication adherence via mobile devices,
Digital education: Providing online training for stress management and self-care (Topol, 2019).

However, maintaining ethical boundaries, data confidentiality, and professional language in digital environments is of primary importance (Yang & Jang, 2025).

10.2. Artificial Intelligence and Empathic Technologies

Advancements in artificial intelligence (AI) systems have provided new opportunities for personalizing therapeutic processes. AI-supported analyses can identify emotional states from patients' speech patterns and alert nurses. These systems enable the early detection of emotional fluctuations (Luxton, 2015).

Clinical Example

In a psychiatric unit, an "emotion analysis algorithm" monitors changes in patients' voice tone to detect signs of depressive relapses. Nurses integrate these data with clinical observations and initiate early supportive sessions. The ethical use of AI must be based on the principle that technology is a complementary tool to the nurse–patient relationship; the goal is not to replace human interaction but to deepen it (Topol 2019).

10.3. Cross-Cultural Therapeutic Approaches

In globalized healthcare systems, cultural sensitivity is a key determinant of treatment effectiveness. The expression of psychological distress, help-seeking patterns, and social support structures vary across cultures. Nurses must recognize that therapeutic interventions implemented without understanding the cultural context may be ineffective or even harmful (Watson et al., 2022).

Clinical Example

A migrant patient's statement "my soul is trapped" may be interpreted as depression in Western diagnostic systems; however, in the cultural context, this expression may signify a spiritual imbalance related to weakened family ties. The nurse evaluates this narrative independently of their own cultural lens and directs the patient to culturally specific support resources. Cross-cultural therapeutic skills broaden nurses' empathic understanding and increase the inclusiveness of care.

10.4. Multidisciplinary Collaboration and Integration

The psychotherapeutic care model of the future will rely on a holistic team approach involving psychiatrists, psychologists, nurses, social workers, physiotherapists, and art therapists. In such teams, nurses serve as a bridge in observation, empathy, emotional regulation, and maintenance of the therapeutic relationship (Forchuk, 2021). This collaboration strengthens the continuity of care and patient safety.

10.5. Trends in Education and Competence Development

In the future, psychotherapeutic skills in nursing education will be supported by simulation-based learning, reflective practice, digital case analysis and supervision-based evaluation models (Salem et al., 2025). These methods enhance nursing students' self-awareness and their therapeutic communication skills.

Clinical Example

In a "reflective awareness program" at a nursing faculty, students watch and analyze recorded simulated patient interviews. This process helps them to recognize their emotional reactions and develop empathy skills.

10.6. Ethical and Legal Dimensions

The digitalization of psychotherapeutic processes has led to new ethical discussions regarding confidentiality, data security, and professional boundaries. Beauchamp and Childress (2019) describe "ethical innovation" as protecting human dignity in technological applications. In digital platforms where nurses provide counseling, professional identity, informed consent, and confidentiality principles have become more important than ever.

10.7. Research and Policy Directions

In the coming years, psychotherapeutic nursing research will focus on the following:

- ✓ The psychological effects of digital therapy and nurse–patient interaction,
- ✓ The impact of empathy-based training on clinical outcomes,
- ✓ The contribution of cultural sensitivity to therapeutic success,
- ✓ Cost-effectiveness of nurse wellness programs.

At the policy level, the international standardization of psychotherapeutic nursing certification will contribute to improvements in the quality of care (Roussel, 2024).

10.8. Conclusion and Practice Recommendations

The future of psychotherapeutic nursing will be grounded in human interaction while using technology ethically.

The following recommendations stand out in this transformation process.

Education: Digital therapeutic communication and cross-cultural psychotherapy modules should be incorporated into nursing curricula.
Research: Multicenter studies assessing the quality of therapeutic relationships in telehealth environments should be conducted in the future.
Practice: Regular supervision and reflective sessions for nurses should be made mandatory in hospital settings.
Ethics: Standards for data confidentiality, informed consent, and professional responsibility in AI applications should be clearly defined and adhered to.

Psychotherapeutic nursing will play a central role not only in mental disorders but also in the management of chronic physical illnesses in the future, becoming a multidimensional healthcare practice that supports biopsychosocial health.

REFERENCES

Altschul, S. (1984). Attachment and Loss, Vol. 3. Loss, Sadness and Depression. By John Bowlby. *Journal of the American Psychoanalytic Association*, *32*(1), 216–218.

American Nurses Association. (2001). Code of ethics for nurses with interpretive statements. Nursesbooks. org.

Bahari, Z., Vosoghi, N., Ramazanzadeh, N., Moshfeghi, S., & Aghamohammadi, M. (2024). Patient trust in nurses: Exploring the relationship with care quality and communication skills in emergency departments. *BMC Nursing*, *23*(1), 595. PMID: 39183274

Beauchamp, T., & Childress, J. (2019). Principles of biomedical ethics: Marking its fortieth anniversary. *The American Journal of Bioethics*, *19*(11), 9–12. PMID: 31647760

Boeldt, D., McMahon, E., McFaul, M., & Greenleaf, W. (2019). Using virtual reality exposure therapy to enhance treatment of anxiety disorders: Identifying areas of clinical adoption and potential obstacles. *Frontiers in Psychiatry*, *10*, 773. PMID: 31708821

Bolton, D. (2023). A revitalized biopsychosocial model: Core theory, research paradigms, and clinical implications. *Psychological Medicine*, *53*(16), 7504–7511. PMID: 37681273

Cuijpers, P., Karyotaki, E., de Wit, L., & Ebert, D. D. (2020). The effects of fifteen evidence-supported therapies for adult depression: A meta-analytic review. *Psychotherapy Research*, *30*(3), 279–293. PMID: 31394976

De Carlo, A., Carluccio, F., Rapisarda, S., Mora, D., & Ometto, I. (2020). Three uses of virtual reality in work and organizational psychology interventions. A dialogue between virtual reality and organizational well-being: Relaxation techniques, personal resources, and anxiety/depression treatments. *TPM. Testing, Psychometrics, Methodology in Applied Psychology*, *27*(1).

Edwards, D., & Burnard, P. (2003). A systematic review of stress and stress management interventions for mental health nurses. *Journal of Advanced Nursing*, *42*(2), 169–200. PMID: 12670386

Forchuk, C. (Ed.). (2021). *From therapeutic relationships to transitional care: A theoretical and practical roadmap*. Routledge.

Ford, D. M., Budworth, L., Lawton, R., Teale, E. A., & O'Connor, D. B. (2023). In-hospital stress and patient outcomes: A systematic review and meta-analysis. *PLoS One*, *18*(3), e0282789. PMID: 36893099

Geller, S. M., & Greenberg, L. S. (2012). *Therapeutic presence: A mindful approach to effective therapy*. American Psychological Association.

Gerges, S., Hallit, R., & Hallit, S. (2023). Stressors in hospitalized patients and their associations with mental health outcomes: Testing perceived social support and spiritual well-being as moderators. *BMC Psychiatry*, *23*(1), 323. PMID: 37161403

Giannetta, N., Villa, G., Pennestrì, F., Sala, R., Mordacci, R., & Manara, D. F. (2021). Ethical problems and moral distress in primary care: A scoping review. *International Journal of Environmental Research and Public Health*, *18*(14), 7565. PMID: 34300016

Haribhai-Thompson, J., McBride-Henry, K., Hales, C., & Rook, H. (2022). Understanding of empathetic communication in acute hospital settings: A scoping review. *BMJ Open*, *12*(9), e063375. PMID: 36171029

Hart, P. L., Brannan, J. D., & De Chesnay, M. (2014). Resilience in nurses: An integrative review. *Journal of Nursing Management*, *22*(6), 720–734. PMID: 25208943

Hawkins, P., & Shohet, R. (2012). *Supervision in the Helping Professions* (4th ed.). Open University Press.

Holmes, J. (1995). Supportive Psychotherapy the Search for Positive Meanings. *The British Journal of Psychiatry*, *167*(4), 439–445. PMID: 8829709

Holmes, J. (1995). Supportive Psychotherapy the Search for Positive Meanings. *The British Journal of Psychiatry*, *167*(4), 439–445. PMID: 8829709

Ingstad, K., Pedersen, M. K., Uhrenfeldt, L., & Pedersen, P. U. (2023). Patients' expectations of and experiences with psychosocial care needs in perioperative nursing: A descriptive study. *BMC Nursing*, *22*(1), 304. PMID: 37670261

International Council of Nurses (ICN). (2021). Guidelines on Mental Health Nursing and Well-Being Support. Geneva: ICN. https://www.icn.ch/resources/publications-and-reports/guidelines-mental-health-nursing

Köbler, P., Krauss-Köstler, E. K., Stein, B., Ficker, J. H., Wilhelm, M., Dechêne, A., & Waller, C. (2022). Specialized biopsychosocial care in inpatient somatic medicine units—A pilot study. *Frontiers in Public Health*, *10*, 844874. PMID: 35493384

Luxton, D. D. (Ed.). (2015). *Artificial intelligence in behavioral and mental health care*.

Markowitz, J. C. (2015). Interpersonal psychotherapy. *Psychiatry*, •••, 1859–1870. PMID: 25677355

Markowitz, J. C., & Weissman, M. M. (2012). Interpersonal psychotherapy: Past, present and future. *Clinical Psychology & Psychotherapy*, *19*(2), 99–105. PMID: 22331561

Maslach, C. (2018). Burnout: A multidimensional perspective. In Professional burnout (pp. 19-32). CRC Press.

McCabe, C. (2004). Nurse–patient communication: An exploration of patients' experiences. *Journal of Clinical Nursing*, *13*(1), 41–49. PMID: 14687292

McDonough, J., Rhodes, K., & Procter, N. (2025). The Impact of Clinical Supervision on the Mental Health Nursing Workforce: A Scoping Review. *International Journal of Mental Health Nursing*, *34*(1), e13463. PMID: 39462993

Moore, C. A. (2025). Early-Career Nurses' Mindfulness and Its Association With Anxiety, Burnout, Perceived Stress, Job Satisfaction, and Intent to Stay: A Descriptive Cross-Sectional Study (Doctoral dissertation, The Ohio State University).

Osman, F. E. S., Sherif, Z. A. E. G., Shalaby, M., & Shaheen, S. H. A. M. (2018). Evaluate the effect of empathy-based training program on psychiatric nurses' communication skills. IOSR Journal of Nursing and Health Science (IOSR-JNHS), 7(3), 32-41.

Peplau, H. E. (1997). Peplau's theory of interpersonal relations. *Nursing Science Quarterly*, *10*(4), 162–167. PMID: 9416116

Peplau, H. E. (1997). Peplau's theory of interpersonal relations. *Nursing Science Quarterly*, *10*(4), 162–167. PMID: 9416116

Ravitz, P., Watson, P., Lawson, A., Constantino, M. J., Bernecker, S., Park, J., & Swartz, H. A. (2019). Interpersonal psychotherapy: A scoping review and historical perspective (1974–2017). *Harvard Review of Psychiatry*, *27*(3), 165–180. PMID: 30883446

Rokach, A. (2016). Psychological, emotional and physical experiences of hospitalized children. *Clinical Case Reports and Reviews*, *2*(4), 399–401.

Roussel, J., Lehwaldt, D., & Rogers, M. (2024). The International Council of Nurses Nurse Practitioner/Advanced Practice Nurse Network. In *Advanced Practice Nurse Networking to Enhance Global Health* (pp. 43–57). Springer International Publishing.

Salem, G. M. M., Hashimi, W., & El-Ashry, A. M. (2025). Reflective mindfulness and emotional regulation training to enhance nursing students' self-awareness, understanding, and regulation: A mixed method randomized controlled trial. *BMC Nursing*, *24*(1), 478. PMID: 40307764

Shore, J. H., Yellowlees, P., Caudill, R., Johnston, B., Turvey, C., Mishkind, M., & Hilty, D. (2018). Best practices in videoconferencing-based telemental health April 2018. *Telemedicine Journal and e-Health*, *24*(11), 827–832. PMID: 30358514

Topol, E. (2019). *Deep medicine: how artificial intelligence can make healthcare human again.*

Van Hees, M. L., Rotter, T., Ellermann, T., & Evers, S. M. (2013). The effectiveness of individual interpersonal psychotherapy as a treatment for major depressive disorder in adult outpatients: A systematic review. *BMC Psychiatry*, *13*(1), 22. PMID: 23312024

Vlake, J. H., Van Bommel, J., Wils, E. J., Korevaar, T. I., Bienvenu, O. J., Klijn, E., & Van Genderen, M. E. (2021). Virtual reality to improve sequelae of the postintensive care syndrome: A multicenter, randomized controlled feasibility study. *Critical Care Explorations*, *3*(9), e0538. PMID: 34549192

Watson, C., Wijesuriya, R., & Bhugra, D. (2022). Culture and mental illness. Oxford Textbook of Social Psychiatry, 83.

Weissman, M. M. (2006). A brief history of interpersonal psychotherapy. *Psychiatric Annals*, *36*(8).

Wheeler, K. (2013). *Psychotherapy for the advanced practice psychiatric nurse: A how-to guide for evidence-based practice*. Springer Publishing Company.

Winston, A., & Schaefer, A. (2023). Supportive psychotherapy. In *Tasman's psychiatry* (pp. 1–27). Springer International Publishing.

Winston, A., & Schaefer, A. (2023). Supportive psychotherapy. In *Tasman's psychiatry* (pp. 1–27). Springer International Publishing.

Wu, Y. (2021). Empathy in nurse-patient interaction: A conversation analysis. *BMC Nursing*, *20*(1), 18. PMID: 33435957

Xiao, X., Song, H., Sang, T., Wu, Z., Xie, Y., & Yang, Q. (2021). Analysis of real-world implementation of the biopsychosocial approach to healthcare: Evidence from a combination of qualitative and quantitative methods. *Frontiers in Psychiatry*, *12*, 725596. PMID: 34764895

Yang, H. M., & Jang, Y. E. (2025). Ethics of nursing in the digital age: Perceptions and challenges among Korean nursing students. *BMC Medical Ethics*, *26*(1), 143. PMID: 41107902

Zhou, H. (2025). Relationship between empathy and burnout as well as potential affecting and mediating factors from the perspective of clinical nurses: A systematic review. *BMC Nursing*, *24*(1), 38. PMID: 39794782

Zhou, H. (2025). Relationship between empathy and burnout as well as potential affecting and mediating factors from the perspective of clinical nurses: A systematic review. *BMC Nursing*, *24*(1), 38. PMID: 39794782

Chapter 7
Multidisciplinary Approach to the Treatment of Cancer Patients

Venelin Terziev
https://orcid.org/0000-0003-1115-8877
Black Sea Institute, Bourgas, Bulgaria

Teodora Petrova
https://orcid.org/0000-0003-4672-1332
Trakia University, Stara Zagora, Bulgaria

Marin Georgiev
https://orcid.org/0000-0002-4530-6471
Vitalis Ruse, Ruse, Bulgaria

ABSTRACT

This study investigates the complex interaction of light with biological tissues, focusing on scattering, absorption, and re-emission mechanisms within quasi-ordered structures. Unlike pharmacological interventions, laser therapy offers a non-invasive, localized approach to normalizing biological processes. However, clinical efficacy is hindered by insufficient data on real-time optical parameter changes. Addressing this gap, the research transitions into a psychosomatic framework, emphasizing that physiological recovery is inextricably linked to the patient's psychological resilience. By analyzing cognitive-behavioral patterns, emotional suppression, and the "internal picture of the disease", the study advocates for a holistic rehabilitative paradigm.

DOI: 10.4018/979-8-3373-6526-8.ch007

1. INTRODUCTION

Fundamental medical research represents a cornerstone of human civilizational advancement. A primary driver of this progress is the reliance of contemporary medical technologies on foundational discoveries within physics, mathematics, biology, and chemistry, as global scientific evolution is dependent upon the integration of diverse, interdisciplinary domains. A prominent modern strategy for enhancing clinical outcomes involves the implementation of laser technologies, which aim to uncover innovative therapeutic pathways for severe pathologies. The utilization of advanced laser systems in healthcare is now pervasive; however, medical lasers differ fundamentally from their industrial or technical counterparts. Each clinical application necessitates the meticulous selection of specific parameters and radiation protocols, including wavelength, exposure duration, output power, and pulse repetition rates.

Owing to their exceptional efficiency, lasers facilitate a diverse array of medical applications. Their integration into various technological frameworks enables the resolution of multi-faceted and complex challenges. A distinctive feature of their clinical use is that during therapeutic interventions on specific organs, the laser's impact may be strategically directed or transferred. In clinical practice, established methodologies utilize laser beams as substitutes for traditional acupuncture. The primary merits of laser-based interventions include the non-contact nature of the procedure with the biological tissue, ensuring a painless, sterile, and highly efficient treatment process (Pletnev, 1996).

The inherent complexity of laser applications in healthcare continues to stimulate research and the engineering of novel technological solutions. A notable contemporary trend is the rapid and dynamic integration of laser-based systems across the medical spectrum. Innovative laser devices are perpetually emerging and undergoing clinical validation. This extensive variety of technologies allows for the successful addressing of specialized tasks in fields such as dermatology, aesthetics, plastic surgery, physiotherapy, otolaryngology, and general surgery. Traditional scalpels are increasingly being replaced by laser-based surgical instruments in modern clinical settings. These "laser scalpels" are often preferred due to their minimally invasive nature, which reduces both physical and psychological trauma while maintaining high procedural efficacy.

The intricate nature of laser-tissue interactions-defined by the simultaneous phenomena of reflection, absorption, and scattering within heterogeneous biological layers-demands a shift from empirical clinical observation toward sophisticated, high-precision modeling. Given the current lack of a comprehensive analytical theory to fully delineate these interactions, the employment of Monte Carlo statistical simulations is indispensable for forecasting energy distribution and subsequent thermal transformations. Nevertheless, this technical endeavor cannot be achieved in a vacuum; it mandates the systematic convergence of physical, biological, and clinical datasets. This requirement for collective professional expertise necessitates a multidisciplinary framework, where the synergy between technical accuracy and a comprehensive understanding of the patient's physiological state forms the foundation for effective oncological interventions, as explored in the subsequent section.

2. LITERATURE REVIEW

The development of modern oncology is undergoing a phase of fundamental reassessment, where the focus is shifting from the isolated treatment of tumor masses toward a comprehensive understanding of the patient as a complex biopsychosocial system. The literature in this field can be classified into two main directions: technological advancement in non-invasive therapies (primarily laser technologies) and the deepening of research into the psychological determinants of the disease.

2.1. Physical and Technological Aspects of Laser Interaction

In the field of medical physics, the literature emphasizes that laser radiation offers unique advantages over traditional pharmacological methods due to its strictly localized focus and non-invasive nature. The primary research interest is directed toward the mechanisms through which light interacts with biological tissues. Researchers investigate the complex processes of scattering and absorption, which depend on the structural organization of the tissues. A frequently highlighted problem is the lack of sufficiently reliable data on changes in the optical parameters of tissues in real-time during therapy. This necessitates the use of statistical models to predict energy distribution and thermal transformations. Despite recent progress, theoretical models still struggle with the heterogeneity of biological layers, making precise dosing a significant challenge. The literature notes that laser systems in medicine differ qualitatively from industrial ones, as they require precise adjustment of wavelength and pulse frequency to achieve a therapeutic effect without thermal damage to surrounding healthy cells.

2.2. The Psychosomatic Paradigm in Oncology

One of the most intriguing areas in contemporary literature is the psychogenesis of cancer. Historically, the connection between emotional status and physical health has been known since antiquity, but modern science frames it within the terms of psychoneuroimmunology. Researchers pay serious attention to the hypothesis that neoplastic cells can exist in the body in a state of dormancy until activated by specific psycho-emotional factors. In this sense, the disease is viewed as a physiological response to deep emotional traumas that have found no other path of expression.

A central place in the literature is occupied by the concept of "shock conflict"-an acute emotional experience that acts as a biological trigger. Studies show that stress itself is not the cause of cancer, but rather the individual's subjective reaction to it. Particular attention is paid to the phenomenon of "learned helplessness", where the patient gives up the struggle and accepts the diagnosis as an inescapable sentence. This psychological capitulation leads to the suppression of the immune system, reduced activity of natural killer cells, and alterations in hormonal balance, creating a favorable environment for tumor growth. Conversely, patients with high emotional vitality and an active stance demonstrate significantly better survival rates.

2.3. Personality Characteristics and Emotional Suppression

The literature identifies specific psychological profiles predisposed to oncological diseases. Frequently described is the model of the "stoic" patient-an individual who systematically blocks the expression of negative emotions such as anger, fear, or sadness in an attempt to meet social expectations. This emotional suppression, combined with a sense of false omnipotence (the belief that one must handle everything alone), is considered a major risk factor. Scientific works emphasize that the patient's ability to externalize suppressed feelings is key to the healing process. Psychotherapy in these cases is not merely supportive but fundamentally transformative, helping the patient take responsibility for their life and health.

2.4. Cognitive-Behavioral and Art-Therapeutic Methods

In the review of psychological rehabilitation methods, Cognitive-Behavioral Therapy (CBT) holds a leading position due to its scientific validity. it is aimed at identifying and correcting destructive thought patterns-for example, the tendency to catastrophize the condition or intrusive thoughts about a fatal outcome. CBT helps patients build new, functional beliefs about themselves and the illness, which directly reflects on their motivation for treatment.

Art therapy is viewed as a powerful auxiliary method, particularly effective for processing traumas that are difficult to access through verbal communication. Through the use of metaphors, symbols, and creative activities (drawing, sculpting, music), patients manage to express subconscious conflicts and release accumulated emotional tension. Visualization is also widely represented in the literature, indicating that creating positive healing images (e.g., imagining the immune system destroying tumor cells) increases the sense of control over the body.

2.5. Multidisciplinary Approach and Complex Rehabilitation

The current literary consensus is that success in oncology is only possible through close cooperation between oncologists, physicists, psychologists, and social workers. Rehabilitation is no longer defined simply as the restoration of physical functions but as the holistic reintegration of the person into social life. The term "prehabilitation" is also introduced-psychological preparation of the patient in the period between diagnosis and the start of active treatment.

The literature pays serious attention to the role of the family. It has been established that a lack of support from relatives is a proven risk factor for relapses. Family members often experience the same stress as the patient, necessitating their inclusion in the therapeutic process. Specialized rehabilitation centers are cited as the best environment for treatment, as they offer continuity of care and an environment of peers, which raises morale and improves discipline in following medical prescriptions.

2.6. Significance of the Internal Picture of the Disease

A critical point in the research is the concept of the "internal picture of the disease"-the subjective experience and intellectual evaluation that the patient gives to their condition. This picture is formed not so much by the stage of the disease as by the individual's personality traits. It includes a sensitive level (physical sensations), an emotional level (distress), an intellectual level (knowledge about the disease), and a volitional level (motivation for recovery). The literature review shows that psychotherapeutic interventions can successfully restructure this internal picture, turning the patient from a passive object of medicine into an active subject of their own healing.

2.7. Integration of Physics and Psychology

In conclusion, authors in the field increasingly point toward the need for a synthesis between high-tech laser methods and humanitarian care. The physical interaction of light with biological tissue does not occur in isolation; its success is inextricably linked to the patient's general physiological and psychological state. Holistic medicine, which combines the precision of optical physics with structured psychorehabilitation, emerges as the only path to the full recovery of the individual. Future research in the literature is directed toward refining tissue models to bridge the gap between theoretical physics and clinical practice, placing the human psyche at the center of the therapeutic process.

A comprehensive analysis of the available literature reveals a significant corpus of research dedicated separately to optical physics and psycho-oncology; however, there remains a notable scarcity of integrated studies that bridge these two domains. While the physical interaction of light with biological tissues is well-documented in technical manuals and biophysical reports, and the psychological impact of cancer is extensively explored in clinical behavioral studies, the synthesis of these findings into a unified rehabilitative framework is less common. Current literary sources increasingly point toward the necessity of a multidisciplinary paradigm that treats the patient not as a series of isolated symptoms, but as a holistic entity. This study, therefore, builds upon these foundational sources by integrating high-precision technological insights with evidence-based psychological strategies, aiming to address the gaps identified in current clinical literature and provide a more cohesive approach to cancer recovery.

3. MULTIDISCIPLINARY APPROACH TO MEDICAL REHABILITATION OF CANCER PATIENTS

It is a biological reality that neoplastic cells may be present within the human organism, often remaining dormant throughout an individual's lifespan without manifesting as a clinical pathology. Similar to the presence of commensal bacteria and various viruses that constitute the human microbiome and serve protective functions, these cells exist in a delicate balance. The critical scientific question arises: what mechanisms trigger the transformation of these cells into malignant tumors, and under what conditions do they evolve into a life-threatening malignancy?

Beyond environmental and external catalysts, it is increasingly recognized that psychological factors may play a fundamental role in the etiology of cancer. Psychosomatic disorders can be interpreted as the physiological manifestation of deep-seated emotional distress and psychological trauma that lack alternative channels for expression. In this context, the disease may be viewed as a somatic "narrative" or a profound "cry" of the psyche.

Pathogenesis often initiates when an individual surpasses their specific physical and emotional threshold. The duration required to reach this critical limit is contingent upon the person's inherent psychological resilience, their bioenergetic reserves, and the frequency with which they have encountered repetitive internal trauma or emotional pain. Consequently, a multidisciplinary approach must account for these complex interactions between the mind and the body during the rehabilitation process.

3.1. Emotional Causes of the Appearance of Cancer

The integration of the soul and the physical body in medical treatment was a principle championed as early as Plato, reflecting the ancient consensus that profound emotional distress could catalyze physical illness. In the second century BC, the prominent Greek physician Galen hypothesized that "black bile" was the primary cause of cancer, suggesting a predisposition among individuals with melancholic temperaments-a view later shared by the Arab physician Avicenna. Similarly, Tibetan Lamaist tradition has long maintained that the individual factor is central to the development of malignant pathologies. Franz Gabriel Alexander, widely regarded as the progenitor of psychosomatics, elucidated in his seminal work, Psychosomatic Medicine, that disease emerges at the intersection of psychological, physiological, and social dimensions.

According to Alexander's framework, pathogenesis occurs when physiological vulnerability (governed by genetics or developmental conditions) converges with specific psychological traits and unresolved internal conflicts. When an unfavorable social environment or a stressful life event is added to this foundation, a symptomatic reaction is triggered. Notably, the initial psycho-emotional conflict often precedes the clinical manifestation of the disease by a significant period. This suggests that individuals may harbor a "latent predisposition" consisting of a weakened organ and a "nuclear conflict". These nuclear conflicts typically originate in childhood, arising from the friction between a child's innate desires and familial expectations. These subconscious patterns may remain dormant until prolonged stress suppresses authentic emotional expression, leading to the onset of somatic illness.

A pivotal contribution to this field was made by the German oncologist Dr. Ryke Geerd Hamer in the late 1970s. Following the tragic loss of his son, Hamer developed cancer, leading him to identify the "shock conflict"-a causal link between acute emotional trauma and severe disease. He proposed that malignancy develops when emotional-mental stressors remain unresolved over extended durations. Hamer hypothesized that the organism possesses an innate capacity for self-healing, provided that:

- The patient receives comprehensive support to "deprogram" the physiological impact of the shock conflict;
- The healing process is not obstructed by the excessive administration of pharmaceuticals.

Hamer's controversial stance suggests that certain conventional oncological interventions may inadvertently exacerbate emotional distress, fostering a sense of helplessness that hinders recovery. He argued that emotional trauma induces a "short circuit" in the brain, which can be visualized via Computed Tomography (CT) scans as concentric wave patterns. According to Hamer, these cerebral pulsations correspond directly to the specific organ where the malignancy develops, providing a physical map of the mind-body connection.

Historical data supports these observations. In the 19th century, British clinical studies-among the first of their kind-revealed that out of 250 observed cancer patients, 156 had experienced significant mental distress, primarily due to the loss of close kin. In 1931, French surgeon Émile Forgue noted that while external carcinogens like radiation and nicotine are critical, emotional factors "prime" the biological terrain for their action. He emphasized that depressive states disrupt endocrine equilibrium, rendering cells more susceptible to malignant transformation.

Although the 20th century saw a shift toward purely organic and viral explanations for cancer, recent decades have seen a resurgence in the study of oncological psychogenesis, enriched by psychoanalytic insights. Hamer's "Iron Rules of Cancer" summarize this perspective:

- Malignancy originates from an acute, isolated conflict shock that manifests simultaneously across the psyche, the brain, and the organ;
- The specific nature of the psychic conflict determines the location of both the cerebral focus and the secondary organic lesion;
- The progression of the psychological conflict is intrinsically linked to the development of the physiological pathology in both the brain and the affected organ.

3.2. Complex Rehabilitation

In contemporary medicine, rehabilitation has emerged as a socially imperative field, undergoing rapid expansion and garnering significant global scholarly interest. This escalating focus is primarily driven by the substantial increase in malignant neoplasm incidence and the corresponding mortality rates observed over the last decade. Projections from the International Agency for Research on Cancer (IARC) suggest that by 2030, the frequency of newly diagnosed oncological cases may more than double. While modern diagnostic and therapeutic modalities have advanced to a stage where five-year survival rates reach approximately 70% (Siegel et al., 2013; Lianos et al., 2015), clinical success should not be measured by survival alone. Rather, the efficacy of the medical intervention is increasingly defined by the patient's ability to reintegrate as a functional member of society (Kulakov et al., 2012).

Standard oncological protocols-including invasive surgery, radiotherapy, chemotherapy, and hormone replacement-frequently result in systemic physiological disruptions, impaired functional capacity, and a diminished quality of life (Balabuha, 2010; Hasanov et al., 2013). Consequently, the ultimate objective of the oncological therapeutic process must transcend clinical remission to encompass the restoration of the patient's prior lifestyle (Tikhonov & Samarsky, 1977; Slepkov et al., 2007). Evidence from European and American longitudinal studies indicates that comprehensive restorative correction of postoperative disorders not only enhances social status and well-being but also significantly mitigates the risks of recurrence and metastasis (Astin et al., 2013; Saotome et al., 2015; Slepkov et al., 2007). This realization has catalyzed the proliferation of specialized oncology rehabilitation centers that prioritize accelerated recovery and social reintegration (Cristian et al., 2012; Ko et al., 2008).

Medical rehabilitation is defined as a multidisciplinary framework of medical and psychological interventions designed to restore impaired functions or compensate for physiological loss. Its scope includes maintaining systemic homeostasis during pathological progression, implementing early diagnostic corrections, and preventing long-term disability (Federal Law, 2011; Tikhonov & Samarsky, 1977). Rehabilitation for oncological patients is characterized by several core principles: it must be staged, continuous, sequential, individualized, and socially oriented, requiring the active engagement of both the patient and their family (Cherkasova et al., 2013; Tikhonov & Samarsky, 1977; Yao et al., 2003).

To implement an effective rehabilitation strategy, goals must be categorized into three distinct levels:

- Restorative: Focused on preserving vocational capacity and ensuring a favorable prognosis;
- Supportive: Aimed at adapting the patient to systemic functional restructuring in cases of partial or total loss of working capacity;
- Palliative: Dedicated to optimizing comfort and life quality during advanced tumor progression and generalization.

Regardless of tumor localization, the rehabilitation process should be structured into four specific phases: the preparatory stage (optimizing the diagnostic and treatment plan), the therapeutic stage (organ-preserving and reconstructive interventions), the early recovery stage (prevention of acute postoperative and radiation-induced complications), and the late recovery stage (self-rehabilitation and social adaptation). This comprehensive care necessitates a multidisciplinary team comprising oncologists, endocrinologists, psychotherapists, physiotherapists, sociologists, and occupational therapists.

Furthermore, the concept of "prehabilitation" has gained prominence in recent literature (Arving et al., 2012; Hasanov et al., 2013; Slepkov et al., 2007; Silver et al., 2013). Prehabilitation occurs in the critical window between diagnosis and the initiation of primary treatment (Slepkov et al., 2007; Silver et al., 2013). This phase is vital for providing immediate psychological support, as the diagnosis of malignancy often triggers acute reactive psychological states (Idrisova et al., 2016). Additionally, the prehabilitation stage allows for early coordination between specialized centers and rehabilitation experts, ensuring that the therapeutic journey is optimized from the outset (Buletov, n.d.; Zhukova & Kolpak, 2013).

3.3. Psychosomatic Medicine: The Key to Effective Rehabilitation in Cancer Patients

Disease should not be perceived merely as a localized somatic pathology, but rather as a holistic disruption involving the body, the intellect, and the emotional spectrum. Emotional and psychological equilibrium significantly influences both susceptibility to oncological diseases and the potential for clinical recovery. Active, positive patient engagement can fundamentally alter the disease trajectory, therapeutic outcomes, and overall quality of life. Increasingly, malignancy is conceptualized through a psychosomatic lens, acknowledging that psychological and psychosocial determinants frequently exert a more profound influence on tumorigenesis than purely physiological factors. A milestone in contemporary medicine is the recognition that individuals can modulate mental states that, in turn, regulate a broad array of biological processes. By strategically intervening in the psyche, it is possible to stimulate systemic physiological recovery, provided specific conditions for successful treatment are met.

Psychoneuroimmunology (PNI) is the scientific discipline dedicated to investigating the interplay between psychological factors, cerebral functional states, and the immune system. It identifies the mechanisms through which personality traits alter immune responses and evaluates their impact on the risk of developing specific pathologies. Animal studies have demonstrated that chronic stress significantly impairs immunocompetence, weakening both cellular and humoral immunity and reducing resistance to infections and tumor growth. Martin Seligman's (Seligman, 1975) seminal research on "learned helplessness" or "capitulation" is particularly relevant here. Capitulation, or demoralization, is defined as a state where an individual feels incapable of overcoming perceived powerlessness, leading to pervasive hopelessness and a loss of existential purpose (Kissane et al., 2001). Experimental data show that animals conditioned to overcome adversity maintain high biological activity and exhibit significantly lower rates of malignancy. Conversely, those that adopt passive, "capitulating" behaviors under identical stressors suffer rapid tumor progression due to immunosuppression. This suggests that the biological decline is triggered not by the stressor itself, but by the psychological reaction of surrender (Baltrusch et al., 1991).

Clinical observations further support this mind-body connection. For instance, a study (Bartrop et al., 1977) of women with cervical cell changes following the loss of a spouse revealed that those exhibiting passive and helpless behaviors showed malignant transformation in 61% of cases, compared to only 24% in the psychologically resilient group. Additionally, breast cancer patients with high emotional vitality demonstrate superior five-year survival rates compared to those who view their diagnosis as an inescapable sentence (Arkhipova et al., 2003; Rotenberg, 2001). Thus, the immune response is often compromised more by the patient's subjective reaction to stress-determined by their life outlook and the significance they assign to events-than by the event itself. Depression and a refusal to seek solutions exacerbate unfavorable prognoses by disrupting hormonal balance and immune function (Malkina-Pykh, 2005). Statistics indicate that 15-30% of cancer patients experience demoralization, and 20% suffer from clinical depression (Lee et al., 2012), yet many demoralized patients who do not fit strict depressive criteria remain without necessary psychological support (Stepanova & Chernavsky, 1983).

The psychophysiological mechanisms facilitating tumor development include complex, interrelated processes:

- Dysregulation of diurnal cortisol rhythms;
- Elevated levels of pro-inflammatory cytokines;
- Diminished activity of Natural Killer (NK) cells;
- Telomere shortening and reduced telomerase activity;
- Glucocorticoid-induced suppression of p53 and BrCA1 gene expression;
- Activation of endothelial growth factor via the sympathetic nervous system (Spiegel, 2013).

Integrating psychotherapy into oncological treatment has been proven to enhance survival. Beyond improving mental status and quality of life, psychotherapeutic interventions bolster immunity, normalize endocrine function, and reduce recurrence risks. Furthermore, these techniques increase patient compliance, thereby optimizing the treatment timeline and prognosis.

The cognitive and emotional state of a patient with a serious illness differs qualitatively from that of a healthy individual. A cancer diagnosis often superimposes a secondary fear of death upon an initial loss of hope, creating a dominant psychological structure that can overwhelm the system if not countered by faith and resilience. Improving the Quality of Life (QOL)-a multifaceted concept encompassing health status, life expectancy, environmental factors, and subjective spiritual satisfaction-is a paramount medical objective. In many societies, cancer is stigmatized as a "sentence" rather than a treatable condition, leading to intense psychological trauma, fear of metastasis, and social isolation. This is particularly evident in gynecological oncology, where specific traumas further impact the psyche (Balabuha, 2010).

A key element in choosing a psychotherapeutic strategy is the Internal Picture of the Disease (IPD). Introduced by R.A. Luria in 1935, IPD refers to the patient's subjective perception and intellectual assessment of their condition. IPD is shaped by personality, age, and social context rather than the disease stage itself. It consists of four interacting levels:

- Sensitive Level: Negative physical sensations resulting from the illness;
- Emotional Level: The affective experiences and distress caused by the diagnosis;
- Intellectual Level: The patient's objective knowledge and rational assessment of the disease;
- Volitional (Motivational) Level: The formation of a proactive attitude toward recovery and conscious lifestyle modifications (Spiegel, 2013).

Psychotherapeutic techniques can target these specific levels to reshape the IPD. While physicians often focus on the sensitive component through pharmacology, a comprehensive multidisciplinary approach allows for intervention at all four levels. The physician's role is critical in instilling hope and convincing the patient of their body's innate capacity to fight the disease, as the patient's belief in the treatment's efficacy significantly dictates the ultimate clinical outcome (Saimonton & Saimonton, 2001).

3.3.1. Psychotherapeutic Frameworks and Patient Attitudes

Within the landscape of oncological rehabilitation, the psychotherapeutic dialogue serves as a fundamental clinical instrument. The initial phase of this intervention involves providing the patient with a lucid explanation of the disease's pathogenesis and symptomatic profile. This clarification is essential to dismantle misconceptions and mitigate the profound sense of insecurity that often breeds debilitating anxiety, which can adversely affect the clinical trajectory. Furthermore, the therapeutic conversation must be tailored to the patient's unique personality, fostering a supportive environment that encourages active engagement in recovery. This relational approach is vital for neutralizing feelings of isolation and ensuring that the patient perceives the physician as a dedicated partner in their health journey.

To address the sensitive dimension of the IPD, patients may be instructed in diaphragmatic breathing, progressive relaxation, and specialized neuro-linguistic programming (NLP) exercises. Conversely, the emotional dimension is typically managed through two primary psychotherapeutic clusters: relaxation and recreation. A key technique, known as "abreaction" or "emotional discharge", involves the controlled, conscious re-experiencing of traumatic events-such as the moment of initial diagnosis-to release suppressed emotions and alleviate psychological tension under professional supervision.

The intellectual (rational) dimension of the IPD is equally critical, as an objective understanding of the pathology dictates therapeutic adherence and compliance. Efficacious interventions here include structured consultations and lectures that elucidate the psychosomatic nature of the illness while detailing treatment protocols, potential side effects, and recovery guidelines. Physicians should address patient inquiries regarding laboratory findings and instrumental examinations with reasoned, empathetic, and accessible language. In cases where maladaptive behaviors impede a realistic perception of the condition, educational efforts alone may be insufficient, necessitating specialized rational psychotherapy. These methods focus on persuasion, reorientation, and psycho-logic to develop functional thinking skills (Egorov, 2003).

The volitional dimension represents the zenith of the IPD structure, emerging from the synergy of the aforementioned levels. This stage governs the individual's behavioral strategy and their capacity for proactive decision-making. In many instances, the patient's willpower must be systematically reconstructed-a task primarily facilitated by the psychotherapist (Bukharov & Golubev, 2007). Central to this process is the concept of somatonosognosia-the personal reaction and attitude toward the illness-which must be accounted for when designing individualized psychotherapeutic programs.

Classification of attitudes toward disease identifies 14 distinct types, categorized by the severity of maladaptive behavior (Lichko, 1980):

1. Adaptive Group (Preserved Social Function): Includes harmonic, ergopathic, and anosognosic types.
2. Maladaptive Group (Significant Behavioral Impairment): Comprises 11 types, such as hypochondriac, anxious-depressive, obsessive-phobic, and melancholic.

Empirical studies indicate that in gynecological oncology, ergopathic and anosognosic types frequently prevail, alongside sensitive and anxious responses; notably, half of the studied population exhibits signs of maladaptive behavior (Sotirov et al., 2019). The ergopathic type is characterized by "work-based avoidance", where professional duties are prioritized over medical care. The anosognosic type involves either the denial of the illness or the dismissal of its severity in the hope of spontaneous remission. Conversely, the sensitive and anxious types are marked by extreme vulnerability and a lack of trust in the medical staff.

These attitudes are not static; they fluctuate based on internal factors (mood, symptom severity) and external factors (prognostic communication, social support, and environment). Research suggests that 10% to 25% of cancer patients experience depression, which can escalate to psychotic levels and significantly diminish motivation and quality of life (Levin & Kissane, 2006). Depression acts as an unfavorable prognostic indicator, particularly in advanced stages (Smulevich et al., 2009).

The diagnosis itself is a traumatic stressor that increases the risk of cardiovascular complications and suicidal ideation (Fang et al., 2012).

Consequently, the integration of social and psychological recovery into oncological rehabilitation is imperative. Timely intervention can reduce comorbidity and mortality related to self-harm. Evidence confirms that psychotherapy is a safe and effective method for mitigating stress and depression in oncology (Sheard & Maguire, 1999). Specifically, supportive-expressive group therapy has been shown to extend the five-year survival rate in metastatic breast cancer patients by an average of 18 months (Spiegel et al., 1989). Such group interventions focus on the verbalization of emotions, the search for existential meaning, and the cultivation of relaxation and visualization skills to restore hope and creative potential.

3.3.2. Clinical Methodologies and Procedural Stages of Psychotherapeutic Rehabilitation

The transition from understanding patient attitudes to the practical implementation of clinical interventions requires a structured multidisciplinary approach. While the classification of disease attitudes provides a diagnostic baseline, the actual rehabilitation process necessitates the deployment of specific psychotherapeutic modalities tailored to the individual's internal picture of the disease. The following section details the specific methodologies, such as cognitive-behavioral and psychodynamic approaches, alongside the chronological stages of oncological rehabilitation and the essential role of familial integration in the healing process.

And individual work with patients is aimed at diagnosing and regulating the psycho-emotional state: to reduce internal tension, which is associated with experiencing negative feelings and emotions, feelings of fear, anxiety, guilt, insult, resentment, and shame; developing skills for processing aggressive feelings; reducing symptoms of apathy and depression; searching for a resource to activate internal energies, the desire for life, for recovery, and faith in recovery; work on accepting one's own body; work on accepting the diagnosis; work on accepting justified medical prescriptions and chemotherapy treatment.

A priority in the work of the psychologist is the use of methodologies and techniques that patients can additionally use independently. The most popular are breathing techniques–visualization, according to Simonton; meditation and relaxation techniques; and art therapy.

According to research conducted among specialists, the most effective are group classes in:

– breathing technique VIVATION. Breathing is directly related to a person's emotional state. During a breathing session, self-regulation mechanisms that

have been blocked for a long time are activated. As a result of this breathing practice, the body begins to regenerate: a person feels calm and rested, the level of anxiety and restlessness decreases, and internal resources appear, which is an important aspect in working with cancer patients;
– art therapy (drawing, sand therapy). It is aimed at finding internal opportunities that contribute to the patient's adaptation process and finding new ways of interacting with the outside world;
– psychodynamics. Provides patients with the opportunity to discuss their current state, share their experiences, and learn to realize and express their feelings and emotions while receiving support.

The effectiveness of the provided psychotherapeutic treatment depends on various factors, such as the qualifications of the doctor, the duration of the course, the method used, and the current condition of the patient. When choosing tactics for providing psychotherapeutic treatment to cancer patients, it is necessary to take into account several of the following conditions:

– scientific validity of the method;
– the availability of developed models and strategies for treating various types of disorders.

It is also possible to significantly change the specific types of psychotherapy depending on the patient's problem. The above criteria, first of all, correspond to the psychodynamic and cognitive-behavioral approaches. As auxiliary methods, the suggestive method can be used, as well as methods that are oriented towards experiences–client–centered therapy and Gestalt therapy, psychodrama, art therapy, and therapy that is oriented towards the body. Personality-oriented or reconstructive psychotherapy is one of the most common methods with a psychodynamic orientation (Ababkov et al., 2000). The main goal of reconstructive psychotherapy is to create a personality that is adapted to resolve internal conflicts by reorganizing the system of human relationships. The main emphasis is on three main aspects of the personality: cognitive, emotional, and behavioral. If necessary, additional therapies, such as communication skills training, etc., can be included in the therapeutic program if there is a need to develop skills for intellectual and emotional understanding. This method can be carried out in three main forms: individual, family, and group. Treatment can be short-term (up to 40 hours) or long-term (up to 1 year or more).

Psychodynamic therapy gives good results in a wide range of mental disorders but is most often used for various borderline mental states. This method demonstrates the greatest effectiveness in various forms of neurosis.

Cognitive-behavioral psychotherapy arose on the basis of behavioral and cognitive psychology. This direction studies the system of thinking and perception of a person and is designed to help him choose the most rational view of the situation and, therefore, to develop the most adequate model of behavior that will help the patient cope with his problems. The therapy process includes correcting the patient's erroneous beliefs, training in control of emotional reactions (including anxiety and depression), and teaching the most successful ways to interpret his own emotions and experiences. The cognitive-behavioral direction of psychotherapy includes a number of techniques, among which the most widespread are cognitive psychotherapy by A. Beck and rational-emotive psychotherapy by A. Ellis, combining the main achievements of other models of cognitive-behavioral therapy. The main thing in these methods is the idea of the important role of thought processes in the development of behavioral and emotional disorders. The main concepts of cognitive psychotherapy include automatic (involuntary) thoughts, cognitive distortions (polarized thinking, negative selection of information, "catastrophizing", personalization, etc.), dysfunctional attitudes and beliefs (about oneself, about one's illness, about other people), and compensatory behavioral strategies (such as avoidance, hyper-responsibility, distancing, etc.). The main methods of this type of therapy include techniques for filling the "gaps", which are aimed at identifying maladaptive cognitions; techniques for assessing and correcting dysfunctional thoughts and beliefs; a system of behavioral techniques for restructuring inadequate compensatory strategies; etc. Cognitive-behavioral psychotherapy has also proven its effectiveness for a wide range of mental disorders, including depression, anxiety disorders, obsessive-compulsive and post-traumatic stress disorders, and somatoform and personality disorders.

Existential and rational approaches are widely used. Within existential psychology, severe somatic disorders are often viewed as an "existential challenge", and full mental health means "enlightened existence" (Bukharov & Golubev, 2007). Two directions of existential psychotherapy are most widespread: existential-humanistic psychotherapy by James Bugental and existential therapy by Irvin Yalom. Existential psychotherapy primarily helps the therapist to cope with the patient's despair, and its main goal is to analyze the values of a person and to help the patient accept the universe, which ultimately leads to a full and meaningful existence. This method of psychotherapy is long-term, since effective therapy requires deep immersion in the patient's worldview. Therapy gives good results for various problems: depression, phobias, addictions, obsessive (compulsive) thoughts and actions, suicidal behavior, crises, and social problems.

The task of rational psychotherapy is to correct misconceptions in the patient's views as a result of motivated and logical influence on the part of the doctor. This method is highly effective, and a positive result can be observed after the first session.

In addition, this approach works best with educated and highly motivated patients who have a high level of intelligence (Abramova, 2003).

In addition to the main methods of psychotherapeutic influence, additional ones are also widely used, among which the most widespread are suggestive methods. While the main principle of rational influence is an appeal to facts and an appeal to the logic and reason of the patient, the method of suggestion is based on suggestive influence, which does not affect the human mind. Suggestion is largely the presentation of information in an imperative mood, which is passively perceived by a person, bypassing his critical assessment. Most often, the doctor appeals to the emotions experienced by the patient. The information received affects neuropsychic and somatic processes in the range of sensations, point of view, emotional states, volitional impulses, and vegetative functions. Historically, suggestive influence combines psychotherapeutic techniques of suggestion and self-hypnosis in the waking state, a state of natural sleep, hypnosis, and narcotic sleep. Current suggestive methods of psychotherapy include various methods of modern hypnotherapy and autogenic training. Suggestive techniques in cancer patients are traditionally applied in the form of emotional–stress psychotherapy, alert hypnosis (a method of influence in panic attacks), autogenic training techniques, etc.

Currently, other alternative methods are used, such as relaxation (including auto-relaxation), art therapy, music therapy, poetry therapy, and body-oriented therapy, as well as synthetic and eclectic trends, including neurolinguistic programming and Gestalt therapy. Other forms of therapy, such as family or group therapy, are also very effective in the rehabilitation of cancer patients.

The appointment of psychotherapy should be carried out in the presence of indications, taking into account possible contraindications (for example, severe mental illness) and the wishes of the patient. If the above factors are not observed, the therapy may not bring the desired effect and may end with premature discontinuation of the course by the patient and the development of negative, pessimistic attitudes towards the treatment being carried out.

In oncology, psychotherapeutic rehabilitation can be divided into three main stages: preoperative, early postoperative, and long-term rehabilitation. In addition to these main stages, there is such a type of rehabilitation as preventive rehabilitation. It pursues two main goals: prevention of the development or delay in time of manifestation of a disease, as well as prophylaxis of the occurrence of regressions during an already existing disease.

In the preoperative period, psychotherapy is reduced to correcting the rational side of the VKZ. Consultation with a doctor is mainly devoted to discussing with the patient issues related to his illness and rationalizing existing knowledge, as well as modeling a new value system. Individual cognitive-behavioral, reconstructive-personality, and rational psychotherapy are suitable for these purposes. At the stage of the early postoperative period, the main task is to prevent the development of an inferiority complex in a patient after traumatic surgery, as well as to create a positive attitude. There are studies that show that psychotherapy can reduce the negative effect of chemotherapy on the patient's condition if it is necessary to do it (Myslivtseva & Zaika, 2014). At this stage, various forms of group therapy are most effective. The period of remote rehabilitation is the longest and most laborious, since the shock of the operation in the early postoperative period can often develop into severe mental disorders if the treatment provided at this stage is not well chosen or does not meet the needs of the patient. The method of therapy in such cases is selected individually, and all treatment should be aimed at returning the patient to an active life after illness. Psychotherapy should be given sufficient attention and applied during all periods of treatment, since the level of mental stability of the patient, especially in the early stages, determines the success of all rehabilitation measures.

When conducting psychotherapy within the framework of complex rehabilitation, it is necessary to take into account such an important factor as the patient's relationship with his family: the patient's family members should be informed about the prognosis of the further course of the disease and about the methods used for rehabilitation and psychotherapy. In some cases, family members should be explained that oncological diseases are not infectious in nature and cannot be infected through household or sexual contact; in addition, it is necessary to convince relatives that treatment is possible and, therefore, they should provide support to the patient. All this is especially important, since insufficient support from relatives is a proven risk factor for complications and relapses, which means that it can lead to an unfavorable outcome (House et al., 1988). Often, not only educational work with the family is necessary, but also the provision of direct psychotherapeutic assistance, since the patient's family may be subjected to psychological stress and depression to the same or even greater extent as the patient himself. This situation can lead to conflicts and family crises. This leads to the creation of a difficult atmosphere for the patient, in which maintaining normal functioning becomes extremely difficult and makes it impossible to share his experiences with loved ones. The problems that arise in such families can be presented in three groups:

– affective reactions of the people caring for the patient, characterized mainly in the form of fear, a sense of helplessness, and hopelessness;

– a change in behavior, which is associated with a change in roles within the family and with possible financial difficulties;

– problems that are related to the service system, arising from a conflict of interests and needs of the patient and his loved ones.

In order to create and maintain a comfortable environment in the patient's family, it is necessary to hold a conversation with all its members, during which they should be motivated to actively participate in the patient's recovery process, provide him with moral support, and create an atmosphere of comfort. At the same time, the patient should not experience a loss of initiative and independence. It is necessary to explain to relatives that attention should be focused on improving self-esteem and changing the patient's thinking, and not on the disease.

The main medical skills that are necessary for the successful rehabilitation of a patientt, and which doctors of any specialization must possess, are the ability to establish contact with both the patient himself and his relatives and to explain in detail and intelligibly to them the features of the disease, the system of treatment and care.

In conclusion, it can be said that psychological factors have a significant impact on the occurrence and development of oncological diseases. Psycho-rehabilitation should be included in the program for complex treatment of patients if we want the treatment to have a positive result. Currently, new, more effective methods and rehabilitation programs are being actively developed, in which the latest methods of physiotherapy replace medical treatment of psychological problems. However, even with the help of a simple psychotherapeutic consultation, much better positive results can be achieved. Psychotherapy helps to reduce the patient's stress and anxiety levels, to realize how thinking and attitude to life led to the oncological disease, which in turn helps to normalize the functioning of the immune system and hormonal levels, and also helps a person realize that life does not end after a terrible diagnosis. The main goal of psychotherapy is to change the patient's attitude to the disease, to help him adapt to the current situation and to express support in the fight against the difficulties that the disease has brought. It is extremely important to start the course as early as possible, since psychotherapeutic assistance significantly increases the likelihood of a positive outcome.

Psychotherapeutic methods of communication with patients should be used by doctors of all specialties during consultations, but they do not always have enough time or the appropriate skills. Therefore, in the vast majority of cases, it is necessary to resort to the help of narrow specialists. The best solution would be to provide psychological support and all types of rehabilitation on the basis of specialized centers. The undoubted advantages of such centers are the concentration of all therapeutic means in one place, which allows to achieve the maximum principle of continuity, and also creates comfort for patients. An environment in which all patients have a similar problem and are united by one goal, contributes to raising their spirits and more strict implementation of doctor's prescriptions, which means it increases the effectiveness of therapy.

Briefly about cancer of various human organs: Thyroid cancer - powerlessness in life; Lung cancer - fear of death or suffocation; Lymphatic system cancer - loss of self-importance; Breast cancer is a conflict of separation; Stomach cancer - accumulated anger, too much negativity is “swallowed”; Pancreatic cancer - family conflicts, including problems with inheritance, constant anxiety, anger; Liver cancer

- fear of starvation; Intestinal cancer - a terrible, "unworked out" conflict; Uterine cancer - sexual conflict; Cervical cancer - very strong disappointment; Bone cancer - inferiority complex; Melanoma/skin cancer - you feel like a dirty person, you lose the integrity of your personality.

Realize that this trauma was far away in childhood, when you could not properly assess the situation. Now you have matured and have the right to become an ordinary person who has the right to release your negative emotions outside. Free yourself from them, let them out – solving all problems by simply suppressing the negative in yourself is not an option. Let your negativity out.

3.4. Psychological Transformation in Oncological Recovery: The Role of Cognitive-Behavioral and Art Therapy

The fundamental premise of psychosomatic oncology is that cancer is frequently rooted in common emotional conflicts, suggesting that psychotherapy is not merely a supportive measure but a critical component of the curative process. The effectiveness of a patient's healing trajectory is largely mediated by their internal psychological constructs-specifically faith, hope, and an active desire for survival. Clinical success requires a profound transition from emotional suppression to expression; patients must be prepared to externalize deeply internalized feelings of fear, anger, sadness, and guilt, which may have been repressed for decades prior to the diagnosis.

Theoretical research by David Kissane regarding breast cancer patients highlights that a profound blocking of emotional expression, coupled with a "narcissistic omnipotence"' -the maladaptive belief that one's problems must be managed in total self-reliance-is a key psychological marker in malignant profiles. This is further substantiated by the studies of S. Levy, which indicate that women with breast cancer who overtly express distress, anger, and fear demonstrate higher survival rates compared to "stoic" or "good" patients who conform to social expectations by suppressing their turmoil. For those seeking to overcome the disease through personality transformation, existential questions regarding the quality of their life and the presence of emotional fulfillment become paramount. Taking responsibility for one's biography allows the patient to shift from a passive role to an active participant in the treatment, where spiritual factors and fundamental questions of identity and purpose come to the fore.

Comprehensive oncological care integrates physiological maintenance with positive thinking, stress-coping mechanisms, and meditative practices. Within this framework, recovery is driven by the synergy between external medical support and the mobilization of internal resources. A vital internal resource is the cognitive ability to view the disease as a natural process with identifiable psychosocial causes. By acknowledging that the disease did not emerge without the individual's own psychological participation, the patient gains a sense of agency and mastery over the situation, facilitating the necessary lifestyle and personality changes. This proactive stance allows the individual to identify specifically what needs to be altered in their life to aid the healing process.

The clinical necessity of this approach is underscored by the high prevalence of psychological comorbidities; studies indicate that 10% to 25% of cancer patients experience depression, ranging from mild distress to psychotic episodes. In the initial year following diagnosis, approximately 10% of patients develop clinical anxiety or depression that significantly impairs motivation, appetite, and overall quality of life, acting as a negative prognostic indicator (Siegel et al., 2013). Consequently, the medical psychologist must prioritize the patient's personality rather than just the somatic symptoms, fostering a therapeutic alliance that allows the patient to confront traumatic life circumstances and discover latent internal resources essential for adaptation (Balabuha, 2010).

In selecting the most appropriate psychotherapeutic tactics, clinicians prioritize methods with high scientific validity and established structural models. Cognitive-Behavioral Therapy (CBT) and Art Therapy are prominent in this regard. CBT is specifically directed at restoring the distorted perceptions involved in the patient's self-assessment and worldview, effectively neutralizing intrusive thoughts and maladaptive cognitive schemas. This approach distinguishes between cognitive and behavioral methods, proving particularly robust in treating the post-traumatic stress symptoms associated with a cancer diagnosis. By deconstructing automatic negative thoughts, CBT aligns the patient's mental state with the goals of recovery, while Art Therapy serves as a powerful auxiliary method for the non-verbal expression of trauma and the discovery of new adaptive pathways.

3.4.1. Cognitive Processing of Traumatic Experiences

Cognitive processing in the context of oncological pathology posits that maladaptive psychological symptoms emerge when the stability of an individual's worldview is shattered by the diagnosis. The conflict between pre-existing life schemas and the new, threatening reality of the disease creates a profound cognitive dissonance. For the oncological patient, this manifests as a direct threat to biological existence, a decline in self-esteem, the forced adoption of new social roles, and a fundamental shift in interpersonal dynamics. These cognitive conflicts often trigger intrusive ideation, chronic physiological arousal, and maladaptive avoidance behaviors. Consequently, therapeutic intervention must focus on identifying and modifying these discrepancies, facilitating the integration of the traumatic information into a revised, functional worldview.

3.4.2. The Visualization Method and Healing Symbolism

As a specialized cognitive-imaginal intervention, visualization involves the deliberate creation of therapeutic mental imagery. Under clinical guidance, the patient is trained to conceptualize internal biological processes through healing symbolism-a subjective set of images designed to enhance coping efficacy. In oncology, the methodology developed by K. Simonton and S. Simonton is prominently utilized. This technique encourages patients to mentally visualize leukocytes actively deconstructing malignant cells and the subsequent systemic removal of necrotic tissue. By visualizing the tumor's regression and the efficacy of medical treatments in reducing pain, the patient cultivates a sense of agency. This mental rehearsal of health and vitality serves as a potent psychological mechanism, restoring the patient's perceived control over the recovery process.

3.4.3. Strategic Goal Setting and Existential Motivation

The formulation of future-oriented goals and tasks is an essential component of oncological psychotherapy, serving as a primary attempt to consciously articulate the patient's "will to live". These objectives function as individual motives for recovery, effectively restoring the patient's existential connection to their own life. Strategic goal setting provides the necessary emotional and intellectual scaffolding for proactive behavior, transforming abstract desires for health into concrete, actionable decisions. This process strengthens the patient's psychological commitment to the treatment protocol and fosters a sense of purpose that is vital for long-term resilience.

3.4.4. The Decatastrophizing Technique

A specific psychological challenge arises when patients in clinical remission exceed their initial medical prognosis. Despite the absence of physical symptoms, the pervasive fear of relapse-the "Sword of Damocles" effect-can induce chronic existential anxiety. The decatastrophizing method is specifically targeted at neutralizing this anticipatory dread. By rationally deconstructing the "worst-case scenario" and evaluating the actual probability of events, the therapist helps the patient move from a state of paralyzed fear toward a more balanced, realistic perspective. This technique is crucial for maintaining psychological stability during the often-uncertain periods of long-term remission.

3.4.5. Expressive Modalities in Art Therapy

Art therapy utilizes creative activity as a non-verbal medium for processing profound traumatic experiences. Recognizing the human tendency to "escape" or suppress overwhelming emotions, this method provides a safe channel for the externalization of distress through drawing, sculpting, or other creative forms. The efficacy of art therapy is rooted in the psychological mechanism of projection; through their artistic output, patients subconsciously communicate experiences that remain inaccessible to verbal expression. This makes art therapy an exceptionally effective tool for the discharge of negative affects, such as suppressed aggression, guilt, and existential pain. The integration of drawing, modeling, music, and literary creativity allows for a multi-sensory response to the disease, facilitating psychological adaptation and significantly improving the patient's overall quality of life.

4. CONCLUSION

The psychological dimension represents a critical determinant in the clinical progression and long-term prognosis of oncological diseases, necessitating the systematic and mandatory integration of psychorehabilitation within the framework of complex multidisciplinary treatment protocols. The efficacy of even fundamental psychotherapeutic counseling should not be underestimated, as targeted interventions possess the capacity to significantly mitigate systemic stress and existential anxiety, which in turn facilitates the biological normalization of the immune system and the restoration of hormonal homeostasis. The primary clinical objective of psychotherapy in this context is to effectuate a transformative shift in the patient's internal perception of the disease, moving from a state of passive victimhood toward proactive adaptation and resilience. Initiating these interventions at the earliest possible diagnostic stage is essential, as early psychological stabilization significantly correlates with improved treatment adherence and an increased likelihood of a positive survival outcome. Furthermore, while the role of the general physician is vital, the inherent constraints of time and specialized training within standard medical consultations underscore the necessity of specialized rehabilitation centers. These facilities offer a concentrated environment where the principle of therapeutic continuity is guaranteed through various restorative modalities, such as expressive arts, movement therapy, and controlled salt rooms. This communal ecosystem, characterized by shared patient experiences and collective existential goals, not only raises morale but also ensures a more rigorous implementation of clinical prescriptions, thereby fundamentally enhancing the overall effectiveness of the rehabilitative process.

Simultaneously, the strategic integration of advanced laser technologies and high-precision dosimetric models marks a transformative milestone in modern oncology, providing a sophisticated technical foundation for the development of non-invasive, targeted therapeutic strategies. However, the physical interactions of light with biological tissues do not occur in a vacuum; their clinical success is inextricably linked to the patient's systemic physiological and psychological state, which dictates the biological response to technological intervention. A truly holistic medical paradigm must therefore bridge the divide between high-tech medical engineering and structured, personality-oriented psychorehabilitation to ensure both the physiological normalization of cellular processes and the total existential recovery of the individual. Future scientific inquiry should focus on the refinement of multi-layered, complex tissue models to bridge the gap between theoretical optical physics and practical clinical application in the ward. By uniting the precision of laser physics with a profound, evidence-based focus on the human psyche, the medical community can ultimately transcend traditional treatment barriers, improving both the subjective quality of life and the statistical probability of a successful outcome for patients facing the profound challenges of oncological disease.

REFERENCES

Ababkov, V. A., Isurina, G. L., Kazakovtsev, B. A., Kulakov, S. A., Nazyrov, R. K., Podsadnyi, S. A., et al. (2000). *Psikhoterapiya. Uchebnik dlya studentov meditsinskii vuzov* [Psychotherapy. A textbook for medical students]. Publisher. (In Russian).

Abramova, G. S. (2003). *Prakticheskaya psikhologiya. Uchebnik dlya studentov vuzov* [Practical psychology. Textbook for university students]. Publisher. (In Russian).

Arkhipova, I. V., Kokorina, N. P., & Magarill, Yu. A. (2003). Psikhogennye faktory i rak molochnoi zhelezy [Psychogenic factors and breast cancer]. In *Aktual'nye problemy raka molochnoi zhelezy* (Vol. 7, pp. 7–8). (In Russian).

Arving, C., Thormodsen, I., & Brekke, G.. (2012). Early rehabilitation of cancer patients – a randomized controlled intervention study. *BMC Cancer, 12*, 13–19.

Astin, J. A., Shapiro, J., & Shapiro, D. H. (2013). Psychological control and morbidity/mortality in breast cancer patients: A 20 year follow-up study. *Behavioral Medicine (Washington, D.C.), 39*, 7–10.

Balabuha, O. S. (2010). Kachestvo zhizni kak osnova program reabilitacii onkologicheskih bol'nyh [Quality of life as the basis of rehabilitation programs for cancer patients] [In Russian]. *Mezhdunarodnyj Medicinskij Zhurnal, 4*, 11–13.

Baltrusch, H. J., Stangel, W., & Titze, I. (1991). Stress, cancer and immunity: New developments in biopsychosocial and psychoneuroimmunologic research. *Acta Neurologica, 13*, 315–327.

Bartrop, R. W., Luckhurst, E., Lazarus, L., Kiloh, L. G., & Penny, R. (1977). Depressed lymphocyte function after bereavement. *Lancet, 1*(8016), 834–836.

Bukharov, Ya. M., & Golubev, M. V. (2007). *Psikhoterapiya v praktike vracha-nepsikhoterapevta* [Psychotherapy in medical practice – neprihotliva]. Publisher. (In Russian).

Buletov, D. A. (n.d.). *Reabilitaciya detej s onkologicheskoj patologiej. Vzglyad onkologa* [Rehabilitation of children with oncological pathology. Oncologist's look]. (In Russian).

Cherkasova, E. A., Krom, I. L., & Novichkova, I. Yu. (2013). Mediko-sociologicheskoe obosnovanie reabilitacii onkologicheskih bol'nyh [Medico-sociological substantiation of rehabilitation of oncological patients] [In Russian]. *Sociologicheskie Nauki, 2*, 10–15.

Cristian, A., Tran, A., & Patel, K. (2012). Patient safety in cancer rehabilitation. *Physical Medicine and Rehabilitation Clinics of North America, 23*(2), 441–456.

Egorov, B. E. (2003). *Ratsional'naya psikhoterapiya: teoriya i praktika. Posobie dlya vrachei* [Rational psychotherapy: Theory and practice. Manual for doctors]. Publisher. (In Russian).

Fang, F., Fall, K., & Mittleman, M. A.. (2012). Suicide and cardiovascular death after a cancer diagnosis. *The New England Journal of Medicine, 366*, 1310–1318.

Federal Law of 21.11.2011 (2011). N° 323-FZ “On the fundamentals of protecting the health of citizens in the Russian Federation”. https://www.rosminzdrav.ru/ (In Russian).

Hasanov, R. Sh., Ozol, S. A., Gilyazutdinov, I. A., & Gataullin, I. G. (2013). Sovremennye principy reabilitacii onkologicheskih bol’nyh [Modern principles of rehabilitation of cancer patients] [In Russian]. *Povolzhskij Onkologicheskij Vestnik, 4*, 49–55.

House, J. S., Landis, K. R., & Umberson, D. (1988). Social relationships and health. *Science, 241*, 540–545.

Idrisova, L. E., Solopova, A. G., Tabakman, Yu. Yu., Makatsariya, A. D., & Surenkov, A. A. (2016). *Osnovnye napravleniya psihologicheskoj reabilitacii onkoginekologicheskih bol’nyh* [The main directions of psychological rehabilitation of oncogynecologic patients]. *Akusherstvo* [In Russian]. *Ginekologiya i Reprodukcija, 4*, 94–104.

Kissane, D. W., Clarke, D. M., & Street, A. F. (2001). Demoralization syndrome – a relevant psychiatric diagnosis for palliative care. *Journal of Palliative Care, 17*, 12–21.

Ko, A. H., Dollinger, M., & Rosenbaum, E. (2008). *Everyone's guide to cancer therapy: How cancer is diagnosed, treated and managed day to day* (5th ed., Vol. 2). Publisher.

Kulakov, A. A., Chuchkov, V. M., & Matyakin, Ye. G.. (2012). Reabilitaciya onkologicheskih bol’nyh s defektom i polnoj vtorichnoj adentiej posle udaleniya obeih verhnih chelyustej [Rehabilitation of cancer patients with a defect and a complete secondary adentia after removal of both upper jaws] [In Russian]. *Opuholi Golovy i Shei, 4*, 34–40.

Lee, C. Y., Fang, C. K., & Yang, Y. C.. (2012). Demoralization syndrome among cancer outpatients in Taiwan. *Supportive Care in Cancer, 20*, 2259–2267.

Levin, T., & Kissane, W. D. (2006). Psychooncology – the state of its development in 2006. *European Journal of Psychiatry, 20*(2).

Lianos, G. D., Mangano, A., Cho, W. C., Dionigi, G., & Roukos, D. H. (2015). Circulating tumor DNA: New horizons for improving cancer treatment. *Future Oncology (London, England)*, *11*(4), 545–548.

Lichko, A. E. (1980). Zhurnal nevrologii i psikhiatrii im. [In Russian]. *S. S. Korsakova*, *8*, 1195–1198.

Malkina-Pykh, I. G. (2005). *Moskovskii psikhologicheskii zhurnal, 12*. (In Russian).

Myslivtseva, A. V., & Zaika, V. G. (2014). *Zhurnal fundamental'noi meditsiny i biologii, 3*, 37–40. (In Russian).

Pletnev, S. D. (1996). Lasers in clinical medicine. *Meditsina = Medicine.*

Rotenberg, V. S. (2001). *Snovideniya, gipnoz i deyatel'nost' mozga* [Dreams, hypnosis and brain activity]. RON. (In Russian)

Saimonton, K., & Saimonton, S. (2001). *Psikhoterapiya raka* [Psychotherapy cancer]. Publisher. (In Russian).

Saotome, T., Klein, L., & Faux, S. (2015). Cancer rehabilitation: A barometer for survival? *Supportive Care in Cancer*, *23*(10), 3033–3041.

Seligman, M. E. P. (1975). *Helplessness: On depression, development, and death.* W. H. Freeman.

Sheard, T., & Maguire, P. (1999). The effect of psychological interventions on anxiety and depression in cancer patients: Results of two meta-analyses. *British Journal of Cancer*, *80*, 1770–1780.

Siegel, R., Naishadham, D., & Jemal, A. (2013). Cancer statistics, 2013. *CA: a Cancer Journal for Clinicians*, *63*(1), 11–30.

Silver, J. K., Baima, J., & Mayer, R. S. (2013). Impairment-driven cancer rehabilitation: An essential component of quality care and survivorship. *CA: a Cancer Journal for Clinicians*, *63*(5), 295–317.

Slepkov, V. A., Suhovolskiy, V. G., & Hhlebopros, Z. G. (2007). Populjacionnaja dinamika v modelirovanii rosta rakovyh opuholej [Population dynamics in the modelling of the growth of cancerous tumors] [In Russian]. *Biophysics*, *52*(4), 733–740.

Smulevich, A. B., Andryushchenko, A. B., & Beskova, D. A. (2009). *Psikhicheskie rasstroistva v obshchei meditsine, 1*, 4–9. (In Russian).

Sotirov, S., Vankova, D., Vasilev, V., & Sotirova, E. (2019). Clustering of intercriteria analysis data using a health-related quality of life data. In *International Conference on Flexible Query Answering Systems* (pp. 242–249). Springer.

Spiegel, D. (2013). Minding the body: Psychotherapy and cancer survival. *British Journal of Health Psychology*, *19*(3), 1–21.

Spiegel, D., Bloom, J. R., Kraemer, H. C., & Gottheil, E. (1989). Effect of psychosocial treatment on survival of patients with metastatic breast cancer. *Lancet*, *334*(8668), 888–891.

Stepanova, N. V., & Chernavsky, D. S. (1983). A mathematical model of immunosuppression by malignant growth. *Mathematical Modelling*, •••, 379–386.

Tikhonov, A. N., & Samarsky, A. A. (1977). *Uravnenija matematicheskoj fiziki* [Equations of mathematical physics]. Nauka. (In Russian)

Yao, W., Gu, L., Sun, D., Ka, W., Wen, Z., & Chien, S. (2003). Wild type p53 gene causes reorganization of cytoskeleton and therefore the impaired deformability and difficult migration of murine erythroleukemia cells. *Cell Motility and the Cytoskeleton*, *56*, 1–12.

Zhukova, I. V., & Kolpak, E. P. (2013). *Matematicheskaja model' solidnoj opuholi* /Mathematical model of solid tumor/. *Natural and Mathematical Science in the Modern World*, *13*, 18–25.

Chapter 8
Trauma-Informed Approaches and Psychotherapy in Nursing Practice

Vesile Adıgüzel
https://orcid.org/0000-0002-9722-3491
Yalova University, Turkey

ABSTRACT

Trauma is defined as a deep emotional wound that emerges when an individual is exposed to events that threaten their life or cause serious psychological harm. In recent years, events such as natural disasters, wars, and sexual abuse have increased the number of individuals in society who are exposed to trauma (Nievergelt et al., 2024). Posttraumatic stress disorder (PTSD) is one of the primary psychological consequences of traumatic experiences. In addition to PTSD, it has been observed that individuals may develop dissociative symptoms after traumatic events, that is, a sense of alienation from oneself or one's surroundings (APA, 2015). In this chapter, the definition of trauma, its common symptoms and effects, the role and importance of stabilization in trauma treatment, the principles of trauma-informed care, and psychiatric nursing practices with individuals who have experienced trauma are discussed.

INTRODUCTION: DEFINITION OF TRAUMA

It is a well-established fact that the frequency of traumatic events has increased significantly in recent years (Dursun & Söylemez, 2020). Since the beginning of

DOI: 10.4018/979-8-3373-6526-8.ch008

humankind, every individual may be exposed to at least one, or multiple, traumatic experiences throughout their lifetime (Ruppert, 2011). Trauma is defined by the American Psychiatric Association as exposure to threatened or actual death, serious injury, or sexual violence (APA, 2013b). Posttraumatic stress disorder (PTSD) is a common mental health problem associated with trauma (APA, 2013b). According to the DSM-5 (APA, 2013b), PTSD is characterized by intrusion symptoms (e.g., nightmares, flashbacks), avoidance (e.g., avoiding thoughts, feelings, places, or people that serve as reminders), negative alterations in cognitions and mood (e.g., self-blame), and alterations in arousal and reactivity (e.g., exaggerated startle response, hypervigilance). These symptoms must persist for at least one month and cause functional impairment (APA, 2013b).

National surveys indicate that trauma affects more than 60% of children in the United States before the age of 18 (Finkelhor, Shattuck, Turner, & Hamby, 2015; McLaughlin et al., 2013). According to the World Mental Health Survey Consortium, 70% of adults across 24 countries have been exposed to at least one traumatic event, and 30.5% have experienced four or more traumatic events (Benjet et al., 2016). Non-interpersonal traumas (e.g., natural disasters) are associated with PTSD prevalence rates of approximately 10%, whereas interpersonal traumas (particularly sexual abuse and assault) are associated with prevalence rates of around 35% (Benjet et al., 2016).

Compared with their non-traumatized peers, young people who have experienced trauma are twice as likely to develop major depressive disorder, externalizing behavior problems, and substance use disorders (LeMoult et al., 2020; Carliner, Gary, McLaughlin, & Keyes, 2017). In a study conducted in Türkiye, 58.6% of participants reported having encountered at least one traumatic experience during their lifetime (Karanci et al., 2012). In another study by Soyer and colleagues (2021), childhood exposure to neglect and abuse and the associated emotional and behavioral problems were examined in 618 adults using a cross-sectional survey design (Soyer, Şenol, & Tümerdem, 2021). The findings indicated that 98.8% of participants had been exposed to physical abuse, 88.8% to emotional abuse, and 17.7% to sexual abuse to varying degrees (Soyer, Şenol, & Tümerdem, 2021). The results of numerous studies conducted both in Türkiye and internationally demonstrate that exposure to at least one traumatic experience is highly prevalent (Soyer, Şenol, & Tümerdem, 2021).

PSYCHOLOGICAL EFFECTS OF TRAUMATIC EVENTS

According to DSM-5, the main psychiatric problems that may be observed in adults following exposure to a traumatic event are classified as Acute Stress Disorder

(ASD), Posttraumatic Stress Disorder (PTSD), Adjustment Disorders, and Prolonged Grief Disorder (APA, 2013b).

Acute Stress Disorder is defined as a mental health condition characterized by avoidance of stimuli related to the event, re-experiencing the event, impairment in functioning, anxiety, emotional numbing, and a state of hyperarousal. These symptoms last for at least 2 and at most 4 weeks and are not attributable to another psychological disorder (APA, 2013a; Engin, 2021). In some individuals exposed to traumatic events, psychiatric symptoms may remit spontaneously without medical intervention (Engin, 2021). However, depending on the person's psychological resilience, age, gender, the severity and type of the traumatic event, and whether it has caused lasting damage, clinical intervention may be required (Büyükbayram, Çam, & Turgut, 2016).

When post-traumatic psychiatric symptoms persist for many years and last for more than one month, this condition is defined as Posttraumatic Stress Disorder (PTSD) according to DSM-5 (APA, 2013b). PTSD symptoms generally emerge within the first few months following the trauma (Engin, 2021). These symptoms include feeling as if the event is being continuously relived (flashbacks), diminished interest in one's surroundings, reduced interpersonal relationships, feeling alienated from other people, and a decrease in the capacity for emotional relationships (Engin, 2021). In addition, increased sensitivity to environmental stimuli, exaggerated startle response, nightmares or night terrors involving the traumatic event, sleep problems, self-blame, uneasiness, reduced work performance, and difficulties with attention and concentration may also occur.

There are three core features in the diagnosis of PTSD (Kaya, 2017):

1. A state of hyperarousal (hyperalertness)
2. A sense that the event is being re-experienced (intrusions)
3. Avoidance of any stimuli related to the event (avoidance)

These symptoms lead to clinically significant distress and negatively affect social and occupational functioning. Typically, symptoms last for at least one month but may continue to affect the individual for many years (Kaya, 2017; Yılmaz, 2016).

Another problem observed in individuals after trauma is Adjustment Disorder. According to DSM-5-TR, adjustment disorders are defined as conditions characterized by emotional or behavioral symptoms that emerge within three months of a triggering event, cause marked distress and a decline in social functioning, and involve depressed mood, anxiety, disturbances of conduct, and/or mixed disturbances of emotions and conduct (APA, 2015).

A further condition seen in adults after trauma is Prolonged Grief Disorder. According to DSM-5-TR, Prolonged Grief Disorder is characterized by the death of a close person at least 12 months previously, intense yearning or longing for the deceased, persistent preoccupation with thoughts or memories of the deceased, difficulty accepting the death, feeling as if a part of oneself has died, intense emotional pain related to the loss, difficulty in resuming social life and daily activities after the death, emotional numbness, a sense that life is meaningless, and profound loneliness (Köroğlu, 2015; APA, 2013b).

In addition to hyperarousal, avoidance, and intrusive thoughts observed in individuals who have experienced trauma, one of the most serious and distressing symptoms is dissociation (Wheeler, 2020). The term dissociation derives from the Greek "dis" (apart) and "sociare" (to join or connect) (Wheeler, 2020). Today, dissociation is used to denote a psychological "splitting" or fragmentation (Duran, 2021). Putnam (1989) offers a particularly influential definition of dissociation: it is "a normal state that is initially used by the individual as a defense mechanism to cope with traumatic symptoms, but subsequently, as the subconscious is pushed into the unconscious, turns into a maladaptive and pathological process" (APA, 2015; Wheeler, 2020). In individuals exposed to traumatic experiences, dissociative symptoms most commonly manifest as depersonalization and derealization (APA, 2015). These two symptoms can be explained in detail as follows:

1. **Depersonalization (Feeling Alienated from Oneself)**

Depersonalization is defined as a state in which an individual feels detached from their own body, thoughts, emotions, or actions, as if observing themselves from the outside (APA, 2022). In this experience, the person may feel unreal or as if they are moving in a mechanical, robot-like manner.

- **Emotional Numbing:** The individual may perceive their feelings or emotional responses as if they are being experienced behind a filter; this may be accompanied by emotional numbing or blunting.
- **Detachment from the Self:** The person may have difficulty recognizing themselves when looking in the mirror, or perceive bodily sensations (e.g., pain, hunger) as distant, as if they belonged to someone else. This process functions as an evolutionarily preserved protective shield used by the brain to keep the traumatic memory or emotional burden away from conscious awareness.

2. **Derealization (Feeling Alienated from the External Environment)**

Derealization refers to a state in which the individual feels alienated from the outside world, including people and objects in their environment, which may appear unreal, foggy, dreamlike, or distorted (APA, 2015). This sense of estrangement indicates a significant alteration in the way the environment is perceived.

- **Perceptual Distortions:** The individual may perceive objects in the environment as larger or smaller than normal (macropsia/micropsia), or may experience alterations in their colors.
- **Environmental Alienation:** Even a familiar place may suddenly appear completely unfamiliar, artificial, or as if it were a stage set. This process aims to facilitate psychological distancing from the environment in which the trauma occurred, thereby reducing the emotional impact of the perceived threat.

Some observable signs of dissociation are as follows:

- Inappropriate responses to stimuli and disorientation (e.g., a collapse-like reaction following a loud noise) (Wheeler, 2020; Schiraldi, 2016; Harnett & Lebois, 2022).
- Delayed and slowed responses to questions or environmental demands (Danböck et al., 2024; Boyd, Lanius, & McKinnon, 2018).
- Flashbacks, that is, reliving the traumatic event or situation accompanied by startle responses, disgust, and heightened arousal (Burback, Brult-Phillips, Nijdam, McFarlane, & Vermetten, 2024).
- Staring fixedly at a particular point as if gazing into space, rapid blinking without clear focus, or maintaining a fixed downward gaze (Wheeler, 2020; Schiraldi, 2016).
- A rigid or frozen bodily posture (Akiki, Averill, & Abdallah, 2017; Menon, 2011).
- Aimless wandering or pacing, episodes of thought blocking and flight of ideas, shifting abruptly to unrelated topics, inattention, and gaps in memory (Herringa, 2017).
- Falling asleep in inappropriate situations or contexts (Wheeler, 2020; Schiraldi, 2016).

TRAUMA STABILIZATION

Stabilization refers to the process of bringing something into a state of balance or steadiness. In the context of psychology and trauma treatment, stabilization generally denotes the process of restoring psychological and emotional equilibrium in an individual (Baranowsky & Gentry, 2023). The aim of stabilization is to reduce the impact of trauma, foster a sense of safety, and employ strategies that help the individual attain a mental state more conducive to therapeutic interventions (Baranowsky & Gentry, 2023). Stabilization occupies a crucial place as one of the initial steps in the treatment process.

Judith Herman, who first introduced the concept of stabilization into the literature in her book *Trauma and Recovery*, emphasized that stabilization constitutes the first stage in the healing of trauma and dissociation and that this process consists of three stages in total (Herman, 1992; Wheeler, 2020; Baranowsky & Gentry, 2023). These stages are:

1. **Safety and Stabilization:** As the most fundamental stage of recovery and the phase that shapes the individual's adaptation to treatment, this stage is characterized by the person's perception that both their body and external environment have betrayed them, a severely disrupted sense of safety, and the presence of the most intense trauma-related symptoms (Ross & Haley, 2004). In order for the individual to manage this period, the primary goals are to help them regain internal and external control, and to develop self-care and self-soothing skills (Baranowsky & Gentry, 2023).
2. **Remembrance and Mourning:** Currently referred to as "working through the trauma," this stage is conceptualized as the phase in which traumatic memories are processed and integrated (Baranowsky & Gentry, 2023). In the trauma-focused phase of treatment, various evidence-based approaches are employed, including Cognitive Behavioral Therapy (CBT), Eye Movement Desensitization and Reprocessing (EMDR), Time-Limited Trauma Therapy (TLTT), and Traumatic Incident Reduction (TIR) (Baranowsky & Gentry, 2023; Lewis et al., 2020; Lewis, Roberts, Gibson, & Bisson, 2020).
3. **Reconnection:** Defined as the final stage of recovery, this phase aims to facilitate the individual's re-engagement with life activities and successful adaptation (Payson, 2023). After completing the second phase of trauma-focused work, the goal of this stage is to expand the person's social and relational connections, support the exploration of broader interests, and create opportunities for new experiences of healing (Baranowsky & Gentry, 2023). In this phase, the individual has developed the capacity to view both the trauma and the self from an external perspective, and this process of liberation fosters an internal motivation that did not previously exist (Payson, 2023).

Findings from numerous scientific studies indicate that, following trauma, individuals may attain a deeper sense of meaning in life and an increased desire to support others who have experienced similar events. In the literature, this phenomenon is referred to as **posttraumatic growth** (Levi-Belz, Krysinska, & Andriessen, 2021; Roepke, 2015; Baranowsky & Gentry, 2023).

POSSIBLE NURSING DIAGNOSES FOR A PATIENT WITH POSTTRAUMATIC STRESS DISORDER (PTSD)

- Disturbed sleep pattern
- Imbalanced nutrition
- Ineffective sexuality pattern
- Impaired memory
- Disturbed self-concept
- Situational / chronic low self-esteem
- Powerlessness
- Hopelessness
- Impaired social interaction
- Ineffective role performance
- Anxiety
- Ineffective individual coping
- Fear
- Post-trauma syndrome / risk for post-trauma syndrome
- Rape-trauma syndrome
- Risk for self-harm
- Risk for suicide
- Risk for violence directed at others
- Dysfunctional grieving
- Risk for loneliness
- Social isolation (Towsend, 2015).

PRINCIPLES OF TRAUMA-INFORMED CARE

When trauma is not treated, individuals may be unable to cope with this stressful experience, may attempt to harm themselves or others, may view harmful substances such as alcohol or drugs as coping mechanisms, and may experience reduced adaptation to daily life, which in turn can lead to functional impairments (Baranowsky & Gentry, 2023). In the effective treatment of trauma, stabilization is one of the most critical steps (Wheeler, 2020). The effects of traumatic experiences on the individual—such as severe stress, difficulties in emotion regulation, and a fragmented sense of self—and the symptoms of dissociative disorders, in which the person feels detached from their own identity or from reality, are addressed through stabilization. Stabilization enables the management of these symptoms and constitutes an important phase that prepares the person for the therapeutic treatment process (Baranowsky & Gentry, 2023; Wheeler, 2020). In the literature, stabilization is described as occurring in five domains: (1) Safety, (2) Body, (3) Cognition, (4) Behavior, and (5) Emotion/Relationship (Baranowsky & Gentry, 2023; Herringa, 2017). Practice protocols related to these domains are discussed sequentially below.

1. Safety

The safety stage evokes Abraham Maslow's hierarchy of needs pyramid (Baranowsky & Gentry, 2023; Punkanen & Buckley, 2021). According to this theory, the lowest level of the pyramid is defined as safety, and the individual cannot move on to higher levels without first meeting safety needs (Wheeler, 2020). Similarly, in the stabilization process, a comprehensive assessment of the person's strengths and available resources should be conducted as a starting point for treatment, and based on this assessment, it should be determined which targets the interventions will focus on in order to build the safety phase (Robinson et al., 2022). Eric Gentry, identified as a trauma specialist, suggests conceptualizing safety at three levels (Baranowsky & Gentry, 2023).

a) **Ensuring safety in the immediate environment:** This level aims to establish a safe environment in terms of physical setting and conditions (Robinson et al., 2022). For example, the person needs to be physically removed from situations such as war, violence, or sexual abuse. At this stage, it may also be observed that the individual remains in a state of hypervigilance despite the absence of an actual external threat, which is one of the manifestations of trauma-related symptoms (Baranowsky & Gentry, 2023; Punkanen & Buckley, 2021). The nurse/therapist must determine whether this hypervigilant state is due to an internal threat or an external threat (Wheeler, 2020; Punkanen & Buckley, 2021). If there is an ongoing external danger, it is not possible to proceed to the subsequent stages of stabilization, and stabilization can only continue once the conditions have improved (Baranowsky & Gentry, 2023; Wheeler, 2020; Punkanen & Buckley, 2021).
b) **Addressing self-harming thoughts and behaviors:** Following a traumatic event, the individual may employ defense mechanisms that turn aggression inward and may blame themselves for what has happened, which can result in self-harming behavior (Robinson et al., 2022). This may manifest as suicide attempts, refusal to eat, addictions, alter-ego states, risk-taking behaviors, and social isolation (Baranowsky & Gentry, 2023; Punkanen & Buckley, 2021). At this stage, the nurse/therapist focuses on ensuring the patient's maximum safety, obtaining consent from the legal guardian if necessary. There are also several psychological techniques that can be employed with the individual during this phase (Reddemann & Piedfort-Marin, 2017; Stige, Rosenvinge, & Træen, 2013).

The first of these is the safety and self-care contract. This method involves a therapeutic agreement with the person to refrain from self-destructive behaviors (Punkanen & Buckley, 2021; Stige, Rosenvinge, & Træen, 2013). Another method is the Safety Net Plan (G-BY), in which, to better manage situations that trigger distress or crisis, the individual prepares in advance a written plan of self-help strategies designed to cope with these difficult moments. In this plan, the individual also includes the telephone and contact details of a person with whom they feel most comfortable and unashamed to reach out, enabling them to navigate crisis episodes in a more planned and manageable way (Baranowsky & Gentry, 2023; Rothschild, 2021).

c) **Transforming from a victim identity to a proactive survivor identity that re-engages with life:** For individuals exposed to trauma, moving beyond the belief that they are being punished by the universe and that the traumatic event has occurred "only to them" signifies reaching a level of posttraumatic growth (Baranowsky & Gentry, 2023; Stige, Rosenvinge, & Træen, 2013). At this stage, daily routines are discussed with the individual; self-care skills are supported; relaxation skills are taught; ineffective coping strategies are replaced with effective coping skills; assertiveness training is provided; and grounding/ containment techniques are introduced.

In addition to these methods, supportive mechanisms made possible by the digital age can also be utilized. Programs such as the "30-Day Stabilization for Unified Online Trauma Therapy," developed specifically for trauma stabilization, can be integrated into treatment, thereby providing patients with structured daily guidance and regulation (Baranowsky & Gentry, 2023).

2. Body

The aim of the body phase is to promote relaxation of the body affected by trauma and dissociation, reduce anxiety, and help the individual feel safe (Rothschild, 2021; Westland, 2020). In this step, which seeks to restore bodily balance and minimize trauma-related pathological responses, body- and energy-oriented interventions are used (Baranowsky & Gentry, 2023; Wheeler, 2020). Several guiding techniques are employed in the implementation of this phase, as outlined below.

a) Establishing a Non-Anxious Posture

This technique aims to ensure that the body is positioned in a safe and comfortable way. The person is encouraged to place their feet firmly on the ground, relax their shoulders, and maintain an upright yet comfortable posture. In this way, bodily relaxation is facilitated and a foundation is created for reducing anxiety (Özden, 2018; Rothschild, 2021; Westland, 2020).

b) **Progressive Relaxation**

In this technique, muscle groups are sequentially tensed and then relaxed. The person works through all major muscle groups, starting from the toes and moving upwards to the head. This process induces bodily relaxation and helps the individual feel calmer (Baranowsky & Gentry, 2023; Ruppert, 2014).

c) **Autogenic Relaxation**

Autogenic relaxation is a technique in which the individual focuses on specific parts of the body and induces sensations of heaviness, warmth, or comfort (Alpay & Çelik, 2022). For example, the person may direct their mind by using statements such as "my arms are getting heavy" or "my feet feel warm and relaxed" (Alpay & Çelik, 2022).

d) **Diaphragmatic Breathing**

This technique encourages breathing from the diaphragm. As the person inhales deeply, the abdomen rises; as they exhale slowly, the abdomen falls again. This type of breathing enhances relaxation and calms the body (Kalaycı, Aygün, & Sayir, 2023).

e) **3–6 Breathing**

In this method, the person inhales through the nose for three seconds and exhales slowly through the mouth over six seconds. This rhythmic breathing pattern helps slow the heart rate and reduce anxiety (Justice, Brems, & Ehlers, 2018).

f) **5–4–3–2–1 Sensory Grounding and Containment**

In this technique, the individual directs their attention to the environment and sequentially identifies 5 things they can see, 4 things they can hear, 3 things they can touch, 2 things they can smell, and 1 thing they can taste. By focusing on the senses, the mind is brought back to the "here and now," which helps the person distance themselves from anxious thoughts (Justice, Brems, & Ehlers, 2018; Baranowsky & Gentry, 2023).

g) **Posture-Based Grounding**

This is a grounding technique performed while the individual is standing or sitting, by firmly pressing the feet or body against the ground or the surface of the chair. By sensing the soles of the feet or the weight of the body, the person reinforces the feeling of "I am here and I am safe" (Reddemann & Piedfort-Marin, 2017; Stige & Binder, 2017).

h) **Anchoring**

Anchoring involves mentally recalling a safe or happy memory and emotionally connecting with that memory so that the person feels stronger and calmer in the present situation. This technique contributes to reducing anxiety and promoting a greater sense of balance (Wheeler, 2020; Lackner, 2023).

i) **9-1-1 Breathing**

This technique, used in emergencies to reduce acute anxiety, involves taking a brief, relatively quick inhalation followed by a slow exhalation. The rhythm of breathing is typically organized so that one full breath cycle is completed approximately every nine seconds (Punkanen & Buckley, 2021).

3. Cognition

The primary aim of the techniques and methods used at this stage is to regulate the individual's mental processes and reduce traumatic and dissociative symptoms (Baranowsky & Gentry, 2023). Some basic techniques applied to help free cognition from trauma- and dissociation-related disturbances are summarized below (Baranowsky & Gentry, 2023; Lackner, 2023; Kluft, 2014).

a) Grounding (Anchoring)

Grounding is a technique that helps the individual feel "here and now." By directing attention to the external world or to bodily sensations, it reduces anxiety and prevents the re-experiencing of past traumatic memories (Baranowsky & Gentry, 2023; Stige & Binder, 2017). For example, the person may be encouraged to focus by touching a physical object or observing their surroundings. Any concrete object in the environment can be used as an anchor in this process (Baranowsky & Gentry, 2023; Stige & Binder, 2017).

b) Safe-Place Imagery

In this technique, the person mentally creates or recalls a safe place. This may be an environment in which they have previously felt at peace or an imagined setting that feels safe. Safe-place imagery contributes to the person's sense of safety and enables them to return to this place mentally during stressful moments to promote relaxation (Stige & Binder, 2017; Lackner, 2023).

c) Positive Self-Talk and Cognitive Restructuring

This technique involves the person using encouraging and positive statements in their inner dialogue (Lackner, 2023). For instance, statements such as "This is a difficult moment, but I can handle it" are used to transform negative thoughts into more positive ones (Lackner, 2023). This approach enhances self-confidence and strengthens the person's capacity to cope with challenging situations. Derived from the cognitive–behavioral therapy framework, it replaces maladaptive cognitions with more adaptive ones, thereby supporting more effective management of the process (Lackner, 2023).

d) Re-Experiencing (Flashback Journal)

Re-experiencing refers to the person reliving traumatic events as if they were happening again. This technique recommends keeping a journal in which such experiences are recorded. By documenting when these episodes occur and which triggers are associated with them, it becomes possible to analyze patterns, which helps the individual be better prepared for these situations (Kluft, 2014; Baranowsky & Gentry, 2023).

e) Thought Stopping

Thought stopping is a technique in which negative thoughts are deliberately interrupted. When the individual notices that they are absorbed in a negative or threatening thought, they consciously say "stop" to block its progression. Alternatively, they may redirect their mind toward a positive or neutral thought (Baranowsky & Gentry, 2023; Valdez & Lilly, 2012).

f) The Buddha Trick

This technique enables the person to observe their emotions and thoughts from an external, non-judgmental perspective (Taute, 2023; Duran, 2021). The individual imagines negative thoughts and feelings in the stream of consciousness as leaves floating down a river, simply watching them pass by. As a mindfulness-based method, it reminds the person that thoughts are transient, thereby helping them to calm down and regain focus (Taute, 2023; Duran, 2021).

4. Behavior

At this stage, the goal is to develop positive behavioral strategies to support the individual's efforts to cope with trauma and dissociation. Techniques that involve behavioral interventions are outlined below (Burback et al., 2024; Taute, 2023).

a) **Rituals**

Rituals, also referred to as routines, are behaviors that the person performs regularly in order to attain a sense of safety, relaxation, or control (Baranowsky & Gentry, 2015). Small but consistent actions that can be integrated into daily life (for example, starting the day with a particular morning routine or practicing a specific relaxation technique before sleep) help the individual feel safe and create structure in daily living. Rituals can assist in soothing the sense of chaos brought on by traumatic experiences (Baranowsky & Gentry, 2015; Burback et al., 2024; Heaney, Conway, & Cormack, 2023).

b) **Safety and Self-Care Contract**

A safety and self-care contract is an agreement in which the individual commits to behaving toward themselves in safe and healthy ways. By making an explicit commitment, the person pledges to refrain from self-harm during traumatic moments and to take good care of their body and mind. This contract reinforces the importance of self-care and supports the individual in changing maladaptive behavioral patterns (Wheeler, 2020; Baranowsky & Gentry, 2023).

c) **Safety Net Plan**

A safety net plan involves the individual identifying people and resources from whom they can seek support during difficult moments (Valdez & Lilly, 2012). This plan specifies those to whom the person can turn when feeling lonely or in crisis (for example, close friends, family members, or a therapist), as well as other potential sources of support. This technique helps the individual feel safer in stressful situations and facilitates drawing on support from their environment (Baranowsky & Gentry, 2023; Valdez & Lilly, 2012).

5. Emotion

The final step in the stabilization of trauma and dissociation focuses on the regulation of emotions. At this stage, the individual is supported in recognizing and sustaining their emotional processes and in coping with trauma-related and dissociative symptoms (Baranowsky & Gentry, 2023). Several effective techniques are employed for managing this emotional phase, including the following:

a) **Transitional Objects**

Transitional objects are special items that help the person feel safe and comfortable and that they tend to keep close to themselves (for example, a necklace, a small toy, or a handkerchief). Such objects can assist the individual in self-soothing during difficult moments and reinforce their sense of safety (Kluft, 2014).

b) **Support Systems**

Support systems comprise the social and emotional networks that the individual needs in order to feel emotionally strong. Close friends, family members, or a therapist can provide support in dealing with distressing emotions and thoughts. These systems enable the person to feel both safe and connected (Lackner, 2023).

c) **Drawing Icons and Envelopes**

The technique of drawing icons or envelopes helps the individual express difficult emotions in a concrete form. The person represents what they are feeling by drawing an icon or an envelope. This creative expression facilitates the identification and management of emotions (Lewis, Roberts, Andrew, Starling, & Bisson, 2020).

d) **Internal Vault**

The internal vault is a technique in which the person creates a safe and solid place in their mind (Lewis, Roberts, Gibson, & Bisson, 2020). Overwhelming or hard-to-manage emotions can be "locked away" in this vault. When experiencing intense emotional states, the individual imagines this vault and temporarily stores these emotions in that secure internal space. This method helps the person feel more in control during periods of emotional intensity (Lewis, Roberts, Gibson, & Bisson, 2020).

e) **Positive Sense of Hope**

This technique supports the individual in focusing on positive and hopeful future experiences. The person imagines pleasant moments they wish to live in the future or uses hopeful statements to maintain a sense of optimism during difficult times. A sense of hope contributes to the individual feeling stronger and more motivated in the aftermath of trauma (Baranowsky & Gentry, 2023).

EXPECTED OUTCOME CRITERIA IN THE CARE OF PATIENTS WITH POSTTRAUMATIC STRESS DISORDER

- The patient should be able to acknowledge and accept the traumatic event they have experienced.
- As acceptance of the traumatic event increases, the frequency and intensity of nightmares and recurrent memories (flashbacks) should decrease.
- The patient should demonstrate the use of adaptive coping strategies (e.g., music, art, relaxation techniques, mental imagery).
- The patient should be able to concentrate and make realistic plans for the future.
- The patient should be able to involve significant others in the treatment process and willingly accept their support.
- The patient should verbalize thoughts related to self-harm.
- Feelings of guilt associated with survival should have been explored and addressed.
- The patient should be able to obtain sufficient sleep in order to reduce the risk of accidents and injury.
- The patient should be able to identify and discuss community resources they can contact during times of stress.
- The patient should participate in support groups composed of individuals who have experienced similar traumas.
- The patient should be able to discuss their desire and efforts to resist and overcome the trauma they experienced in the past and throughout their life course (Büyükbayram, Çam, & Turgut, 2016).

PSYCHIATRIC NURSING INTERVENTIONS WITH INDIVIDUALS WHO HAVE EXPERIENCED TRAUMA

Trauma is among the most common mental health–related problems in the general population (Benjet et al., 2016; Heaney, Conway, & Cormack, 2023). One specific form of trauma, posttraumatic stress disorder, leads to serious difficulties in individuals following traumatic experiences (Punkanen & Buckley, 2021; Benjet et al., 2016). Nurses, who provide services to all age groups and work in a wide range of roles and settings, are among the most accessible health professionals and thus bear major responsibilities in recognizing, managing, and appropriately referring trauma-related symptoms (Reddemann & Piedfort-Marin, 2017; Wheeler, 2020; Rothschild, 2021).

A key component of these responsibilities is the recognition and stabilization of traumatic manifestations and dissociative symptoms (Westland, 2020; Baranowsky & Gentry, 2023). When nurses are actively involved in the stabilization phase and support the patient in completing this phase, it becomes easier to progress to subsequent stages of trauma treatment, and the patient's adherence to treatment improves (Wheeler, 2020; Taute, 2023). In this way, the individual is prepared for the interventions included in later phases of care—such as psychotherapeutic treatments and recovery processes—and their mental state is stabilized (Robinson et al., 2022).

Above, stabilization techniques that can be implemented by nurses, therapists, psychologists, and other mental health professionals have been discussed in detail. In addition to these, there are specific interventions that are particularly important for nurses in stabilizing the patient. These can be classified under three main headings.

1. Mindfulness

In individuals experiencing trauma and dissociation, mindfulness practices help reduce dissociative symptoms by directing attention to the "here and now" and to one's bodily/mental experiences (Boyd, Lanius, & McKinnon, 2018; Mattheß et al., 2019; Wiltshire, 2024). Mindfulness contributes to the alleviation of anxiety and dissociative symptoms by weakening the link with past traumatic memories (Wiltshire, 2024; Wheeler, 2020). Practical applications for nurses include the following.

The first is **sensory grounding exercises** (Wheeler, 2020). Sensory grounding exercises are recommended to help individuals with dissociation feel that they are "here and now" (Boyd, Lanius, & McKinnon, 2018). Nurses can ask patients to notice five objects they can see in their environment, four sounds they can hear, three tactile sensations they can feel (for example, their clothes or the chair), two smells, and one taste (Roepke, 2015). This technique helps the person feel better in the moment.

Another practice is the **body scan exercise** (Wheeler, 2020; Westland, 2020). Body scan can be used to increase bodily awareness and reduce dissociative symptoms in individuals who have experienced trauma (Baranowsky & Gentry, 2023). Nurses may ask the patient to slowly focus on each part of their body, starting from the toes and moving upward (Mattheß et al., 2019). During this process, attention is directed to the body, and the person observes whether there is tension or relaxation in each region (Wiltshire, 2024). This exercise supports reconnection with the body during moments of dissociation (Mattheß et al., 2019; Westland, 2020).

Another mindfulness-based technique is **breath-focused awareness**. Nurses can teach simple breathing exercises to individuals experiencing dissociation or intense anxiety, enabling them to focus on their breathing (Taute, 2023). For example, inhaling for 4 seconds, holding the breath for 7 seconds, and then exhaling over 8 seconds through pursed lips establishes a rhythmic breathing pattern that calms the mind and soothes dissociation (Wiltshire, 2024; Stige, Rosenvinge, & Træen, 2013).

2. Sleep Hygiene

Individuals with traumatic experiences frequently suffer from sleep problems; improving sleep quality is therefore important in reducing trauma-related and dissociative symptoms (Shortland, 2016). By providing sleep hygiene guidance, nurses can help regulate patients' sleep patterns and thus contribute to the alleviation of these symptoms. Practical applications for nurses regarding sleep hygiene include:

Establishing relaxing pre-sleep routines: Nurses can support patients in developing a bedtime routine that facilitates relaxation before sleep (Westland, 2020). For example, taking a warm shower, doing slow breathing exercises, or listening to calm music can ease the transition to sleep. In addition, limiting caffeine and fluid intake before bedtime, ventilating the bedroom, and going to bed only when feeling sufficiently sleepy help create a safe and soothing pre-sleep environment (Westland, 2020; Baranowsky & Gentry, 2023).

Anchor objects against nightmares: Anchor objects can be recommended for individuals who experience traumatic nightmares and flashbacks. Nurses may suggest that patients keep a comforting object they can immediately hold upon waking (for example, a small pillow, prayer beads, or a soft piece of cloth) (Baranowsky & Gentry, 2023). This object helps reduce dissociative feelings after awakening from a nightmare and supports the restoration of a sense of safety (Lackner, 2023).

Arranging a low-stimulus sleep environment: For individuals with posttraumatic symptoms, the sleep environment becomes especially important. Nurses can recommend that patients create a dark, quiet, and cool bedroom (Lewis, Roberts, Andrew, Starling, & Bisson, 2020). Dimming the lights before bedtime and avoiding electronic devices can prevent the triggering of traumatic reminders and enhance sleep quality (Westland, 2020).

3. Psychoeducation

Psychoeducation is an easily accessible and simple-to-implement intervention. It is a component that can be integrated into all stages of managing trauma and dissociative symptoms (Whitworth, 2016; Demirci, Bilge, Emiral, & Şen, 2024). Providing individuals with information about trauma and the neurobiology of trauma, helping them understand that they are not to blame for what happened, clarifying anxiety, fear, and posttraumatic symptoms, and supporting the development of effective coping strategies all become possible through psychoeducation (Brouzos, Vatkali, Mavridis, Vassilopoulos, & Baourda, 2022; Wheeler, 2020). With these educational interventions, individuals who have experienced trauma can learn that their reactions are normal and develop a more self-compassionate attitude toward themselves (Brouzos, Vatkali, Mavridis, Vassilopoulos, & Baourda, 2022; Wheeler, 2020; Whitworth, 2016).

To ensure that psychoeducation is implemented effectively, practical strategies for nurses include:

Providing information about trauma symptoms: Nurses can inform individuals who have experienced trauma about dissociative symptoms and the effects of trauma (Brouzos, Vatkali, Mavridis, Vassilopoulos, & Baourda, 2022). This information helps individuals understand the origin of their symptoms and learn that these reactions are normal (Shortland, 2016). For example, knowing that dissociation is a defense mechanism may bring relief to the individual.

Teaching safe-place imagery: Nurses can teach patients to imagine a safe place during times of stress or dissociation (Wheeler, 2020). This safe place may be a location where they felt happy in the past or an imagined peaceful setting. In individuals who have experienced trauma, safe-place imagery facilitates calming during difficult moments and contributes to the reduction of dissociative symptoms (Tripp, Potash, & Brancheau, 2019).

Explaining the importance of support systems: The power of social support in the posttraumatic period is substantial. Nurses can encourage individuals to reach out to people or groups from whom they can receive support (Stige & Binder, 2017). The importance of participating in psychotherapy or support groups can be emphasized; this helps individuals realize that they are not alone and that others have had similar experiences (Shortland, 2016).

CONCLUSION

This section has comprehensively addressed the profound emotional impact of trauma, its common psychiatric consequences, and, in particular, the importance of stabilization as one of the most critical stages in the treatment process. Trauma is defined as a deep emotional wound arising from events that threaten an individual's life and has increasingly become a societal problem with the growing prevalence of natural disasters, wars, and various forms of abuse. Among the most common mental health problems that emerge following exposure to traumatic events are Posttraumatic Stress Disorder (PTSD), Acute Stress Disorder (ASD), Adjustment Disorder, and Prolonged Grief Disorder. PTSD, in particular, is characterized by intrusions (nightmares, flashbacks), avoidance, negative alterations in cognition and mood, and hyperarousal. In addition to these symptoms, dissociation—defined as a sense of detachment from oneself and from others—appears as a defense mechanism against trauma, yet may gradually evolve into a pathological process.

Stabilization is the first and most critical step in achieving effective outcomes in trauma treatment. As emphasized in Judith Herman's three-stage recovery model, stabilization (safety and remobilization) is the foundational phase that shapes treatment adherence and aims to restore the individual's internal and external sense of control.

The five core domains of stabilization examined in detail in this chapter (Safety, Body, Cognition, Behavior, and Emotion) constitute the essential principles of trauma-informed care. These principles range from ensuring physical safety (e.g., securing the immediate environment) to implementing interventions aimed at preventing suicide and self-harm. Techniques such as the Safety Net Plan and safety/self-care contracts, in particular, provide crucial support for managing crisis situations.

Psychiatric nurses occupy a critical position as the most accessible health professionals in the recognition and management of trauma-related symptoms. Nursing interventions have been grouped under three main headings: Mindfulness (e.g., sensory grounding, body scan), Sleep Hygiene (e.g., relaxing routines, anchor objects against nightmares), and Psychoeducation (e.g., providing information about trauma symptoms and the importance of support systems). These practices facilitate the individual's engagement with the treatment process and help them prepare for subsequent phases of recovery.

In conclusion, stabilization constitutes the cornerstone of rebuilding psychological resilience in the aftermath of trauma. This process secures the person's safety, and supports bodily and emotional regulation, ultimately aiming to promote readaptation to daily life activities and even to reach a level of posttraumatic growth (greater access to meaning in life and an enhanced desire to be of help to others). In the care of trauma survivors, a multidisciplinary approach and the presence of health professionals who can effectively implement stabilization techniques are of vital importance in supporting the individual's journey toward recovery.

REFERENCES

Akiki, T. J., Averill, C. L., & Abdallah, C. G. (2017). A network-based neurobiological model of PTSD: Evidence from structural and functional neuroimaging studies. *Current Psychiatry Reports, 19*, 81. DOI: 10.1007/s11920-017-0840-4

Alpay, H., & Çelik, D. (2022). Complex post-traumatic stress disorder: A review. *Psikiyatride Güncel Yaklasimlar, 14*(4), 589–596. DOI: 10.18863/pgy.1050659

APA. (2013a). *Diagnostic and statistical manual of mental disorders* (5. baskı). American Psychiatric Association.

APA. (2013b). Diagnostic and Statistical Manual of Mental Disorders DSM-V. Translated by P. D. E. Köroğlu.

Baranowsky, A. B., & Gentry, J. E. (2015). *Trauma practice: Tools for stabilization and recovery*. Hogrefe Publishing.

Baranowsky, A. B., & Gentry, J. E. (2023). *Trauma practice: A cognitive behavioral somatic therapy*. Hogrefe Publishing GmbH.

Benjet, C., Bromet, E., Karam, E. G., Kessler, R. C., McLaughlin, K. A., Ruscio, A. M., Shahly, V., Stein, D. J., Petukhova, M., & Hill, E. (2016). The epidemiology of traumatic event exposure worldwide: Results from the World Mental Health Survey Consortium. *Psychological Medicine, 46*(2), 327–343. DOI: 10.1017/S0033291715001981

Boyd, J. E., Lanius, R. A., & McKinnon, M. C. (2018). Mindfulness-based treatments for posttraumatic stress disorder: A review of the treatment literature and neurobiological evidence. *Journal of Psychiatry & Neuroscience : JPN, 43*(1), 7–25. DOI: 10.1503/jpn.170021

Brouzos, A., Vatkali, E., Mavridis, D., Vassilopoulos, S. P., & Baourda, V. C. (2022). Psychoeducation for adults with post-traumatic stress symptomatology: A systematic review and meta-analysis. *Journal of Contemporary Psychotherapy, 52*(2), 155–164. DOI: 10.1007/s10879-021-09526-3

Burback, L., Brult-Phillips, S., Nijdam, M. J., McFarlane, A., & Vermetten, E. (2024). Treatment of posttraumatic stress disorder: A state-of-the-art review. *Current Neuropharmacology, 22*(4), 557–635. DOI: 10.2174/1570159X21666230428091433

Büyükbayram, A., Çam, O., & Turgut, E. Ö. (2016). Mental health and psychiatric nursing approach after trauma. Anadolu Nursing and Health Sciences Journal, 19(3).

Carliner, H., Gary, D., McLaughlin, K. A., & Keyes, K. M. (2017). Trauma exposure and externalizing disorders in adolescents: Results from the National Comorbidity Survey Adolescent Supplement. *Journal of the American Academy of Child and Adolescent Psychiatry*, *56*(9), 755–764.e3. DOI: 10.1016/j.jaac.2017.06.006

Danböck, S. K., Duek, O., Ben-Zion, Z., Korem, N., Amen, S. L., Kelmendi, B., Wilhelm, F. H., Levy, I., & Harpaz-Rotem, I. (2024). Effects of a dissociative drug on fronto-limbic resting-state functional connectivity in individuals with posttraumatic stress disorder: A randomized controlled pilot study. *Psychopharmacology*, *241*(2), 243–252. DOI: 10.1007/s00213-023-06479-4

Demirci, H., Bilge, Y., Emiral, E., & Şen, S. (2024). Enhancing recovery in post-earthquake adolescents: Examining the impact of a psychoeducational intervention on traumatic stress symptoms and coping strategies. *Current Psychology (New Brunswick, N.J.)*, *43*(33), 26983–26996. DOI: 10.1007/s12144-024-06333-6

Duran, B. (2021). Trauma and dissociation. In Güler, K. (Ed.), *A clinical perspective on trauma* (pp. 94–112). Eğiten Kitap.

Dursun, P., & Söylemez, İ. (2020). Post-traumatic growth: A comprehensive assessment with the latest revised model. *Turkish Journal of Psychiatry*, *31*(1), 57–68. DOI: 10.5080/u23694

Engin, E. (2021). Trauma and stressor-related disorders. In Olcay Çam, E. E. (Ed.), *The art of psychiatric nursing care in mental health and diseases* (3rd ed., pp. 274–287). Istanbul Medical Bookstores.

Finkelhor, D., Shattuck, A., Turner, H., & Hamby, S. (2015). A revised inventory of adverse childhood experiences. *Child Abuse & Neglect*, *48*, 13–21. DOI: 10.1016/j.chiabu.2015.07.011

Harnett, N. G., & Lebois, L. A. M. (2022). Leveraging resting-state neurophenotypes to identify susceptibility to and heterogeneity of posttraumatic stress disorder. *Neuropsychopharmacology: Official Publication of the American College of Neuropsychopharmacology*, *47*(1), 403–404. DOI: 10.1038/s41386-021-01134-y

Heaney, F., Conway, Y., & Cormack, S. (2023). Principles of trauma care. In *Orthopaedic and trauma nursing: An evidence-based approach to musculoskeletal care* (ss. 215-239).

Herman, J. L. (1992). *Trauma and recovery*. Basic Books.

Herringa, R. J. (2017). Trauma, PTSD, and the developing brain. *Current Psychiatry Reports*, *19*, 69. DOI: 10.1007/s11920-017-0825-3

Justice, L., Brems, C., & Ehlers, K. (2018). Bridging body and mind: Considerations for trauma-informed yoga. *International Journal of Yoga Therapy*, *28*(1), 39–50. DOI: 10.17761/2018-00017R2

Kalaycı, T., Aygün, Ü., & Sayir, F. (2023). Multiple trauma approach in earthquake. *Ağrı Medical Faculty Journal*, *1*(2), 22–25.

Karanci, A. N., Işıklı, S., Aker, A. T., Gül, E. İ., Erkan, B. B., Özkol, H., & Güzel, H. Y. (2012). Personality, posttraumatic stress and trauma type: Factors contributing to posttraumatic growth and its domains in a Turkish community sample. *European Journal of Psychotraumatology*, *3*(1), 17303. DOI: 10.3402/ejpt.v3i0.17303

Kaya, H. (2017). Psychological traces of terrorism: A review of direct and indirect exposure. Master's Thesis, Ankara University Institute of Health Sciences, Department of Interdisciplinary Forensic Sciences.

Kluft, R. (2014). Stabilization basics. In M. L. Brand, R. A. Lanius, U. Schnyder, & R. P. Frewen (Eds.), *Neurobiology and treatment of traumatic dissociation: Towards an embodied self* (ss. 319-338).

Köroğlu, E. (2015). *Klinik Psikiyatri*. Boylam Psikiyatri Enstitüsü.

Lackner, R. (2023). *Stabilization in trauma treatment: A holistic cross-method practical guide*. Springer Nature.

LeMoult, J., Humphreys, K. L., Tracy, A., Hoffmeister, J.-A., Ip, E., & Gotlib, I. H. (2020). Meta-analysis: Exposure to early life stress and risk for depression in childhood and adolescence. *Journal of the American Academy of Child and Adolescent Psychiatry*, *59*(7), 842–855. DOI: 10.1016/j.jaac.2019.10.011

Levi-Belz, Y., Krysinska, K., & Andriessen, K. (2021). “Turning personal tragedy into triumph”: A systematic review and meta-analysis of studies on posttraumatic growth among suicide-loss survivors. *Psychological Trauma: Theory, Research, Practice, and Policy*, *13*(3), 322–335. DOI: 10.1037/tra0000977

Lewis, C., Roberts, N. P., Andrew, M., Starling, E., & Bisson, J. I. (2020). Psychological therapies for post-traumatic stress disorder in adults: Systematic review and meta-analysis. *European Journal of Psychotraumatology*, *11*(1), 1729633. DOI: 10.1080/20008198.2020.1729633

Lewis, C., Roberts, N. P., Gibson, S., & Bisson, J. I. (2020). Dropout from psychological therapies for post-traumatic stress disorder (PTSD) in adults: Systematic review and meta-analysis. *European Journal of Psychotraumatology*, *11*(1), 1709709. DOI: 10.1080/20008198.2019.1709709

Mattheß, C., Farrell, D., Mattheß, M., Bumke, P., Sodemann, U., & Mattheß, H. (2019). The therapeutic value of trauma stabilisation in the treatment of post-traumatic stress disorder – A Southeast Asian study. *Asian Journal of Psychiatry, 41*, 45–49. DOI: 10.1016/j.ajp.2018.09.010

McLaughlin, K. A., Koenen, K. C., Hill, E. D., Petukhova, M., Sampson, N. A., Zaslavsky, A. M., & Kessler, R. C. (2013). Trauma exposure and posttraumatic stress disorder in a national sample of adolescents. *Journal of the American Academy of Child and Adolescent Psychiatry*, *52*(8), 815–830.e14. DOI: 10.1016/j.jaac.2013.05.011

Menon, V. (2011). Large-scale brain networks and psychopathology: A unifying triple network model. *Trends in Cognitive Sciences*, *15*(10), 483–506. DOI: 10.1016/j.tics.2011.08.003

Nievergelt, C. M., Maihofer, A. X., Atkinson, E. G., Chen, C. Y., Choi, K. W., Coleman, J. R. I., & Koenen, K. C. (2024). Genome-wide association analyses identify 95 risk loci and provide insights into the neurobiology of post-traumatic stress disorder. *Nature Genetics*, *56*(5), 792–808. DOI: 10.1038/s41588-024-01707-9

Özden, M. Ş. (2018). Trauma and dissociative disorders: A general overview. *Bartın University Faculty of Literature Journal*, *3*(3), 71–76.

Payson, H. (2023). Reconnecting: Trauma, addiction, and group EMDR therapy. In Luber, M. (Ed.), *EMDR group therapy: Emerging principles and protocols to treat trauma and beyond* (p. 233).

Punkanen, M., & Buckley, T. (2021). Embodied safety and bodily stabilization in the treatment of complex trauma. *European Journal of Trauma & Dissociation = Revue Européenne du Trauma et de la Dissociation*, *5*(3), 100156. DOI: 10.1016/j.ejtd.2020.100156

Reddemann, L., & Piedfort-Marin, O. (2017). Stabilization in the treatment of complex post-traumatic stress disorders: Concepts and principles. *European Journal of Trauma & Dissociation = Revue Européenne du Trauma et de la Dissociation*, *1*(1), 11–17. DOI: 10.1016/j.ejtd.2017.01.009

Robinson, L. K., Sterling, L., Jackson, J., Gentry, E., Araujo, F., LaFond, C., Jacobson, K. C., & Lee, R. (2022). A secondary traumatic stress reduction program in emergency room nurses. *SAGE Open Nursing*, *8*, 23779608221094530. DOI: 10.1177/23779608221094530

Roepke, A. M. (2015). Psychosocial interventions and posttraumatic growth: A meta-analysis. *Journal of Consulting and Clinical Psychology*, *83*(1), 129–142. DOI: 10.1037/a0036872

Ross, C. A., & Haley, C. (2004). Acute stabilization and three-month follow-up in a trauma program. *Journal of Trauma & Dissociation*, *5*(1), 103–112. DOI: 10.1300/J229v05n01_06

Rothschild, B. (2021). *Revolutionizing trauma treatment: Stabilization, safety, & nervous system balance*. W. W. Norton & Company.

Ruppert, F. (2011). *Travma, bağlanma ve aile konstelasyonları: Ruhun yaralarını anlamak ve iyileştirmek*. Kaknüs Yayınları.

Schiraldi, G. R. (2016). *The self-esteem workbook* (2nd ed.). New Harbinger Publications.

Shortland, A. (2016). Working with trauma. In ... *Clinical practice at the edge of care: Developments in working with at-risk children and their families* (ss. 153-174).

Soyer, M. K., Şenol, A., & Tümerdem, B. Ç. (2021). An examination of childhood trauma experiences in a group of adults in terms of various variables. *Humanistic Perspective*, *3*(2), 324–343.

Stige, S. H., & Binder, P.-E. (2017). From painstaking work to a new way of meeting the world—Trauma clients' experiences with skill training in a stabilization group approach. *Psychotherapy Research*, *27*(5), 571–582.

Stige, S. H., Rosenvinge, J. H., & Træen, B. (2013). A meaningful struggle: Trauma clients' experiences with an inclusive stabilization group approach. *Psychotherapy Research*, *23*(4), 419–429. DOI: 10.1080/10503307.2013.778437

Taute, C. (2023). Learning to cope with trauma and moving forward. *Psychology (Irvine, Calif.)*, *14*(6), 1033–1037. DOI: 10.4236/psych.2023.146055

Towsend, M. C. (2015). Trauma-and stressor-related disorder. In *Psychiatric mental health nursing: Concepts of care in evidence-based practice* (8. Baskı, ss. 559-578).

Tripp, T., Potash, J. S., & Brancheau, D. (2019). Safe place collage protocol: Art making for managing traumatic stress. *Journal of Trauma & Dissociation*, *20*(5), 511–525. DOI: 10.1080/15299732.2019.1597813

Valdez, C. E., & Lilly, M. M. (2012). Thought control: Is it ability, strategies, or both that predicts posttraumatic symptomatology in victims of interpersonal trauma? *Journal of Psychopathology and Behavioral Assessment*, *34*, 531–541. DOI: 10.1007/s10862-012-9300-y

Westland, G. (2020). Healing trauma through embodied relating. In *Trauma in the creative and embodied therapies: When words are not enough*.

Wheeler, K. (2020). *Psychotherapy for advanced practice in psychiatric nursing* (A. A. Özbaş & N. Gürhan, Çev.; K. Wheeler, Ed.; C. 2). Springer Publishing Company.

Whitworth, J. D. (2016). The role of psychoeducation in trauma recovery: Recommendations for content and delivery. *Journal of Evidence-Informed Social Work, 13*(5), 442–451. DOI: 10.1080/23761407.2016.1166852

Wiltshire, J. T. (2024). The role of mindfulness and embodiment in group-based trauma treatment. *Psychotherapy and Counselling Journal of Australia, 12*(1). Advance online publication. DOI: 10.59158/001c.94979

Yılmaz, S. (2016). Trauma and stressor-related disorders. In Gürhan, N. (Ed.), *Mental health and psychiatric nursing* (1st ed., pp. 815–843). Nobel Medical Bookstore.

Chapter 9
Nurses' Therapeutic Roles in Digital Environments

G. SudhaAnanthi
https://orcid.org/0009-0001-5062-5311
Winners Academy, India

ABSTRACT

The evolution of nursing in digital environments represents a profound transformation in healthcare delivery, professional practice, education, and patient engagement. The integration of digital technologies—such as electronic health records (EHRs), telehealth systems, artificial intelligence (AI), wearable sensors, and mobile health (mHealth) applications—has redefined the roles, responsibilities, and competencies of nurses in the 21st century. This digital transformation has enabled nurses to transcend traditional clinical boundaries, providing care that is more data-driven, patient-centered, and accessible. In the early stages, nursing's interaction with technology was largely administrative, focusing on documentation and record-keeping. However, as digital health infrastructures matured, the scope of nursing practice expanded dramatically, aligning with global movements toward digital health transformation. The modern nurse now operates in a hybrid environment that combines human compassion with technological precision.

THE EVOLUTION OF NURSING IN DIGITAL ENVIRONMENTS

The evolution of nursing in digital environments represents a profound transformation in healthcare delivery, professional practice, education, and patient engagement. The integration of digital technologies—such as electronic health records (EHRs),

DOI: 10.4018/979-8-3373-6526-8.ch009

telehealth systems, artificial intelligence (AI), wearable sensors, and mobile health (mHealth) applications—has redefined the roles, responsibilities, and competencies of nurses in the 21st century. This digital transformation has enabled nurses to transcend traditional clinical boundaries, providing care that is more data-driven, patient-centered, and accessible. In the early stages, nursing's interaction with technology was largely administrative, focusing on documentation and record-keeping. However, as digital health infrastructures matured, the scope of nursing practice expanded dramatically, aligning with global movements toward digital health transformation. The modern nurse now operates in a hybrid environment that combines human compassion with technological precision, requiring the seamless integration of clinical judgment and digital literacy (Ackerman et al., 2018). Digital environments have fundamentally reshaped the nurse-patient relationship. Virtual consultations, remote monitoring, and digital communication platforms allow nurses to deliver care to patients regardless of geographical location, particularly benefiting those in rural or underserved areas. Telehealth nursing, or telenursing, has emerged as a vital extension of nursing practice, enabling remote assessment, triage, education, and chronic disease management. Through secure video conferencing and mobile platforms, nurses can provide personalized advice, monitor treatment adherence, and respond to emergencies in real time.

The digital evolution has also introduced advanced data analytics and artificial intelligence into nursing practice, enabling more precise and predictive forms of care. AI-driven systems assist nurses in early diagnosis, risk assessment, and personalized treatment planning by analyzing vast amounts of clinical data. Decision-support tools integrated into EHR systems help nurses detect patient deterioration, identify potential medication errors, and streamline workflows. Predictive algorithms can flag early warning signs of sepsis or falls, empowering nurses to take preemptive actions that improve patient safety outcomes. In critical care units, AI-enhanced monitoring devices continuously track vital signs, alerting nurses to deviations that require immediate intervention (Bolier et al., 2014). These technologies augment the cognitive capacity of nurses, allowing them to focus more on direct patient care and empathetic interactions rather than repetitive administrative tasks. However, the integration of AI also necessitates ethical vigilance—nurses must ensure that algorithms do not perpetuate bias, compromise patient privacy, or undermine professional judgment. Thus, nursing in digital environments requires not only technological competence but also ethical literacy and critical reflection.Education and professional development have similarly undergone significant transformation in the digital era. Nursing education increasingly incorporates digital simulation, virtual reality (VR), and online learning platforms to enhance clinical training and theoretical understanding. Virtual simulation laboratories allow students to practice critical decision-making in realistic, risk-free environments, while e-learning tools support continuous professional development and upskilling.

BENEFITS OF DIGITAL NURSING

The rise of digital nursing represents one of the most transformative developments in modern healthcare, offering a broad spectrum of benefits that enhance accessibility, efficiency, safety, and personalization in patient care. As healthcare systems worldwide undergo digital transformation, the integration of technologies such as telehealth, electronic health records (EHRs), mobile health (mHealth) applications, artificial intelligence (AI), and wearable devices has redefined the nursing profession. Digital nursing bridges geographical, temporal, and systemic barriers, ensuring that patients receive timely and high-quality care regardless of location or circumstance (Carolan et al., 2017). It enhances the capacity of nurses to deliver patient-centered care while optimizing healthcare outcomes through data-driven insights. The benefits of digital nursing extend beyond clinical outcomes—they encompass professional empowerment, operational efficiency, patient engagement, and the democratization of healthcare delivery. This digital evolution enables nurses to merge traditional caregiving values with cutting-edge technologies, creating a synergistic model of compassionate, connected, and intelligent healthcare. Digital tools have expanded the reach of nurses far beyond the walls of hospitals and clinics, enabling them to provide remote consultations, monitor patients in their homes, and offer continuous support to those in rural, isolated, or underserved regions. Through telehealth platforms, nurses can conduct virtual assessments, manage chronic conditions, and provide patient education without requiring physical presence.

Digital technologies empower nurses with real-time access to comprehensive patient data, allowing for individualized treatment plans that reflect each patient's health status, preferences, and history. Wearable sensors, mobile health trackers, and connected medical devices continuously record physiological data such as heart rate, glucose levels, blood pressure, and oxygen saturation. This wealth of information enables nurses to detect subtle health changes and intervene proactively before complications arise. AI-driven analytics further enhance personalization by identifying patterns in patient data, predicting risks, and recommending tailored interventions. For example, predictive algorithms can alert nurses to early signs of sepsis, dehydration, or medication nonadherence, enabling timely corrective actions. This shift from reactive to proactive care significantly improves patient outcomes while fostering trust and engagement (Doran et al., 2010). Personalized care also strengthens the therapeutic relationship between nurses and patients, as digital tools provide insights that enable nurses to respond with empathy and precision to individual needson paperwork and allowing them to focus more on direct patient care. Automation tools assist in medication administration, scheduling, and inventory management, minimizing human error and improving accuracy. Digital communication platforms facilitate seamless coordination among multidisciplinary teams, ensuring that critical information is shared promptly and securely. In busy hospital environments, such systems enhance patient throughput and reduce duplication of efforts. Additionally, mobile devices and handheld applications allow nurses to access patient records at the bedside, improving decision-making and response times. By leveraging data analytics, healthcare organizations can identify workflow bottlenecks and implement process improvements, ultimately enhancing efficiency and patient safety.

TELECONSULTATION AND REMOTE MONITORING

Teleconsultation and remote monitoring represent two of the most significant advancements in contemporary nursing practice, redefining the way nurses deliver, coordinate, and evaluate patient care. These digital modalities have revolutionized healthcare accessibility, continuity, and efficiency by enabling nurses to assess, guide, and monitor patients beyond traditional clinical boundaries. Teleconsultation involves the use of telecommunications technology to conduct virtual consultations between nurses, patients, and other healthcare professionals, while remote monitoring refers to the continuous or periodic observation of patients' physiological parameters using connected digital devices. Together, they form the backbone of modern telehealth systems, promoting a shift from episodic, in-person encounters to continuous, technology-mediated care (Drissi et al., 2021). The integration of teleconsultation and remote monitoring in nursing practice has improved health outcomes, optimized resource utilization, and empowered both patients and healthcare professionals in managing health proactively.The concept of teleconsultation in nursing emerged from the need to overcome geographical barriers and ensure equitable access to healthcare services. By using video conferencing, mobile health applications, and secure messaging platforms, nurses can conduct real-time consultations with patients regardless of physical distance. This capability has proven invaluable in rural and underserved regions where healthcare professionals are scarce. Through teleconsultation, nurses can perform initial assessments, follow-up evaluations, chronic disease management, medication counseling, and patient education—all without requiring patients to travel. The virtual environment allows for immediate communication, timely interventions, and ongoing support.

Teleconsultation also fosters interdisciplinary collaboration among healthcare providers. Nurses can consult with physicians, specialists, and allied health professionals through virtual case discussions and digital documentation systems (Dutton & Kozachik, 2020). This enhances care coordination and ensures that complex cases are managed comprehensively. In acute care or emergency settings, teleconsultation enables nurses to seek immediate guidance from specialists located in distant facilities, facilitating timely decision-making and life-saving interventions. For example, tele-intensive care units (tele-ICUs) allow critical care nurses to collaborate with off-site intensivists who monitor patients through high-resolution cameras and real-time data feeds. This model extends expert oversight to remote hospitals and strengthens the capacity of local nursing staff. Moreover, teleconsultation is invaluable for mental health nursing, where therapeutic communication and counseling can be conducted effectively through digital platforms, expanding access to psychological support for patients who may otherwise face stigma or logistical barriers in seeking care.Remote monitoring, as a complementary practice, has transformed how nurses track and manage patient health status over time. Through wearable sensors, mobile apps, and Internet of Things (IoT)-enabled devices, nurses can continuously observe vital signs, activity levels, and other physiological indicators such as blood pressure, oxygen saturation, heart rate, or glucose levels. Data collected from these devices are transmitted securely to healthcare databases or dashboards, where nurses analyze trends, identify anomalies, and intervene proactively. This continuous flow of health data allows for early detection of deterioration, preventing complications and hospital readmissions. For example, a nurse monitoring a patient with chronic heart failure can receive automated alerts if weight gain or heart rate fluctuations indicate fluid retention, prompting early intervention before hospitalization becomes necessary. Remote monitoring also supports post-operative care by ensuring adherence to recovery protocols and detecting potential infections or complications early. These systems provide a safety net that extends nursing care into patients' daily lives, reinforcing preventive health and long-term condition management.The synergy between teleconsultation and remote monitoring creates a comprehensive digital care ecosystem. Patients can communicate with nurses virtually while simultaneously transmitting health data through connected devices.

DIGITAL PATIENT EDUCATION

Digital patient education has become a transformative force in modern healthcare, reshaping how patients access, understand, and apply health information. Through the integration of digital platforms such as mobile health (mHealth) applications, online learning portals, virtual simulations, and social media, healthcare systems have entered an era of continuous, interactive, and patient-centered education. Nursing professionals play a pivotal role in designing, delivering, and evaluating digital education interventions that empower patients to manage their own health effectively. The shift from traditional, face-to-face instruction to technology-enabled learning environments represents more than just a change in medium—it signifies a paradigm shift toward participatory, data-driven, and lifelong health education. Digital patient education empowers individuals by promoting self-care, enhancing health literacy, and facilitating informed decision-making, ultimately leading to better health outcomes and stronger partnerships between patients and nurses (Engström et al., 2009). Through web-based portals, mobile applications, and virtual counseling sessions, nurses can deliver educational content to patients regardless of location or physical ability. For individuals in rural or underserved communities, digital tools offer vital access to evidence-based health information that might otherwise be unavailable. Multilingual content, audio-visual aids, and adaptive interfaces make digital education accessible to people with varying literacy levels and disabilities. For instance, mobile applications can include voice-guided instructions or interactive infographics that explain medication regimens or self-care procedures. Furthermore, digital resources can be accessed on demand, allowing patients to learn at their own pace and revisit information whenever necessary. This flexibility not only enhances comprehension but also promotes patient autonomy and confidence in managing health conditions.artificial intelligence (AI), and electronic health records (EHRs), nurses can design customized educational interventions that reflect a patient's medical history, demographic background, and behavioral patterns.

This collective learning not only enhances motivation but also reduces isolation and stigma, particularly for patients managing chronic or stigmatized conditions. Nurses, as facilitators in these communities, provide guidance, ensure information accuracy, and promote safe and respectful dialogue. Empowerment through education transforms the nurse-patient relationship from a hierarchical model to a collaborative partnership, emphasizing shared decision-making and mutual respect. Animations, quizzes, and simulations enhance comprehension and retention by appealing to different sensory modalities. Virtual reality (VR) and augmented reality (AR) technologies provide immersive learning experiences—for instance, simulating insulin injection techniques, wound care, or physical rehabilitation exercises. These interactive tools allow patients to practice skills in a safe, controlled environment before performing them independently. Gamification strategies, such as achievement badges or progress tracking, further increase motivation and adherence to educational programs (Gál et al., 2021). For pediatric and adolescent patients, gamified learning can make health education engaging and age-appropriate, reducing anxiety and encouraging healthy habits.

VIRTUAL SUPPORT GROUPS

Virtual support groups have emerged as an essential component of contemporary nursing practice, reflecting the ongoing digital transformation of healthcare delivery and patient engagement. These online communities—facilitated through video conferencing platforms, social media networks, and specialized health forums—create spaces for patients, caregivers, and healthcare professionals to connect, share experiences, and provide mutual support. For nurses, virtual support groups offer a powerful avenue to extend care beyond the clinical environment, fostering emotional well-being, knowledge sharing, and social connection among patients (Guru Basava Aradhya et al., 2025). The concept aligns closely with the holistic philosophy of nursing, which emphasizes not only physical health but also psychological and social well-being. As healthcare systems increasingly incorporate digital tools, nurses have assumed new roles as moderators, educators, and facilitators in these virtual environments, using technology to build trust, empathy, and resilience within diverse patient populations. The rise of virtual support groups marks a paradigm shift in nursing practice—one that bridges technology and compassion, enabling more inclusive, accessible, and patient-centered care.geography, scheduling, and mobility barriers. Virtual platforms, however, transcend these constraints, allowing patients from different regions or countries to participate from the comfort of their homes. This accessibility is particularly valuable for individuals with chronic illnesses, disabilities, or limited transportation options. For example, a patient undergoing chemotherapy can join an online cancer support group without the physical strain of hospital visits. Similarly, caregivers who cannot leave their dependents can engage in virtual meetings to seek guidance and share coping strategies. The asynchronous nature of many online groups—through discussion boards, chat rooms, or mobile applications—also accommodates participants across various time zones and personal schedules. Nurses who facilitate virtual groups use empathy, active listening, and evidence-based communication strategies to nurture supportive, nonjudgmental spaces where participants feel heard and validated. This peer interaction helps normalize experiences of pain or uncertainty, reducing psychological distress. Research has shown that patients who engage in online peer support communities experience improved coping mechanisms, reduced loneliness, and a greater sense of control over their health. Virtual support groups also promote the exchange of practical coping strategies, lifestyle adaptations, and self-care routines that may not always be discussed during clinical appointments (Havale et al., 2026).

Nurses play a central role in curating evidence-based resources, correcting misinformation, and ensuring that discussions remain factual and constructive. In many cases, these groups serve as informal learning environments where patients and caregivers acquire practical skills that empower them to make informed health decisions. For instance, a cardiac rehabilitation support group may include educational modules on medication adherence, diet modification, and stress reduction, all facilitated through digital content such as videos or infographics. This continuous flow of knowledge complements clinical care by extending learning beyond hospital visits. Moreover, digital platforms enable the storage and retrieval of educational materials, allowing participants to revisit resources at their convenience (Hersch et al., 2016). The result is a sustainable model of patient education that is both participatory and adaptive to individual needs. Nurses also benefit professionally from participating in or moderating virtual support groups. These platforms provide opportunities to develop advanced communication, digital literacy, and leadership skills while expanding the scope of nursing practice. Nurses can use virtual environments to monitor patient progress, identify psychosocial needs, and tailor care interventions based on ongoing interactions. They also gain valuable insights into patient experiences, preferences, and cultural contexts that may inform clinical decision-making. Virtual support groups can serve as early warning systems for deteriorating mental or physical health, as nurses may recognize changes in patient engagement or tone during discussions.

DIGITAL LITERACY IN NURSING

Digital literacy has become an essential competency in modern nursing practice, representing a fundamental shift in how nurses deliver care, communicate, and engage with patients in technology-driven healthcare environments (Higgins & Green, 2011). As digital transformation reshapes every aspect of healthcare—from electronic health records (EHRs) and telehealth services to artificial intelligence (AI)-assisted diagnostics and wearable health technologies—nurses are increasingly required to possess not only clinical expertise but also strong digital capabilities. Digital literacy in nursing refers to the ability to effectively locate, evaluate, use, and communicate information through digital tools and technologies. It encompasses proficiency in using healthcare information systems, understanding data privacy and security principles, engaging in virtual communication, and critically evaluating digital information sources. In the evolving digital healthcare landscape, nurses' digital literacy directly influences the quality, safety, and efficiency of patient care, as well as their ability to adapt to new technologies and maintain professional relevance. Monitoring systems, and clinical decision-support tools have become integral to daily nursing activities, and proficiency in these systems ensures accurate documentation, timely interventions, and effective coordination among healthcare teams. For example, nurses who are digitally literate can efficiently access patient data, identify abnormal trends in vital signs, and communicate critical information to physicians in real-time. They can also leverage clinical information systems to ensure medication accuracy, reduce duplication of tests, and enhance continuity of care across departments. Poor digital literacy, on the other hand, can result in documentation errors, miscommunication, and workflow inefficiencies that compromise patient safety. AI-powered literature search engines provide nurses with instant access to global knowledge resources. Digitally literate nurses can critically appraise research, integrate findings into practice, and use data analytics to evaluate patient outcomes. This capability transforms the nursing role from one of task execution to one of informed decision-making and professional leadership. For example, a nurse who can navigate PubMed, interpret data from digital dashboards, and use statistical software can make evidence-driven judgments that enhance patient care quality. In this way, digital literacy supports lifelong learning, professional growth, and the advancement of the nursing discipline as a whole. As healthcare becomes more consumer-oriented, patients increasingly seek information about their conditions online.

Figure 1. Defining digital nursing

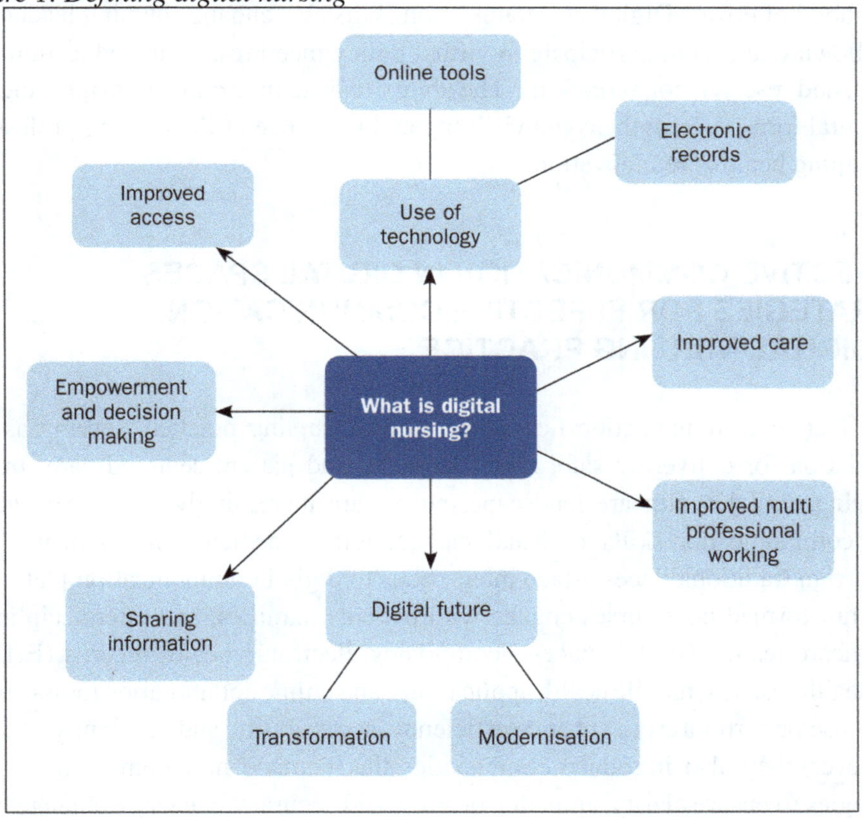

Understanding how to interpret, secure, and ethically use this data is central to responsible nursing practice. Digital literacy equips nurses to comply with privacy regulations such as the Health Insurance Portability and Accountability Act (HIPAA) or the General Data Protection Regulation (GDPR), ensuring the confidentiality and integrity of patient information. Moreover, nurses must be able to recognize cybersecurity threats—such as phishing, malware, or unauthorized data sharing—and take appropriate precautions to safeguard sensitive health data. Ethical considerations, including informed consent in telehealth, data transparency, and equitable technology use, also fall within the domain of digital literacy (Higgins et al., 2003). A nurse who is aware of these principles contributes With the increasing reliance on digital platforms for coordination—such as teleconferencing tools, digital dashboards, and shared care records—nurses must be adept at communicating effectively through digital channels. Digital fluency enables them to exchange information with physicians, pharmacists, and allied health professionals in real time, regardless of location. For example, during a telemedicine session, a nurse may collect patient data, update the EHR, and share clinical notes with multiple team members instantly. This seamless information flow improves decision-making speed and reduces the likelihood of errors. Digital communication skills also enhance nursing leadership by allowing nurses to participate in virtual policy meetings, online education sessions, and research collaborations. The ability to articulate clinical insights clearly in digital forums strengthens the visibility and influence of the nursing profession in shaping healthcare innovation.

EFFECTIVE COMMUNICATION IN DIGITAL SPACES: STRATEGIES FOR EFFECTIVE COMMUNICATION IN DIGITAL NURSING PRACTICE

Effective communication lies at the core of nursing practice, serving as the foundation for delivering safe, compassionate, and patient-centered care. In the evolving digital healthcare landscape, nurses are increasingly required to adapt their communication skills to virtual and technology-mediated environments. The shift from traditional face-to-face interactions to digital communication platforms has transformed how nurses engage with patients, families, and interdisciplinary healthcare teams. Digital spaces—comprising electronic health records (EHRs), telehealth systems, mobile health applications, and online collaboration tools—offer immense opportunities to enhance efficiency, accessibility, and continuity of care. However, they also introduce complexities that demand new competencies and strategies to ensure clarity, empathy, privacy, and accuracy in every exchange. The ability to communicate effectively in these digital contexts is not merely a technical skill but a professional imperative that directly influences patient safety, satisfaction, and clinical outcomes. Therefore, understanding and implementing best practices in digital communication is essential for nurses to navigate modern healthcare settings effectively. Nurses must maintain the same ethical standards, empathy, and professionalism online as they do in face-to-face interactions. This includes using clear, respectful language, maintaining appropriate tone in written communication, and ensuring that all digital correspondence aligns with institutional policies and patient confidentiality regulations such as the Health Insurance Portability and Accountability Act (HIPAA).

Digital literacy encompasses not only the ability to operate devices and software but also an understanding of data security, online etiquette, and accessibility considerations. Nurses should be trained to use clinical documentation systems accurately, ensuring that all patient data is entered, stored, and shared appropriately. In telehealth settings, for example, nurses must ensure that audiovisual technology functions properly, that communication channels are secure, and that patients are guided in using digital tools confidently. Providing pre-session instructions, testing audio and video quality, and maintaining a distraction-free environment all contribute to more meaningful virtual interactions. Moreover, familiarity with assistive technologies and accessibility features enables nurses to accommodate patients with disabilities, language barriers, or limited technological experience, thus ensuring equity and inclusiveness in digital care delivery.active listening, and the intentional use of verbal cues to convey empathy and understanding. In teleconsultations, nurses can employ techniques such as maintaining eye contact through the camera, nodding, and using affirming verbal responses to replicate the warmth and attentiveness of in-person interactions. They must also be sensitive to the emotional cues expressed through tone, pauses, and patient word choice, responding in ways that validate patient feelings and foster trust.

BEST PRACTICES FOR MANAGING AND SECURING PATIENT DATA IN DIGITAL ENVIRONMENTS

In the contemporary healthcare landscape, data management and security have become integral pillars of nursing practice, underpinning the ethical, legal, and professional responsibilities of healthcare providers. The digital transformation of healthcare—driven by electronic health records (EHRs), telehealth services, mobile health applications, wearable devices, and cloud-based systems—has revolutionized how patient information is collected, stored, and shared. However, this digital expansion also presents unprecedented challenges related to data protection, privacy, and cybersecurity. As nurses increasingly engage with digital technologies, their role in ensuring the integrity, confidentiality, and availability of patient data becomes more critical than ever. Effective data management not only supports clinical decision-making and continuity of care but also builds patient trust and safeguards the reputation of healthcare organizations (Jakel et al., 2016). To achieve these goals, nurses and healthcare institutions must adhere to rigorous best practices in data governance, cybersecurity protocols, and ethical standards that align with global regulations such as the Health Insurance Portability and Accountability Act (HIPAA) in the United States, the General Data Protection Regulation (GDPR) in the European Union, and similar frameworks worldwide. Data governance encompasses the policies, procedures, and standards that define how patient information is created, stored, accessed, and shared within healthcare systems. Effective governance requires a clearly defined structure that assigns accountability for data handling, establishes data quality standards, and enforces compliance with privacy regulations.

Nurses, as primary users of patient information, must understand the principles of data stewardship—ensuring that data are accurate, complete, timely, and relevant. Accurate documentation in EHRs, for example, supports safe clinical decisions and effective interprofessional communication. Data governance also involves data classification and retention policies that dictate how long patient records are maintained and when they should be securely disposed of. This helps reduce the risk of data breaches caused by improper handling of obsolete records. Furthermore, incorporating metadata standards and data interoperability protocols ensures that information can be safely exchanged between systems while maintaining consistency and integrity. Including ransomware, phishing, and malware intrusions, every nurse must be equipped with fundamental cybersecurity knowledge and vigilance. Human error remains a significant vulnerability in data security, making continuous education and awareness training essential. Nurses should be trained to recognize suspicious emails, avoid clicking on unknown links, use strong and unique passwords, and log out of systems after each use. Multi-factor authentication (MFA) and role-based access controls are best practices that limit system access only to authorized personnel, thereby minimizing risks of unauthorized data exposure (Kloos et al., 2019). Regular system audits, intrusion detection mechanisms, and encrypted communication channels are also critical measures for preventing data breaches. Institutions should implement advanced firewalls, antivirus software, and security monitoring systems, complemented by clear incident response plans that guide staff on how to act in case of a suspected security breach. These proactive strategies not only mitigate potential threats but also enhance institutional resilience against cyber vulnerabilities.

Nurses should be aware of whether their systems use encryption protocols such as SSL/TLS for web-based communications and AES (Advanced Encryption Standard) for stored data. Cloud-based healthcare platforms, though efficient, require strict vetting of third-party vendors to ensure compliance with security certifications and data protection standards. Secure backup and disaster recovery systems are also essential components of data management. Regularly backing up patient data—preferably in multiple secure locations—ensures that critical information remains available in the event of hardware failure, system outage, or cyberattack. Additionally, data integrity checks and version controls help detect unauthorized modifications or corruption of records, maintaining the authenticity and reliability of digital patient data are foundational ethical principles that must be upheld in every aspect of data handling. Nurses must ensure that patients understand how their personal information will be used, shared, and stored, especially when digital technologies such as telehealth or remote monitoring devices are involved. Informed consent should not be a one-time event but an ongoing dialogue, particularly when new technologies or data uses are introduced. Patients have the right to access their own health data, request corrections, and control the sharing of their information.

THE APPLICATION OF CBT IN DIGITAL NURSING PRACTICE

Cognitive-Behavioral Therapy (CBT) has long been recognized as a highly effective, evidence-based psychotherapeutic intervention for a wide range of mental health conditions, including anxiety, depression, post-traumatic stress disorder (PTSD), and chronic pain. Traditionally delivered in face-to-face settings, CBT focuses on identifying and modifying maladaptive thoughts, emotions, and behaviors through structured, goal-oriented interventions. In recent years, the digital transformation of healthcare has expanded the reach and accessibility of CBT, enabling its integration into digital environments such as telehealth platforms, mobile applications, online therapy portals, and virtual support programs. Digital CBT offers unique advantages, including increased flexibility, accessibility for underserved populations, cost-effectiveness, and the potential for real-time monitoring and feedback. For nurses, particularly those engaged in mental health care, chronic disease management, and patient support, understanding how to effectively apply CBT in digital contexts is critical. It requires not only mastery of core CBT principles but also proficiency in digital tools, awareness of ethical and legal considerations, and the ability to foster therapeutic rapport in virtual spaces (Marvaldi et al., 2021). The application of CBT in digital nursing practice represents a convergence of psychological expertise, technological competence, and patient-centered care, underscoring the evolving role of nurses as facilitators of mental well-being in the digital age. Core CBT interventions—such as cognitive restructuring, behavioral activation, exposure therapy, and skills training—can be effectively translated into digital formats with careful planning and structured protocols.

Active listening, reflective questioning, validation of emotions, and consistent feedback are critical in fostering trust and promoting adherence to therapy. Nurses must also consider patient preferences, technological comfort levels, and potential barriers to engagement, such as limited internet access, privacy concerns, or cognitive and sensory impairments. By creating a safe, supportive, and user-friendly digital environment, nurses can enhance the therapeutic alliance, which is a key predictor of CBT effectiveness and positive clinical outcomes or the Generalized Anxiety Disorder (GAD-7) scale for anxiety, can be administered electronically, allowing for continuous monitoring of symptom severity and treatment response. Mobile applications and online platforms often incorporate real-time data tracking, mood diaries, thought records, and behavioral logs, which provide nurses with rich information to guide therapeutic interventions. These tools facilitate timely identification of patient progress or setbacks, enabling adaptive modifications to the CBT plan. Automated feedback and analytics can supplement nurse guidance, offering patients personalized recommendations, reminders, and reinforcement strategies (Yildiz & Yildiz, 2022). However, nurses must remain vigilant in interpreting data accurately, contextualizing quantitative metrics within qualitative patient experiences, and ensuring that technology augments rather than replaces clinical judgment. CBT platforms often provide patients with tools to practice skills independently, encouraging active participation in their mental health care.

THE ROLE OF MINDFULNESS IN PROMOTING DIGITAL WELLNESS IN NURSING PRACTICE

In the contemporary nursing environment, digital technologies play a pivotal role in patient care, documentation, communication, and professional development. Electronic health records (EHRs), telehealth systems, mobile health applications, wearable monitoring devices, and digital collaboration platforms have transformed the scope and efficiency of nursing practice. While these advancements enhance accessibility, streamline workflows, and facilitate patient engagement, they also introduce challenges associated with information overload, digital fatigue, reduced attention span, and increased stress levels among nursing professionals. The constant interaction with screens, notifications, and multitasking demands can lead to cognitive and emotional strain, negatively impacting clinical performance, decision-making, and overall well-being. In response to these challenges, the integration of mindfulness practices has emerged as a valuable strategy for promoting digital wellness among nurses. Mindfulness, defined as the intentional, nonjudgmental awareness of the present moment, offers nurses a framework to cultivate self-regulation, resilience, and emotional balance in environments dominated by rapid technological interactions (Ye, 2021). By fostering a conscious, reflective approach to digital engagement, mindfulness supports sustainable, effective, and patient-centered nursing practice. navigate multiple digital platforms simultaneously—updating EHRs, responding to messages, coordinating care, and monitoring patient data. These tasks, if performed without conscious attention, can lead to automatic, distracted behavior that increases the risk of errors, miscommunication, and cognitive overload. Mindfulness practices encourage nurses to pause, focus attention on the task at hand, and approach each interaction with deliberate intention. For instance, before entering patient information into an EHR or sending a telehealth communication, a nurse can take a brief mindful pause to center attention, ensure accuracy, and cultivate clarity. This intentional approach enhances the quality of digital documentation, reduces mistakes, and promotes thoughtful, patient-centered communication. Over time, incorporating mindfulness into routine digital tasks cultivates sustained concentration, reduces reactive behavior, and strengthens the nurse's ability to manage high-demand, technology-intensive workflows without succumbing to fatigue or distraction.

Notifications, alerts, and data monitoring can contribute to feelings of overwhelm, anxiety, and cognitive saturation. Mindfulness interventions, such as breathing exercises, body scans, and focused attention techniques, provide nurses with tools to regulate emotional responses and maintain equanimity amidst digital and clinical pressures (WHO, 2022a). By recognizing and accepting internal experiences without judgment, nurses develop resilience to stressors, preventing digital fatigue and burnout. Mindfulness also supports reflective practice, enabling nurses to process challenging patient encounters, ethical dilemmas, or technological frustrations in a constructive manner. This emotional stability directly benefits patient care, as nurses who maintain calm, present, and regulated states are better equipped to make accurate clinical decisions, communicate effectively, and demonstrate empathy. Devices in healthcare can blur the lines between work and personal life, contributing to chronic stress and decreased well-being. Mindfulness encourages nurses to establish intentional boundaries regarding device usage, work-related communications, and digital accessibility. Strategies such as scheduled email or messaging check-ins, designated "digital-free" periods, and conscious disengagement from non-urgent notifications help nurses reclaim focus and energy for restorative activities. By cultivating awareness of their physiological and emotional states, nurses can recognize signs of digital fatigue early and implement restorative practices such as brief mindfulness pauses, guided meditation, or short walks. These practices not only protect nurses' health but also enhance cognitive clarity, productivity, and presence in patient care activities. Mindful boundary setting promotes sustainable engagement with digital tools, ensuring that technology serves as an enabler rather than a source of stress or distraction.

BUILDING AND MAINTAINING THERAPEUTIC RELATIONSHIPS IN DIGITAL ENVIRONMENTS

Therapeutic relationships are foundational to nursing practice, underpinning effective patient care, trust, collaboration, and positive health outcomes (van der Meer et al., 2020). Traditionally, these relationships have been developed and nurtured through direct, face-to-face interactions, where nurses rely on verbal and non-verbal cues, empathy, active listening, and personal presence to establish rapport (Vallières et al., 2016). However, the rapid digitization of healthcare has introduced new platforms for patient engagement, including telehealth consultations, mobile health applications, virtual support groups, patient portals, and online care coordination systems. These digital environments offer significant benefits, such as increased accessibility, continuity of care, and flexible communication, particularly for patients in remote or underserved areas. Yet, they also present unique challenges for the formation and maintenance of therapeutic relationships, as traditional relational cues may be absent or altered. In digital nursing practice, cultivating effective therapeutic relationships requires intentional strategies that integrate professional competence, digital literacy, empathy, ethical awareness, and cultural sensitivity. Nurses must adapt traditional relational skills to virtual contexts, ensuring that technology enhances rather than undermines the humanistic essence of care. Nurses must employ precise, empathetic language in written communications and maintain professional demeanor in video or audio interactions. Trust is further reinforced by transparency regarding confidentiality, data security, and the limits of digital interactions, such as the response time for messaging or the scope of care provided virtually. Patients are more likely to engage fully and adhere to care recommendations when they perceive their nurse as competent, attentive, and trustworthy in the digital space. Strategies such as structured introduction messages, clear explanations of care plans, and the use of consistent communication channels can help establish this foundational trust, creating a sense of safety and psychological security for patients.

In text-based interactions, clarity, tone, and responsiveness are crucial, as the absence of visual cues increases the risk of misinterpretation. Nurses should use concise, patient-centered language, avoid jargon, and employ reflective or summarizing statements to ensure mutual understanding. Techniques such as open-ended questions, validation of emotions, and structured follow-up messages foster active dialogue, reinforce engagement, and demonstrate respect for the patient's perspective (Tufanaru et al., 2020). Moreover, nurses must be mindful of timing, frequency, and method of communication to align with patient preferences, ensuring that digital interactions are supportive, non-intrusive, and tailored to individual needs of patient experiences, and responsive listening techniques to create a sense of connection. Emotional attunement in digital spaces requires heightened sensitivity to subtle indicators of patient distress, frustration, or confusion, which may manifest through tone, pacing, choice of words, or behavioral patterns in the digital environment. Nurses should actively interpret these cues, ask clarifying questions, and provide supportive feedback, ensuring that patients feel heard, validated, and emotionally supported. By intentionally integrating empathy into digital interactions, nurses preserve the relational essence of care, mitigating the risk of depersonalization and fostering a sense of therapeutic alliance personalization of care. Nurses can leverage digital tools to provide patients with access to educational resources, self-management applications, symptom tracking systems, and virtual coaching. Integrating these resources into the therapeutic relationship encourages patients to take an active role in their health, promotes adherence to care plans, and facilitates informed decision-making. Personalized communication strategies, such as tailoring messages to patient literacy levels, cultural context, and learning preferences, reinforce engagement and demonstrate respect for individual needs. Nurses' ability to guide patients through digital tools, interpret data, and provide timely, meaningful feedback strengthens both the relational and functional aspects of care, ensuring that technology serves as a facilitator of connection rather than a barrier.

ETHICAL CONSIDERATIONS IN DIGITAL NURSING

The integration of digital technologies into nursing practice has revolutionized healthcare delivery, offering opportunities to enhance patient care, improve communication, and facilitate data-driven decision-making. However, the adoption of digital tools in nursing also introduces a complex landscape of ethical considerations that necessitate careful reflection and proactive management to ensure that technology supports patient-centered care without compromising moral, legal, or professional standards. Ethical considerations in digital nursing encompass a wide array of issues, including patient privacy and confidentiality, informed consent, data security, equity of access, professional boundaries, accountability, and the potential impact of artificial intelligence (AI) and algorithm-driven decision-making on clinical judgment. Patient privacy and confidentiality remain foundational ethical obligations in nursing practice, yet the digitalization of health records, telehealth consultations, and mobile health applications poses significant risks for unauthorized access, data breaches, and inadvertent disclosure of sensitive information (Motamed-Jahromi et al., 2017). Nurses must therefore adhere to stringent protocols for data protection, comply with regulatory frameworks such as the Health Insurance Portability and Accountability Act (HIPAA) in the United States or the General Data Protection Regulation (GDPR) in Europe, and ensure that patients are adequately informed about how their data will be collected, stored, shared, and utilized.

Informed consent in digital nursing also requires nuanced attention, as patients must understand not only the clinical aspects of their care but also the technological dimensions, including the potential risks and benefits associated with telehealth platforms, wearable devices, remote monitoring systems, and AI-assisted interventions. Nurses are ethically obligated to provide clear, comprehensible explanations and to verify that patients have the capacity and resources to make informed decisions, particularly when dealing with vulnerable populations such as older adults, individuals with cognitive impairments, or those with limited digital literacy. Equity and accessibility constitute another central ethical concern, as the digital divide may disproportionately affect marginalized or underserved populations, leading to disparities in access to digital health services and information. Ethical nursing practice requires advocacy for inclusive design, equitable access, and interventions that minimize disparities, ensuring that technological advancements enhance rather than undermine health equity. Professional boundaries in digital nursing also demand careful attention, particularly when communication extends beyond traditional face-to-face interactions to virtual platforms, social media, and mobile messaging. Nurses must navigate the complexities of maintaining therapeutic relationships, avoiding dual relationships or over-familiarity, and ensuring that digital communication upholds professional integrity and respect.

Accountability and transparency in digital nursing practice are equally crucial, especially in the context of AI-driven decision-making, predictive analytics, and algorithm-based clinical recommendations. While these technologies can enhance efficiency and support clinical judgment, they also raise questions about responsibility when errors occur, the potential for bias in algorithmic outputs, and the need for human oversight to safeguard patient welfare. Ethical principles such as beneficence, nonmaleficence, autonomy, and justice must guide nurses in evaluating the appropriateness of digital interventions, balancing innovation with the imperative to do no harm, respect patient autonomy, and promote fair and equitable care. Data security, including encryption, secure authentication, and robust cyber hygiene practices, forms a critical component of ethical digital nursing, as breaches can result in tangible harm to patients, loss of trust, and legal liabilities. Nurses must remain vigilant in monitoring security protocols, educating patients about safe use of digital tools, and advocating for institutional policies that prioritize the protection of digital health information. In addition to technological considerations, ethical challenges in digital nursing extend to the social and psychological impacts of digital care delivery (Popay et al., 2006). The impersonal nature of virtual interactions, potential depersonalization of care, and reliance on automated systems may affect patient engagement, satisfaction, and emotional support.

Ethical practice requires nurses to maintain empathy, presence, and responsiveness even within virtual environments, ensuring that technology complements rather than replaces the humanistic elements of nursing care. Furthermore, continuous professional development and ethical training in digital competencies are essential, enabling nurses to navigate emerging technologies responsibly, identify potential ethical dilemmas, and implement strategies that uphold professional and moral standards. Multidisciplinary collaboration is also critical, involving ethicists, IT specialists, healthcare administrators, and policymakers to develop guidelines, protocols, and frameworks that address ethical concerns systematically and comprehensively. Research ethics in digital nursing constitutes an additional dimension, particularly as data from electronic health records, wearable devices, and mobile applications are increasingly utilized for research and quality improvement initiatives. Nurses involved in research must ensure informed consent, data anonymization, protection against re-identification, and transparency regarding the purpose, scope, and potential outcomes of digital research. Legal and regulatory compliance intersects with ethical obligations, reinforcing the need for nurses to remain informed about evolving standards, reporting requirements, and professional codes of conduct that govern digital practice. Ethical considerations in digital nursing also extend to global perspectives, recognizing cultural sensitivities, differing regulatory environments, and varying expectations of privacy, autonomy, and professional accountability across regions. Nurses must be culturally competent and adaptable, ensuring that digital interventions are ethically aligned with the values and norms of diverse patient populations.

MAINTAINING BOUNDARIES IN DIGITAL ENVIRONMENTS

The increasing integration of digital technologies in nursing practice has transformed the ways in which nurses interact with patients, colleagues, and interdisciplinary teams, offering unprecedented opportunities for communication, collaboration, and care delivery. Telehealth platforms, electronic messaging systems, social media, and mobile health applications facilitate real-time engagement, remote monitoring, and personalized patient support, enhancing efficiency and accessibility (Page et al., 2021). However, the shift to digital environments also presents significant challenges in maintaining professional boundaries, a cornerstone of ethical and safe nursing practice. Professional boundaries refer to the limits that define the therapeutic nurse-patient relationship, ensuring that interactions remain focused on patient well-being, respect autonomy, and prevent exploitation, over-involvement, or conflicts of interest. In digital contexts, these boundaries can be blurred due to the immediacy, informality, and omnipresence of digital communication tools, which may lead to dual relationships, over-familiarity, unsolicited contact, or inappropriate disclosure of personal information (Sasikala et al., 2026). Maintaining boundaries in digital nursing practice requires a comprehensive understanding of both ethical principles and practical strategies that safeguard the professional integrity of nurses while supporting patient-centered care. One key strategy involves establishing clear communication guidelines and protocols for digital interactions, including defining appropriate channels, response times, and acceptable content for messaging, email, video consultations, and social media engagement. Nurses must ensure that these guidelines are consistently communicated to patients, caregivers, and colleagues to manage expectations, prevent misunderstandings, and reinforce professional roles.

The use of professional accounts and institutional platforms, rather than personal devices or social media profiles, further delineates boundaries, reducing the risk of informal or dual relationships and preserving privacy for both patients and nurses (Nguyen et al., 2021). Confidentiality and privacy considerations are integral to boundary maintenance, as digital communication can inadvertently expose sensitive patient information through unencrypted messages, screenshots, or shared devices. Nurses must adhere to data protection regulations, utilize secure platforms, and educate patients about safe communication practices, including avoiding the sharing of personal contact information or private social media accounts. Self-disclosure represents another area where boundaries may be challenged in digital environments; while some degree of professional transparency can foster trust and rapport, excessive sharing of personal information may compromise professional judgment, blur relational limits, and shift focus from patient needs to the nurse's personal narrative. Establishing explicit policies regarding appropriate self-disclosure and model professional behavior in all interactions are critical components of maintaining ethical boundaries. Digital environments also necessitate careful attention to time management and availability, as patients may expect continuous access to nursing support through text messages, emails, or telehealth platforms. Setting clear boundaries regarding response times, consultation schedules, and after-hours availability preserves work-life balance for nurses and prevents burnout while maintaining consistency and predictability in patient care.

Training and professional development in digital communication skills, boundary management, and ethical decision-making are essential to equip nurses with the competencies to navigate the complexities of online interactions (Satyanarayana et al., 2026). These programs should incorporate scenario-based learning, reflective practice, and discussion of case studies that illustrate potential boundary violations and strategies to prevent them. Interdisciplinary collaboration is equally important, involving requires adherence to organizational social media policies, avoiding personal engagement with patients online, and exercising caution when sharing educational content to prevent misinterpretation or unintended disclosure. Reflective practice is a vital strategy for sustaining professional boundaries, allowing nurses to critically examine their interactions, identify areas of vulnerability, and implement corrective measures proactively. Regular supervision, (Porter & Wang, 2022) peer consultation, and mentorship provide additional support in navigating complex digital interactions, ensuring that decisions align with professional ethics and patient-centered care principles. The integration of emerging technologies, such as AI-driven chatbots, virtual reality platforms, and remote patient monitoring systems, introduces additional boundary considerations, including automated interactions, data interpretation, and the potential for over-reliance on digital tools. Nurses must maintain oversight of these technologies, ensuring that they complement rather than replace therapeutic relationships, preserve human connection, and uphold ethical standards. Legal and regulatory frameworks further reinforce the importance of maintaining boundaries in digital nursing practice.

EMERGING TRENDS IN DIGITAL NURSING

The rapid advancement of digital technologies is profoundly transforming nursing practice, giving rise to innovative approaches that enhance patient care, optimize clinical workflows, and expand the scope of healthcare delivery. Emerging trends in digital nursing encompass a range of technological, procedural, and he constraints of physical proximity. This trend has been accelerated by the COVID-19 pandemic, which highlighted the need for flexible, technology-enabled care delivery and demonstrated the potential of virtual platforms to maintain patient engagement, reduce hospital readmissions, and enhance overall health outcomes. Alongside telehealth, mobile health (mHealth) applications and wearable devices are revolutionizing patient self-management and monitoring, allowing nurses to track vital signs, activity levels, medication adherence, and symptom progression in real-time. These technologies enable proactive intervention, personalized care plans, and data-driven decision-making, fostering patient empowerment and enhancing the nurse's ability to deliver individualized care. Artificial intelligence (AI) and machine learning represent another transformative trend, offering tools for predictive analytics, clinical decision support, and automated documentation. AI algorithms can analyze large volumes of patient data to identify patterns, predict health risks, and generate recommendations that assist nurses in early detection of complications, prioritizing interventions, and optimizing resource allocation. While these technologies augment nursing practice, they also require critical oversight to ensure ethical use, prevent bias, and maintain patient-centered care.

Robotics and automation are emerging in clinical and community settings, streamlining repetitive tasks, supporting rehabilitation, and assisting with mobility and medication administration. The use of robotic devices not only improves efficiency but also enables nurses to focus on complex, cognitively demanding tasks, enhancing both productivity and quality of care (Sreekanthaswamy et al., 2026). Virtual reality (VR) and augmented reality (AR) are gaining traction as tools for patient education, pain management, and clinical training. VR simulations allow patients to engage in immersive learning experiences, such as managing chronic disease symptoms or preparing for surgical procedures, while AR applications provide nurses with real-time visual overlays that facilitate complex interventions, procedural guidance, and remote mentorship. Blockchain technology is emerging as a promising solution for secure, transparent, and interoperable management of health records, enabling nurses to verify patient information, track care transitions, and enhance data integrity across multiple healthcare organizations. This trend aligns with growing concerns about cybersecurity, privacy, and the ethical stewardship of patient data, highlighting the intersection of technology, ethics, and clinical practice. Another notable trend is the adoption of digital therapeutic interventions and virtual care programs, including cognitive-behavioral therapy apps, mindfulness platforms, and remote rehabilitation services (Munn et al., 2014). These interventions expand nursing roles into health promotion, mental health support, and chronic disease management, leveraging technology to deliver evidence-based care in accessible, scalable formats. Interprofessional collaboration is also being reshaped by digital platforms, allowing nurses to coordinate care seamlessly with physicians, pharmacists, social workers, and other healthcare professionals through integrated electronic health records (EHRs), secure messaging, and collaborative dashboards. This integration improves communication, reduces errors, and enhances efficiency in care delivery, supporting holistic, patient-centered approaches.

CONCLUSION

The successful implementation of digital nursing practices in healthcare settings requires a strategic, evidence-based approach that integrates technology, clinical workflows, staff competencies, patient engagement, and organizational policies. As healthcare systems increasingly adopt telehealth platforms, electronic health records (EHRs), mobile health applications, wearable devices, and data analytics tools, establishing best practices for digital nursing implementation is essential Change management strategies are also essential, as transitioning from traditional to digital workflows can encounter resistance due to fear of technology, concerns about increased workload, or uncertainty regarding professional roles. Best practices include providing clear communication about the purpose and benefits of digital initiatives, setting realistic timelines for adoption, and creating structured support mechanisms that guide staff through the transition. Education and training are central to successful implementation, as nurses must develop competencies in digital literacy, data security, telehealth communication, and device operation. Ongoing professional development programs, simulation-based learning, and mentorship opportunities enable nurses to gain confidence in using digital tools, troubleshoot technical issues, and apply technology effectively to patient care. Incorporating standardized protocols and guidelines for digital nursing practice ensures consistency, safety, and quality of care across the organization. These protocols may include procedures coordinated care delivery. Evaluation and continuous improvement mechanisms are critical for sustaining the effectiveness of digital nursing practices. Metrics such as patient satisfaction, clinical outcomes, workflow efficiency, error rates, and staff adoption levels provide insights into the impact of digital interventions and inform iterative refinements. Feedback loops involving nurses, patients, and interdisciplinary teams enable organizations to address challenges, optimize functionality, and adapt to evolving technological advancements. Leadership support is a key determinant of successful implementation, as nurse leaders and administrators play a pivotal role in securing resources, advocating for policy development, fostering a culture of innovation, and reinforcing accountability.

Organizational culture that values digital competence, ethical practice, and patient-centered care facilitates the acceptance and sustainability of new technologies. Ethical considerations should be embedded throughout implementation, ensuring equitable access to digital tools, preventing disparities, and maintaining professional boundaries in virtual care environments. Addressing the digital divide requires proactive strategies, such as providing devices for underserved populations, ensuring reliable internet access, and offering training to enhance digital literacy among patients and caregivers. Collaboration with technology vendors, IT specialists, and academic institutions supports the development of user-centered design, intuitive interfaces, and evidence-based digital interventions that are adaptable to diverse healthcare settings. Standardizing policies for data governance, consent, documentation, and telehealth interactions ensures compliance with legal and professional standards while promoting transparency and trust. Simulation and pilot testing prior to full-scale deployment allow organizations to identify technical issues, workflow bottlenecks, and usability challenges, mitigating risks before broader implementation. Integrating artificial intelligence, predictive analytics, and decision-support tools requires careful evaluation of algorithmic accuracy, bias, and ethical implications, with nurses maintaining oversight to contextualize recommendations and ensure patient safety.

Continuous professional development and competency assessment ensure that nurses remain proficient in emerging technologies, understand updates in digital systems, and can apply evidence-based practices effectively. Cross-disciplinary collaboration and interprofessional training reinforce team-based care, enhance communication, and optimize coordination in digital environments. Incorporating patient feedback in evaluating digital nursing initiatives ensures that tools are accessible, comprehensible, and culturally sensitive, fostering trust, satisfaction, and adherence to care plans. Scalability and sustainability planning are essential, allowing digital nursing practices to adapt to changing patient needs, technological advancements, and organizational growth. Resource allocation, technical support, and maintenance protocols must be established to ensure the long-term effectiveness and reliability of digital interventions. Finally, fostering a culture of innovation and reflective practice empowers nurses to contribute to digital transformation, identify opportunities for improvement, and advocate for patient-centered technology integration. an increasingly digital world. Best practices in digital nursing implementation, therefore, encompass a holistic approach that integrates technology, ethics, human factors, education, policy, and continuous improvement, ensuring that digital innovations are effectively translated into meaningful, sustainable improvements in healthcare delivery and patient outcomes.

REFERENCES

Ackerman, C. E., Warren, M. A., & Donaldson, S. I. (2018). Scaling the heights of positive psychology: A systematic review of measurement scales. *International Journal of Wellbeing*, *8*, 1–21.

Bolier, L., Ketelaar, S. M., & Nieuwenhuijsen, K.. (2014). Workplace mental health promotion online to enhance well-being of nurses and allied health professionals: A cluster-randomized controlled trial. *Internet Interventions : the Application of Information Technology in Mental and Behavioural Health*, *1*, 196–204.

Carolan, S., Harris, P. R., & Cavanagh, K. (2017). Improving employee well-being and effectiveness: Systematic review and meta-analysis of web-based psychological interventions delivered in the workplace. *Journal of Medical Internet Research*, *19*, e271. PMID: 28747293

Doran, D. M., Haynes, R. B., & Kushniruk, A.. (2010). Supporting evidence-based practice for nurses through information technologies. *Worldviews on Evidence-Based Nursing*, *7*, 4–15. PMID: 20028493

Drissi, N., Ouhbi, S., & Marques, G.. (2021). A systematic literature review on e-Mental health solutions to assist health care workers during COVID-19. *Telemedicine Journal and e-Health*, *27*, 594–602. PMID: 32970532

Dutton, S., & Kozachik, S. L. (2020). Evaluating the outcomes of a web-based stress management program for nurses and nursing assistants. *Worldviews on Evidence-Based Nursing*, *17*, 32–38. PMID: 31912984

Engström, M., Scandurra, I., & Ljunggren, B.. (2009). Evaluation of OLD@HOME virtual health record staff opinions of the system and satisfaction with work. *Telemedicine Journal and e-Health*, *15*(1), 53–61. PMID: 19199848

Gál, É., tefan, S., & Cristea, I. A. (2021). The efficacy of mindfulness meditation apps in enhancing users' well-being and mental health related outcomes: A meta-analysis of randomized controlled trials. *Journal of Affective Disorders*, *279*, 131–142. PMID: 33049431

Guru Basava Aradhya, S., Chithambar Gupta, V., Selvakumar, P., Raman, M. S., Singh, J., Manjunath, T. C., & Sharma, M. (2025). Health Crises and Digitalization: Digital Health. In Yıldırım, S. Y., & Kandpal, V. (Eds.), *Sustainable Digitalization Strategies in Business and Healthcare* (pp. 171–198). IGI Global Scientific Publishing., DOI: 10.4018/979-8-3373-5087-5.ch007

Havale, D. S., Patole, J., Anute, N., Rane, D. P., Shah, A. H., & Selvakumar, P. (2026). Digital Tools and Resources for Teaching Sustainability. In Hans, E., & Hans, A. (Eds.), *Harnessing E-Learning to Create a Sustainable Future* (pp. 45–74). IGI Global Scientific Publishing., DOI: 10.4018/979-8-3373-0112-9.ch003

Hersch, R. K., Cook, R. F., & Deitz, D. K.. (2016). Reducing nurses' stress: A randomized controlled trial of a web-based stress management program for nurses. *Applied Nursing Research, 32*, 18–25. PMID: 27969025

Higgins, J., & Green, S. (2011) Combining groups. In: Cochrane Handbook for Systematic Reviews of Interventions Version 5.1.0, p. 7.7.3.8. Available at: https://training.cochrane.org/handbook/archive/v5.1/ (accessed 11 August 2022).

Higgins, J. P. T., Thompson, S. G., & Deeks, J. J.. (2003). Measuring inconsistency in meta-analyses. *British Medical Journal, 327*, 557–560. PMID: 12958120

Jakel, P., Kenney, J., & Ludan, N.. (2016). Effects of the use of the provider resilience mobile application in reducing compassion fatigue in oncology nursing. *Clinical Journal of Oncology Nursing, 20*, 611–616. PMID: 27857259

Kloos, N., Drossaert, C. H. C., & Bohlmeijer, E. T.. (2019). Online positive psychology intervention for nursing home staff: A cluster-randomized controlled feasibility trial of effectiveness and acceptability. *International Journal of Nursing Studies, 98*, 48–56. PMID: 31295708

Marvaldi, M., Mallet, J., & Dubertret, C.. (2021). Anxiety, depression, trauma-related, and sleep disorders among healthcare workers during the COVID-19 pandemic: A systematic review and meta-analysis. *Neuroscience and Biobehavioral Reviews, 126*, 252–264. PMID: 33774085

Motamed-Jahromi, M., Fereidouni, Z., & Dehghan, A. (2017). Effectiveness of positive thinking training program on nurses' quality of work life through smartphone applications. *International Scholarly Research Notices, 2017*, 1–6. PMID: 28589174

Munn, Z., Tufanaru, C., & Aromataris, E. (2014). Data extraction and synthesis. *The American Journal of Nursing, 114*, 49–54. PMID: 25742352

Nguyen, O. T., Shah, S., & Gartland, A. J.. (2021). Factors associated with nurse well-being in relation to electronic health record use: A systematic review. *Journal of the American Medical Informatics Association : JAMIA, 28*, 1288–1297. PMID: 33367819

Page, M. J., McKenzie, J. E., & Bossuyt, P. M.. (2021). The PRISMA 2020 statement: An updated guideline for reporting systematic reviews. *BMJ (Clinical Research Ed.), 372*(71). PMID: 33782057

Popay, J., Roberts, H., Sowden, A., ... (2006) Guidance on the conduct of narrative synthesis in systematic reviews – a product from the ESRC Methods Programme. https://www.lancaster.ac.uk/media/lancaster-university/content-assets/documents/fhm/dhr/chir/NSsynthesisguidanceVersion1-April2006.pdf

Porter, M., & Wang, J. (2022). Personal resources and work engagement: A literature review. *Journal of Continuing Education in Nursing*, *53*, 115–121. PMID: 35244461

Sasikala, K., Dahiya, R., Selvakumar, P., Sudheer, P., Rajagopalan, K. K., Manjunath, T. C., & Sharma, M. (2026). Reducing Carbon Footprint With AI-Driven Logistics Planning. In Chahal, B., David, A., Singh, A., Madaan, G., & Singh, G. (Eds.), *Impact of Generative AI on Food Supply Chain Management* (pp. 189–216). IGI Global Scientific Publishing., DOI: 10.4018/979-8-3693-9856-2.ch007

Satyanarayana, P., Anute, N., Ghewari, A., Chahande, S., Sharma, A., Selvakumar, P., & Manjunath, T. C. (2026). Interdisciplinary Applications of AI and AR in Research. In Vrba, J., & Huynh, T. (Eds.), *Revolutionizing Academic Research With AI and Augmented Reality* (pp. 283–310). IGI Global Scientific Publishing., DOI: 10.4018/979-8-3373-1414-3.ch009

Sreekanthaswamy, N., Chib, S., Maddel, M., Khande, R., Kalshetti, P., Selvakumar, P., & Manjunath, T. C. (2026). AI Smart-Enabled and Machine Learning Intensifies Smart Multimedia Platforms. In van Wyk, M. (Ed.), *AI Smart-Enabled Architecture and Infrastructure for Higher Education* (pp. 29–54). IGI Global Scientific Publishing., DOI: 10.4018/979-8-3693-8915-7.ch002

Tufanaru, C., Munn, Z., Aromataris, E., ... (2020) Chapter 3: Systematic reviews of effectiveness. In: JBI Manual for Evidence Synthesis, pp. 71–133.

Vallières, F., Mcauliffe, E., & van Bavel, B.. (2016). There's no app for that: Assessing the impact of mhealth on the supervision, motivation, engagement, and satisfaction of community health workers in Sierra Leone. *Annals of Global Health*, *82*, 936–949. PMID: 28283148

van der Meer, C. A. I., Bakker, A., & van Zuiden, M.. (2020). Help in hand after traumatic events: A randomized controlled trial in health care professionals on the efficacy, usability, and user satisfaction of a self-help app to reduce trauma-related symptoms. *European Journal of Psychotraumatology*, *11*, 1717155. PMID: 32284818

WHO. (2022a) Mental Health and COVID-19: Scientific brief. Available at: https://www.who.int/publications/i/item/WHO-2019-nCoV-Sci_Brief-Mental_health-2022.1 (accessed 23 April 2022).

Ye, J. (2021). Advancing mental health and psychological support for health care workers using digital technologiesand platforms. *JMIR Formative Research*, *5*, e22075. PMID: 34106874

Yildiz, B., & Yildiz, T. (2022). A systematic review and meta-analytical synthesis of the relationship between work engagement and job satisfaction in nurses. *Perspectives in Psychiatric Care*, *58*, 3062–3078. PMID: 35383388

Chapter 10
Psychotherapy Authority and Boundaries in Psychiatric Nursing Within Comparative Legal Framework

Harun Mirsad Günday
https://orcid.org/0000-0001-9429-393X
Faculty of Law, Erciyes University, Turkey

ABSTRACT

This study examines the evolving role of mental health and psychiatric nursing, focusing on the authority and boundaries of advanced practice nursing in psychotherapy. Within a comparative legal framework, the transition from Peplau's interpersonal process to structured modalities is analyzed across diverse jurisdictions, including the US, the UK, and various EU countries. The research highlights the critical importance of title protection, professional competence, and the scope of practice in defining the nurse psychotherapist's role. Significant attention is given to the legal liability and ethical boundaries associated with autonomous practice, particularly in therapeutic risk management and informed consent. By comparing international regulatory standards, such as those of the ANA and NMC, the study addresses the legislative gaps and the necessity for clear statutory bases for psychiatric nurses. Ultimately, it emphasizes that establishing robust legal and ethical frameworks is essential for ensuring patient safety and professional accountability in psychiatric care.

DOI: 10.4018/979-8-3373-6526-8.ch010

INTRODUCTION

Throughout its history, mental health and psychiatric nursing has undergone a fundamental paradigm shift. Within this framework, mental health and psychiatric nursing has evolved from a role defined by custodial care and monitoring into an autonomous discipline grounded in evidence-based therapeutic interventions and advanced practice roles. This evolution is reflected in nurses' ability to independently implement specialized techniques, such as guided imagery, to effectively manage complex patient symptoms like anxiety and pain (Topan et al., 2025). At the center of this evolution lies the theoretical framework established by Hildegard Peplau in 1952, which defines nursing as a "significant, therapeutic, and interpersonal process." In this context, Peplau characterized nursing as an "educative instrument" and a "maturing force." She proposed that the interaction between nurse and patient is, in itself, a therapeutic modality (Peplau, 1952), a principle that remains valid today through modern psychotherapy trainings delivered even via virtual platforms (Gülırmak Güler et al., 2024).

When looking at the current field of mental health, it is evident that mental health and psychiatric nursing has evolved into a model that goes beyond general therapeutic communication. Indeed, today, mental health and psychiatric nursing encompasses not only general therapeutic communication but also the delivery of structured psychotherapy modalities such as Cognitive Behavioral Therapy (CBT) and Psychodynamic Therapy. While this development can be considered positive for mental health and psychiatric nursing, it undoubtedly brings with it certain debates, particularly regarding authority, competence, and legal boundaries. This situation becomes much more understandable when considering the global burden of disease. Indeed, according to the World Health Organization (WHO), mental disorders constitute a significant portion of the global burden of disease. However, the availability of qualified mental health professionals remains insufficient to meet this demand (WHO, 2022). Ultimately, this imbalance forces health systems to adopt "task shifting" strategies. Consequently, this necessitates that mental health and psychiatric nurses take an active role in psychotherapeutic interventions alongside pharmacological management. In the end, this necessity emerges as an area requiring intervention by legislators.

In today's world, legal systems are seeking different solutions to the aforementioned problems. In this context, regulatory bodies such as the Nursing and Midwifery Council (NMC) in the United Kingdom (UK) and the American Nurses Association (ANA) in the United States (US) exist. These institutions have established clear pathways for Advanced Practice Nurses (APNs) to obtain certification and authority to practice psychotherapy (ANA, 2014; NMC, 2018). In contrast, a very different situation is encountered when looking at European Union (EU) member states and Turkey. Indeed, the answer to the question of whether mental health and psychiatric nurses in these regions have the authority to conduct psychotherapy is virtually uncertain. The issue of whether mental health and psychiatric nurses have the authority to practice psychotherapy, or what the boundaries of such authority are if it exists, constitutes a gray area due to deficiencies and ambiguities in legal regulations. However, in our opinion, it is unacceptable for a legal system to have such uncertainty regarding psychotherapy practices, which constitute a medical intervention.

Indeed, psychotherapy is not merely a medical intervention. By its very nature, it involves a psychological intervention directed at the most intimate and vulnerable aspects of the patient. Therefore, the issue here is not simply a question of who can practice psychotherapy. In our view, addressing the issue in this manner and reducing it to professional titles is nothing more than oversimplifying the subject. The real issue here is establishing demonstrable competence and the determination of the applicability of standards in psychotherapy practices.

In this context, the involvement of mental health and psychiatric nurses in the psychotherapeutic process raises two distinct questions: where "using oneself therapeutically" ends and where "formal psychotherapy" begins. At this point, Barker (2009) argues that the essence of psychiatric nursing is to understand the patient's worldview and accompany them. However, he suggests that transforming this interaction into a systematic psychotherapy session is a separate clinical competency requiring specialized training and clinical supervision. Therefore, he states that failing to make this distinction clearly in legal regulations paves the way for ethical violations such as malpractice, role confusion, boundary violations, and usurpation of authority. Indeed, it seems possible to say at this point that the biomedical ethical principles of beneficence, non-maleficence, autonomy, and justice, as defined by Beauchamp and Childress (2019), create complex dilemmas for nurses practicing psychotherapy.

This study aims to examine the authority and boundaries of psychotherapy in mental health and psychiatric nursing within the context of comparative law by analyzing the Turkish, Anglo-Saxon, and EU legal systems. In this context, this study is divided into four main sections. The first section examines the historical development and theoretical foundations of the concept of psychotherapy in mental health nursing. The second section addresses the psychotherapeutic competence, educational standards, and legal boundaries of nurses through a comparative legal methodology. The third section discusses the ethical standards and existing dilemmas in psychotherapy practices. This study aims to draw attention to the legal and ethical gaps in the field of mental health and psychiatric nursing and to provide policymakers with an evidence-based perspective.

THE CONCEPT OF PSYCHOTHERAPY IN MENTAL HEALTH NURSING AND ITS HISTORICAL EVOLUTION

The incorporation of psychotherapy into the nursing profession necessitates a significant departure from the traditional biomedical approach. Indeed, in this scenario, the mental health and psychiatric nurse is no longer merely someone who executes the physician's instructions. On the contrary, they attain the position of an autonomous therapeutic subject. Therefore, determining the legal and ethical boundaries mentioned in this study primarily requires defining what constitutes psychotherapy and examining the historical process that legitimizes this role.

Defining the Scope: Therapeutic Alliance vs. Formal Psychotherapy

There is a critical distinction between "therapeutic communication" and the advanced practice role of "psychotherapy" in mental health and psychiatric nursing. Therapeutic communication involves the use of specific techniques that foster a professional relationship characterized by mutual respect and goal-directed interaction (Travelbee, 1971; Unhjem & Hem, 2025). In contrast, psychotherapy involves a structured interaction aimed at alleviating psychological distress through specific psychological techniques (Wheeler, 2014). Here, the fundamental aim is simply to endow the individual with the capacity for reasonable thinking (Günday, 2015). Competence in psychotherapy generally requires education at the master's or doctoral level, beyond undergraduate nursing (Bilkay et al., 2025; García-Sastre et al., 2024).

According to the American Psychiatric Nurses Association (APNA, 2019), psychotherapy lies at the core of the role possessed by mental health and psychiatric nurses, particularly APNs (García-Sastre et al., 2024). Unlike general counseling, psychotherapy involves a theory-based process. Therefore, it is imperative for the practitioner to understand and navigate complex psychodynamics, as well as transference and counter-transference phenomena. For this reason, mental health and psychiatric nurses, particularly those with advanced education and experience, possess the skills to offer such interventions (Bilkay et al., 2025).

Nursing's approach to psychotherapies has a holistic outlook. At this point, the field of nursing combines the biopsychosocial model of medicine with nursing's caring sciences (Bilkay et al., 2025; García-Sastre et al., 2024). In this framework, psychiatric nurses serve as both practitioners and coordinators in the delivery of psychosocial therapies, ensuring that evidence-based interventions like CBT and milieu therapy are integrated into the patient's daily recovery process (Albayrak Günday & Gülırmak Güler, 2025). Thus, what emerges is virtually a hybrid model. This hybrid model allows the 'Nurse Psychotherapist' to uniquely address both the neurobiological aspects of mental illness and psychosocial determinants, leveraging the prescriptive authority already established for the Psychiatric-Mental Health Nurse Practitioners (PMHNP) in 26 US states. Ultimately, this ensures the emergence of a comprehensive treatment modality (Delaney, 2023; García-Sastre et al., 2024). Indeed, it is argued that nurse psychotherapists possess expertise that includes a holistic perspective on patients, crisis management skills, and a comprehensive understanding of health issues. It is suggested that this distinguishes them from non-medical therapists and non-therapy-oriented medical practitioners (García-Sastre et al., 2024). However, despite this, the full utilization of the psychotherapeutic skills of mental health and psychiatric nurses is often underestimated. Consequently, psychotherapy practices are hindered in many regions due to restrictive policies and a lack of professional recognition (Bilkay et al., 2025; García-Sastre et al., 2024). As a natural result of this, there is a call for improved leadership, advocacy, and official regulation to fully integrate psychotherapeutic nursing into healthcare systems (García-Sastre et al., 2024).

Major Psychotherapeutic Modalities in Nursing Practice

Evidence-based and applicable psychotherapy approaches are utilized in the field of mental health and psychiatric nursing. Understanding the intrinsic nature of these relevant psychotherapy approaches is of significant importance. This is because the determination of the "standard of care" from a legal perspective necessitates establishing the nature of the approaches in question. Otherwise, one would be attempting to find the answer to how something should be performed without knowing what it actually is. This is logically impossible in terms of legal reasoning.

Various psychotherapy approaches are encountered in the field of mental health and psychiatric nursing. Cognitive Behavioral Therapy (CBT), motivational interviewing, family therapy, psychoanalytic, and humanistic theories appear as approaches that can be enumerated in this field (Bilkay et al., 2025; García-Sastre et al., 2024). Among these, CBT constitutes the approach with the most widespread use and empirical support. The point of departure for this approach is the cognitive model, in which distorted thoughts influence emotion and behavior. For this reason, mental health and psychiatric nurses use this approach to restructure automatic negative thoughts (Wright et al., 2009). Indeed, it is stated that CBTs conducted under the leadership of mental health and psychiatric nurses are generally successful in improving various problems, including depressive symptoms and quality of life (Bilkay et al., 2025; Yoshinaga et al., 2022). However, the applicability of the CBT approach is ultimately a significant matter requiring additional certification or graduate education (Bilkay et al., 2025).

Psychodynamic psychotherapy appears as an approach focusing on unconscious processes (such as transference and defense mechanisms) and past experiences. In practice, it is stated to be a fundamental approach, particularly for APNs (Scheydt & Hegedüs, 2021). Similarly, Dialectical Behavior Therapy (DBT) is addressed as an approach combining mindfulness and acceptance strategies with CBT. It is accepted as a gold standard for Borderline Personality Disorder (Jones et al., 2023). Finally, Humanistic and Person-Centered Approaches, which shift nursing to a person-centered model, emphasize empathy and unconditional positive regard (Scanlon, 2006; Zhu et al., 2022).

These approaches are significant for mental health and psychiatric nursing. However, this importance is not limited solely to "what these approaches are." Another crucial issue here is the clarification of the therapeutic roles of mental health and psychiatric nurses in the implementation of these approaches. In other words, it is the simultaneous creation of clear frameworks that define the scope of practice and current legal regulations aimed at recognizing and developing professional competence (Bilkay et al., 2025). This is because one of the conditions that can give rise to legal liability for mental health professionals appears as "error in undertaking" (*Übernameverschulden*). That is, if a mental health professional applies a specific therapy approach without possessing the necessary knowledge, experience, and prerequisites to apply that approach, this application constitutes an assumption error. As a natural consequence of this, legal liability arises if other conditions of liability are also present (Günday, 2015). For example, this is the case if a "so-called" CBT approach is conducted in the absence of the aforementioned additional certification or required training regarding CBTs.

Historical Development of Psychotherapy in Nursing and the Peplau Paradigm

The history of psychotherapy in nursing essentially represents the history of the profession's struggle for autonomy. Indeed, prior to the mid-20th century, mental health and psychiatric nursing was characterized by "custodial care," which managed the physical needs and safety of institutionalized patients under the strict hierarchy of the asylum system. During this period, somatic treatments (insulin shock, hydrotherapy) held a dominant position in mental health practices. Therefore, the role of nurses was physiological rather than psychological in nature.

A paradigm shift occurred in the 1900s with Hildegard Peplau's book, *Interpersonal Relations in Nursing*, published in 1952. The foundation of this paradigm shift was the idea put forward by Peplau in the relevant work, arguing that the nurse-patient relationship was not merely a context but the therapy itself. This idea advocated that nursing is "doing *with* the patient" rather than "doing *to* the patient."

Thus, it elevated nurses to the position of an active "counselor" in the therapeutic process. This provided a scientific foundation for the nursing profession (Peplau, 1952; Forchuk, 2021).

By the 1960s, following Peplau, the Deinstitutionalization Movement shifted care from mental hospitals to the community. This created a void (service gap) that psychiatrists alone could not fill (Hein & Schärer, 2014; Júnior et al., 2017; Niles, 2013). At this point, this gap was filled by graduate education programs initiated under Peplau's leadership, and thus the Clinical Nurse Specialist (CNS) role gained official status (O'Brien, 2001). Subsequently, this process, reinforcing its legitimacy with certification and reimbursement rights in the US, evolved over time into the PMHNP model (Phoenix & Chapman, 2020; Scheydt & Hegedüs, 2021). These PMH advanced practice nurses are today trained to provide services similar to psychiatrists, including psychotherapy (Delaney, 2023). However, when looking at Europe and Turkey, it is observed that medical hegemony has kept nurses mostly in supportive roles and delayed the integration of psychotherapy education into the profession.

Current Perspective: Task Shifting and Global Status

It is possible to state that the concept of the "nurse psychotherapist" is now well-established. However, in our view, it is not possible to assert that the role corresponding to this concept is uniform worldwide. Indeed, in countries practicing Anglo-Saxon law, such as the USA and the UK, this role has been placed on a legal footing with titles such as "Psychiatric-Mental Health Nurse Practitioner" or equivalent designations. Conversely, when examining Continental European and Turkish legal systems, it is observed that this development has not been fully realized, and a state of "lagging behind" is evident. The historical divergence between these legal systems constitutes the fundamental cause of this gap (disparity) in practice. For instance, while it may be legally possible for a nurse in New York to open a private psychotherapy clinic, it does not appear legally feasible for a nurse with identical experience in Istanbul to do so.

By the 21st century, the driving force behind this role has ceased to be a purely theoretical debate and has evolved into a practical necessity (WHO, 2008). Indeed, the World Health Organization has recognized "task shifting" as a crucial strategy to address the global mental health treatment gap, particularly in low- and middle-income countries (Aurizki & Wilson, 2022; Günday & Albayrak Günday, 2025; Lange, 2021; Pepfar, 2007; Purgato et al., 2020). The task shifting referred to here entails the delegation of tasks, such as the delivery of psychotherapeutic interventions, from highly trained professionals (such as psychiatrists) to non-specialist health workers with shorter training and fewer qualifications, including nurses (Aurizki & Wilson, 2022; Lange, 2021; Purgato et al., 2020). In this context, it is acknowledged that nurses possess the capacity to deliver psychosocial interventions normally provided by mental health specialists, provided they receive appropriate training and supervision (Aurizki & Wilson, 2022; Bolton et al., 2023; Rocha et al., 2020). Thus, the aim is to utilize existing human resources more efficiently and to alleviate bottlenecks in service delivery (Lange, 2021). At this juncture, it is evident that nurses have the potential to contribute significantly to mental health services through psychotherapy (Albayrak & Asi Karakaş, 2022). Nevertheless, despite this potential, their roles and skills are not fully utilized or appreciated in the international arena. Consequently, it is argued by some authors in the doctrine that further research, education, political advocacy, and advanced leadership are necessary to achieve official regulation and accreditation (Bilkay et al., 2025; García-Sastre et al., 2024; Hurley et al., 2022).

COMPETENCE AND LIMITATIONS IN PSYCHOTHERAPY PRACTICE: A COMPARATIVE LEGAL ANALYSIS

The legal authority of nurses to practice psychotherapy varies significantly worldwide. The fundamental reason underlying this variation is the differences in the legal systems possessed by countries. More specifically, the distinction between Common Law (Anglo-Saxon) systems, which possess a system based on regulatory flexibility and case law, and Civil Law (Continental European) systems, which are characterized by rigid codification and inherently tend to be less prescriptive, plays a determining role at this point (Beis et al., 2022). Within this framework, it is, in our opinion, quite important to address the EU law and national differences in the context of the Anglo-Saxon system, which includes the USA and the UK, and the Continental European legal model. Finally, examining the issue within the context of Turkish law appears as another subject that needs to be addressed.

The Anglo-Saxon Model: Advanced Practice and Autonomy (USA and UK)

In both the US and the UK, the legal framework has evolved to recognize the "Advanced Practice Nurse" as an independent provider (Phoenix & Chapman, 2020; Scheydt & Hegedüs, 2021). Therefore, in these legal systems, psychotherapy practices are not a type of medical intervention reserved solely for physicians. At the same time, they appear as a competency that nurses can also legally perform, provided they meet certain education and certification standards (Delaney, 2023).

The United States: Statutory Authority and The "LACE" Consensus

The US offers the most structured and legally protected pathway for nurse psychotherapists. Here, the legal authority for nurses to practice psychotherapy stems from Nurse Practice Acts enacted by state legislatures. Indeed, the evolution of Advanced Practice Registered Nurse (APRN) education and regulation has been significantly shaped by the APRN Consensus Model introduced in 2008, which aimed to establish a uniform framework for licensure, accreditation, certification, and education across states (Cahill et al., 2014; Davis et al., 2024). Similarly, the LACE initiative aimed to align APRN education programs and accreditation with professional certification options, particularly for the purpose of legal regulation (Fulton, 2019). In this aspect, the APRN Consensus Model guides states in implementing and overseeing the practice of APRNs in various areas of specialization.

When examining the US legal system, it is observed that a significant condition is required for nurses to have the authority to practice psychotherapy. That is, the nurse wishing to practice psychotherapy must have earned the title of PMHNP (ANCC, 2020). Indeed, MH-APRNs are skilled and qualified nurses specifically trained to increase access to mental health services (Delaney, 2023). However, this does not mean that APRNs have absolute freedom in practice. Indeed, scopes of practice that are national in character for APRNs have been put forth by professional organizations such as the American Psychiatric Nurses Association (APNA, 2019). within this framework, it is stated that the scope of practice of APRNs includes the diagnosis and management of mental disorders, the prescribing and management of psychotropic treatments, the conduct of psychotherapeutic interventions, and the making of outcome evaluations as professional activities (Delaney, 2023). Ultimately, with the receipt of the certificate and the earning of the PMHNP title, various matters are included within the scope of the PMHNP's practice authority. It is possible to list these as the authority to conduct psychotherapy, diagnose, and prescribe.

The requirements sought for obtaining the PMHNP title are a matter necessitating high standards at the federal level. However, despite this, the answer to the question of what the scope of the PMHNP's practice authority is largely depends on state laws and shows variability (Oleck et al., 2011). In this framework, for example; it is possible to say that nurse psychotherapists have full independence in states such as Oregon, Washington, and New York. This is because in the said states, it is possible for nurse psychotherapists to perform many various procedures, including conducting assessments, diagnosing, ordering and interpreting tests, initiating and managing treatment including prescribing medication, or billing insurance companies, without the need for a physician's supervision (Delaney, 2023; Slade et al., 2024). In other words, in these jurisdictions, so to speak, full practice authority exists. Indeed, as of 2024, approximately 26 US states and the District of Columbia have granted full practice authority to PMHNPs (Delaney, 2023). In contrast, when looking at other different jurisdictions, it is observed that reduced or restricted practice authority is encountered. In these states, it is stated that PMHNPs are subject to restrictions regarding the prescribing of certain medications or have obligations to collaborate with other providers regarding the provision of care (Delaney, 2023). Based on the year 2023, it is seen that reduced or restricted practice authority exists in approximately thirteen states, including states such as Alabama, Utah, Mississippi, and Kentucky (Delaney, 2023). In parallel with this, it is stated that the practice authority of APRNs in the US continues to be unnecessarily restricted (Phoenix & Chapman, 2020).

These restrictive state regulations pose an obstacle to the full utilization of PMH-APRNs, thereby weakening the health system's ability to meet the increasing demand for behavioral health services (Martin et al., 2020). Since PMHNPs in the US have independent licensure, they carry their own malpractice liability. With increasing clinical responsibilities, psychiatric nurse practitioners must be familiar with the legal issues surrounding their practice to ensure best practices and avoid malpractice lawsuits and licensing issues (Balestra, 2018). Indeed, PMHNPs are held directly liable in a lawsuit involving psychotherapy errors (Buppert, 2017), similar to other independent healthcare providers.

The United Kingdom: Competency Frameworks and the NHS Model

When looking at the English legal system, one encounters an image where the title of "Psychotherapist" is not legally protected, unlike in the US where "Psychotherapist" is generally a protected title tied to licensure. That is, the title "Psychotherapist" does not possess the same legal protection as a "Nurse" or "Doctor." However, this situation does not mean that psychotherapy activities can be conducted completely arbitrarily. Because psychotherapy activity within the National Health Service (NHS) is strictly regulated. Indeed, due to the importance of expanding the health workforce capacity in England, the issue of developing and implementing advanced nurse practitioner roles in mental health services is receiving increasing attention (Oliphant, 2023).

One of the things that needs to be mentioned in this regard in England appears as the NMC. The NMC is a statutory regulator. In this aspect, the NMC Code issued by the NMC is another matter that needs to be mentioned. The manner in which the limits of competence are addressed in the NMC Code is quite interesting. Because in the Code, an approach has been adopted where "proficiency" is placed at the focal point rather than including specific "permitted" procedures. As a result of this, it is legally possible for nurses to perform any activities for which they are deemed competent (Bífárìn et al., 2024). Thus, an attitude allowing for fluid role expansion provided that nurses meet professional standards has been adopted (Bífárìn et al., 2024).

The legal integration of nurses into psychotherapy in England is exemplified by the Improving Access to Psychological Therapies (IAPT) program (now known as NHS Talking Therapies). In this context, nurses are frequently trained as "High Intensity Therapists" delivering evidence-based psychological therapies. Ultimately, a nurse in this role continues their work under the NHS legal framework. They also have the authority to independently administer CBT, DBT, or EMDR. However, regarding English nurses working in the NHS, the principle of vicarious liability applies. That is, the NHS Trust (Dimond, 2015) assumes responsibility for the nurse's actions provided the nurse acts within the scope of employment and competence. In this aspect, an opposite solution path completely diverging from the independent US contractor model has been adopted. However, when the issue is viewed in the context of prescribing authority, a completely different approach exists.

Indeed, when looking at the English model, the "V300 Independent Prescribing" qualification appears as a unique power. This is because a British mental health and psychiatric nurse with this qualification possesses legal rights to prescribe medication and practice psychotherapy reflecting the US model within the context of a national health system. At this point, it must be said that prescribing practices in England are governed by numerous laws and case law covering controlled drugs, unlicensed medicines, and addressing negligence (Rae, 2024). Furthermore, mental health nurses in England can also assume roles such as Approved Mental Health Professionals, which allows them to make applications for compulsory detention, a responsibility previously held by social workers (Coffey & Hannigan, 2013).

Synthesis of the Anglo-Saxon Approach

When looking at the US and UK legal systems, it is seen that there is a common point in these legal systems regarding psychotherapy practices. That is, psychotherapy has been separated from the exclusive domain of medicine. In this context, it is observed that mental health and psychiatric nurses can conduct psychotherapy practices. At this point, it is beneficial, in our opinion, to draw attention to three different issues regarding nurses. These are autonomy, standardization, and accountability.

Firstly, in US and UK law, it is possible for nurses to perform assessments, diagnose, and treat without the need for a physician's presence (in most US states and the UK). This issue also appears consistent with the recommendation that nurses practice to the full extent of their education and training (Phoenix & Chapman, 2020). Indeed, this situation was emphasized in the Institute of Medicine's landmark report, The Future of Nursing (Phoenix & Chapman, 2020).

Secondly, the existing system in the US and UK possesses a certain standardization. This is because the legal systems of both countries have standardized graduate education regarding the authority to apply psychotherapeutic interventions. In other words, it is mandatory for the psychotherapy practitioner to have education at the master's level. Thus, the provision of a specialized knowledge base to the psychotherapy practitioner regarding advanced practice roles is guaranteed (Sastre-Fullana et al., 2014).

Finally, in US and UK law, nurses have legal responsibilities due to psychotherapeutic interventions. More clearly, nurse psychotherapists are not treated as assistants in these legal systems; on the contrary, they are treated as independent practitioners. In this aspect, as discussed in the further parts of the study; it forms a sharp contrast with Continental European Legal systems where legal frameworks are generally more prescriptive, the nurse's role is often defined as "dependent on physician orders," and there is difficulty in defining roles outside these boundaries (Beis et al., 2022).

The Civil Law Model: The European Union and National Divergences

The Continental European approach has a historical tendency towards rigid codification and medical hegemony (Beis et al., 2022). For this reason, it has an appearance quite different from the Anglo-Saxon model, which has tended towards regulation based on professional autonomy and competence. This difference is not only in the form of differentiation from the Anglo-Saxon model; it also has a meaning containing differentiations within itself. Indeed, within the EU, the legal authority of nurses to practice psychotherapy is not uniform but regulated in different ways. In this framework, there is virtually a mosaic of fragmented regulations ranging from strict prohibition to developing advanced practice roles. As a result of this, there is no uniform legal definition for psychological interventions and psychotherapy in health services across Europe. This hinders quality control of training programs and services provided and complicates care coordination (Broeck & Lietaer, 2008). This lack of uniform regulation becomes even more complex due to the fields of mental health and law approaching the subject from different angles (disciplinary differences) (Cohen et al., 2022).

The Supranational Framework: Absence of a Unified "Scope of Practice"

The EU presents a regulatory paradox regarding the nursing profession. Indeed, the EU, unlike the federalized legal structures found in the US, does not possess a legal regulation equivalent to a "European Nursing Practice Act" defining the scope of clinical practice. The reason for this is the regulation contained in Article 168 of the Treaty on the Functioning of the EU, which grants member states broad autonomy over the organization and delivery of health services (European Union, 2012). Therefore, there is no legal regulation at the EU level that explicitly grants nurses the authority to practice psychotherapy or prohibits this authority. This situation results in reliance on broader professional acceptance and national regulatory mechanisms instead of the Union's central laws regarding legal recognition.

One of the fundamental regulations addressing the activities of professionals in the health field in the EU region is Directive 2005/36/EC on the Recognition of Professional Qualifications (European Commission, 2005). This Directive serves the harmonization of minimum training requirements for "General Care Nurses" (Ypma et al., 2020). However, it does not explicitly include a regulation regarding advanced practice roles of nurses or whether psychotherapy practices can be performed by them. For this reason, there is a significant gap in the recognition and regulation of advanced nursing roles (Paul et al., 2023). This has naturally led to the emergence of efforts to fill this gap in practice.

Indeed, the academic world has attempted to fill this gap through the Bologna Process and the European Qualifications Framework due to the absence of a legal directive for advanced practice roles of nurses (EFN, 2015; Horatio, 2018). At this point, the Bologna process has specifically aimed to harmonize study processes (Laireiter & Weise, 2019; Možina, 2024). In general, these initiatives aim to standardize higher education across Europe, including nursing degrees, to facilitate cross-border mobility and mutual recognition of qualifications (Antão et al., 2025; Palese et al., 2014). However, despite this, significant differences still exist among European countries in graduate education and practical studies in clinical psychology. This naturally affects the standardization of psychotherapy education and regulation (Laireiter & Weise, 2019; Možina, 2024). Indeed, in a mapping study conducted by the European Federation of Nurses Associations, attention was drawn to the existence of significant differences in the definition, recognition, regulation, and education of advanced practice nursing (APN) across Europe (Paul et al., 2023). Whereas, specialist nurse roles, regulations, and competencies have been extensively discussed since the beginning of the 21st century. Studies in this field also show that further harmonization is needed to improve quality practice and mobility (Decock et al., 2022).

National Regulatory Landscapes: A Spectrum of Autonomy

As previously stated, there is no specific and binding legal regulation regarding nursing practice within the EU. Consequently, the limits of authority for nurse psychotherapists exhibit significant differences among member states. This has resulted in a fragmented mosaic of regulations, ranging from strict prohibitions to developing advanced practice roles. In our opinion, it is possible to categorize this mosaic into three distinct legal archetypes: the regulated dual-title model, the delegated medical act model, and the emerging advanced practice model.

Type I: The Regulated "Dual-Title" Model

According to this model, found in countries such as France and Austria, there is a strict separation between the nursing profession and the practice of psychotherapy. In this system, a nursing license is insufficient to practice therapy. A nurse wishing to practice psychotherapy must obtain a completely separate and secondary license education (Broeck & Lietaer, 2008).

The French legal system constitutes one of the pioneers of this restrictive model. The legal situation in France underwent a significant transformation with the entry into force of the Decree of May 20, 2010. Indeed, with this regulation, the title of "psychotherapist" gained official status, and the accompanying special training requirements mandated that professionals wishing to work in this field often possess two separate qualifications (dual titles) (Debout et al., 2012; Légifrance, 2010). Although APN has been introduced through legal frameworks in France, it faces various obstacles in implementation. Moreover, this model does not make a distinction between Nurse Practitioners and CNSs (Devictor et al., 2022). On the other hand, a much more complex situation exists for nurses wishing to practice psychotherapy. Competence in nursing does not provide a direct legal basis or advantage for these individuals to automatically obtain the title of "Psychotherapist." Instead, separate and specialized training is required. This requirement is fully consistent with the "dual-title" approach in France (Broeck & Lietaer, 2008).

Similarly, Austria possesses one of the strictest regulatory frameworks in Europe due to the *Psychotherapiegesetz* (Psychotherapy Act) (BMSGPK, 2021) currently in force. Indeed, this law defined psychotherapy as an autonomous profession in 1991. In this aspect, it actually ensured a significant increase in the number of psychotherapists and improved access to psychotherapy services (Možina, 2024). The education process to become a psychotherapist has a highly academic appearance; there are postgraduate programs, and more recently, undergraduate psychotherapy programs have been included in universities (Možina, 2024). The authority to practice psychotherapy (legal recognition) is generally granted to professionals who have completed the necessary specialized training in this field, such as clinical and health psychologists and psychiatry specialists (Možina, 2024).

Regarding nurses, the issue requires separate consideration. Indeed, Advanced nursing practice has begun to develop in Austria with master's level education in accordance with the International Council of Nurses core curriculum. However, national implementation and evaluation strategies are still in the development phase (Glarcher & Lex, 2020). As a result of this situation, nurses are not explicitly listed among the professions directly recognized as psychotherapists in Austria. Therefore, for a nurse to practice psychotherapy, they would likely need to obtain a separate psychotherapy qualification (Možina, 2024).

Type II: The "Delegated Medical Act" Model

Germany presents a unique and somewhat paradoxical legal anomaly within the European context, largely due to the coexistence of modern nursing laws and archaic health regulations. In the German hospital system, the standard psychiatric nurse (*Fachkrankenpfleger*) operates strictly under the principle of physician delegation. In this framework, the legal authority to treat flows from the physician to the nurse, leaving very little room for autonomous psychotherapeutic practice within the clinical hierarchy (Burgi & Igl, 2021; Scheydt & Hegedüs, 2021). Therefore, it is possible to say that nurses cannot intervene therapeutically (e.g., psychotherapy practice) with the patient on their own initiative. On the other hand, it is stated that Germany lags behind international standards in nursing education and training. There is particular uncertainty regarding the employment of academically qualified nurses (Scheydt et al., 2025). This situation limits the independent scope of nursing practice, especially for psychotherapeutic interventions that generally require authorization from a physician or psychotherapist (Scheydt & Hegedüs, 2021). In other words, the nursing profession does not possess an authority framework to conduct such advanced interventions on its own and with legal autonomy.

However, a separate legal pathway exists in Germany through the *Heilpraktikergesetz* (Natural Health Practitioners Law), which allows individuals, including nurses, to work as "natural health practitioners" (Gaebel et al., 2020). Indeed, this law allows persons who pass a specific exam to offer certain therapeutic services, including psychotherapy. Although *Heilpraktikers* are recognized by the state, they are not regulated health professionals in the traditional sense, as training in this field is evaluated in a completely separate status from traditional medicine or nursing education (Hoffmeister et al., 2021; Krug et al., 2016). The implication of this for nurses is as follows: A nurse may obtain the *Heilpraktiker* title to offer psychotherapy independently. However, this pathway is completely independent of the nursing license. Therefore, this authority does not directly expand nursing's own psychotherapeutic scope of practice. In other words, the authority gained belongs to the *Heilpraktiker* status, not the nursing profession.

On the other hand, another important regulation that should be mentioned in this regard in German law is the *Psychotherapists Law*. This law primarily regulates psychological psychotherapists and child/adolescent psychotherapists. These professions are established as "autonomous professions" with highly regulated education and licensing processes (Melcop et al., 2019; Možina, 2024). Indeed, with significant amendments made to this law in 2019/2020, a new and academic educational pathway allowing for independent practice for psychotherapists was created.

Unfortunately, nurses were not included within the scope of this new regulation. In other words, the relevant regulation did not integrate nursing into this autonomous psychotherapeutic role (Melcop et al., 2019; Možina, 2024).

Type III: The Emerging Advanced Practice Model

When examining Ireland and the Scandinavian countries, legal frameworks exhibit a tendency to align with the Anglo-Saxon tradition, in contrast to the restrictive continental models. Consequently, the Advanced Practice Nurse has been able to find a place directly within nursing legislation and has been recognized. According to this model, psychotherapeutic competence is not addressed as a separate profession. On the contrary, it constitutes an integral part of advanced nursing (Paul et al., 2023). Indeed, with the enactment of the Nurses and Midwives Act 2011 in Ireland, the Advanced Nurse Practitioner (ANP) gained a statutory basis (NMBI, 2017). Furthermore, the APN role in Ireland has developed significantly since 2001, driven by the need for highly skilled nursing professionals to address complex health demands and improve patient outcomes (Doody et al., 2025).

In Ireland, the psychiatric and mental health specialization mandates education requiring the completion of 120 ECTS credits. On the other hand, specific specializations in this field necessitate recognized titles and additional registration for nurses (Dury et al., 2014). More clearly, this education implies the necessity of a formal registration added on top of the nurse's basic license registration, which legally provides autonomous practice authority in this field of specialization. In this framework, adequate legal regulations have been established for roles regarding APNs. This has naturally brought about results providing positive contributions in individual, familial, and societal terms (Ladd et al., 2020; Poghosyan & Maier, 2022).

In Sweden, it is also observed that psychotherapy education is directly integrated into advanced nursing education. Indeed, firstly, psychotherapy was accepted as an autonomous profession in Sweden in 1985 (Možina, 2024). In Swedish law, a two-stage education is envisaged for nurses to practice psychotherapy. In this context, nurses are first subjected to a three-year basic training program involving psychotherapy under supervision. After this basic training is completed, there is a transition to a specialist training involving more comprehensive supervised practice and personal experience (Možina, 2024). To use the title of "Psychotherapist," a license issued by the National Board of Health and Welfare is required after these trainings are completed (Možina, 2024).

Finally, in Finland, the title of "psychotherapist" has been recognized as an independent profession since 1994, and legal regulations guaranteeing this are included. The training programs required to obtain the psychotherapist title are multiprofessional. That is, they are not open only to a single health group, but rather to professionals with different basic professional backgrounds. In this context, those who have completed certain master's degrees or nurses specialized in the field of psychiatry (those who have received post-secondary nursing education) can be included in these programs (Možina, 2024). This structure demonstrates that there is a clear and structured pathway for nurses to gain psychotherapeutic competence and practice autonomously. Thus, it reflects a comprehensive approach to advanced nursing care involving psychotherapy (García-Sastre et al., 2024). Indeed, Iceland is also developing advanced practice mental health nursing programs with a clinically focused Master's program initiated in 2022. With this development, it is possible to say that the region is making a strong movement towards the Emerging Advanced Practice Model (Pedersen et al., 2022).

The "Competence vs. Title" Conflict in Europe

The most critical legal hurdle faced by APNs in EU countries has been the issue of title protection rather than the questioning of their professional competence (Paul et al., 2023). This discrepancy regarding title and authority, namely the precedence of legal recognition over professional qualification, constitutes a significant challenge to the recognition and effective utilization of APNs across Europe (Decock et al., 2022).

It is, in our opinion, possible to say that the difference in titles lies at the basis of the competence and title conflict within the EU. Indeed, while the US directly recognizes "Nurse Psychotherapists" (a nursing specialty), laws in many EU countries view the title of "Psychotherapist" strictly as a protected title belonging to psychologists or psychiatrists. In the doctrine, it is argued that this legal rigidity in Continental Europe leads to a "waste of human capital" (García-Sastre et al., 2024). This is because highly experienced psychiatric nurses are legally restricted from utilizing their full therapeutic potential, despite possessing practical skills. This view also appears consistent with broader discussions on the underutilization of psychotherapeutic skills possessed by psychiatric nurses. The reason for this underutilization is cited as nursing roles being viewed as undervalued and misunderstood in various contexts (García-Sastre et al., 2024).

On the other hand, the lack of standardized prescribing authority for nurses across Europe (Maier, 2019) is another important point deepening this conflict. Indeed, nurse prescribing is showing an increase worldwide and in many European countries (e.g., the UK, Finland, Norway). Despite this, significant differences exist in legal regulations, including requirements for collaborative agreements with physicians (Escardívol et al., 2024; Maier, 2019). The complexity and lack of uniformity in legal regulations show that legal regulations lag behind and fail to keep up with the proven competencies of nurses, particularly in specialized fields like mental health where psychotropic medication management is often intertwined with psychotherapeutic interventions (Phoenix & Chapman, 2020). More clearly, the law seems to have failed to follow the developing world and keep pace with the era. As a result of this, various restrictive policies have played a role in limiting nurses' ability to provide psychotherapy. This simultaneously hinders nurses' professional identities, competencies, and autonomy (García-Sastre et al., 2024).

The Legal Framework in Turkey: Regulatory Ambiguities and the "Physician's Shadow"

The Turkish legal system falls within the Continental European Law tradition. In this aspect, it possesses a complex landscape struggling between a historical medical hegemony and modern aspirations for autonomy regarding the nursing profession. Indeed, the issue of whether psychiatric nurses have the authority to conduct psychotherapy is within a significant dilemma. In this framework, while current statutory regulations adopt a fundamentally restrictive solution; lower-ranking regulations in terms of hierarchy and also draft legal regulations have preferred more inclusive solution paths. Due to this existing uncertainty and the lack of clearly establishing professional frameworks, the issue of whether psychiatric nurses can fully assume psychotherapy roles is significantly complicated (Bilkay et al., 2025).

The Existing Statutory Paradox: Law No. 6283 and the 2011 Regulation

The fundamental legal regulation regarding the nursing profession in Turkish law is the Nursing Law No. 6283. Article 4/I of the Law No. 6283 defines the nurse essentially as health personnel authorized and tasked with planning, implementing, supervising, and evaluating nursing care. However, ultimately, the nurse acts dependent on the supervision and instructions of a physician, especially regarding the implementation of medical treatments (Solak & Kayaer, 2024).

The authority for mental health and psychiatric nurses to diagnose mental illnesses or independently administer psychotherapeutic treatments does not yet exist in Turkish law. In this aspect, the solution path adopted by the Nurse Practice Acts in the US has not been preferred in Turkey. Furthermore, Article 4/g of the Patient Rights Regulation (PRR) of 1998 defined medical intervention as physical and psychological interventions applied by persons authorized to practice the profession. Likewise, Article 13 of the Medical Deontology Regulation of 1960 counted only physicians and dentists among the persons who would diagnose and apply treatment in accordance with scientific requirements. Psychotherapy practices are ultimately medical interventions and are psychological attempts directed at the patient's bodily integrity (Günday, 2015). This being the case, it is clear that they must be applied by "persons practicing the medical profession." Naturally, these persons are none other than physicians.

On the other hand, it is argued in the literature that a significant "gray area" emerged with the 2011 Regulation on the Amendment of the Nursing Regulation. The reason for this is the inclusion of duties such as "creating a therapeutic environment," "providing psycho-education," and conducting "individual and group counseling" in the section where the specific roles of the "Psychiatric Clinical Nurse" are defined (Bilkay et al., 2025). However, our opinion is that this regulation does not give rise to a gray area. At least, as discussed below, when examining the regulations in Article 2/ı and j of the Proposed Mental Health Law (PMHL 2023), it is clearly seen that the terms psychotherapy and mental intervention possess meanings different from each other. In this context, while psychotherapy is a medical intervention; mental intervention is a concept covering a much broader range of interventions, including psychotherapies, provided they are within the mental health professionals' own scope of authority. Therefore, the duty of "creating a therapeutic environment" in the Regulation does not, in our opinion, absolutely make possible the interpretation that nurses can also practice psychotherapy. Nevertheless, the "obligation to assess suicide risk," which is evaluated within the scope of the psychiatrist's diagnosis and treatment obligation (Günday, 2015), is clearly mentioned within the duties and authorities of the psychiatric clinical nurse in the Regulation. The same situation exists regarding anamnesis, which is a diagnostic activity (Günday, 2015). In our opinion, these should be the regulations in the Regulation that need to be criticized primarily. Because the authority to independently conduct diagnosis and treatment activities belongs only to physicians authorized to practice the medical profession.

Consequently, there is no clear statutory basis for nurses to practice psychotherapy in Turkish law. It is stated in the literature that this situation causes highly educated psychiatric nurses to use the title of "psychotherapist" in clinical settings or to perform therapy-like interventions *de facto* rather than *de jure* without legal basis (Bilkay et al., 2025). In fact, in practice, even young individuals who have merely completed a four-year undergraduate education in psychology are encountered engaging in activities they call so-called psychotherapy, which in our opinion can be nothing more than sophistry and ordinary conversation.

This gap is challenging and, in our opinion, quite meaningless when international standards requiring master's level education compatible with the psychiatric nurse's educational background as a prerequisite in foreign legal systems are considered (Bilkay et al., 2025). When the costs of certificate trainings regarding psychotherapy approaches and inadequate physical conditions in clinics are added to this situation, the obstacles nurses face regarding practicing psychotherapy grow even larger (Bilkay et al., 2025).

The Proposed Mental Health Law: Reinforcing the Medical Hierarchy

The tension regarding professional boundaries and scope of practice is explicitly addressed in the PMHL and reinforces the existing medical hierarchy. Although the PMHL states that it philosophically aims for person-centered and community-based services, in its implementation articles, it builds mental health services upon a rigid "medical model" and codifies this model.

The Legal Status of Psychotherapy: Positioning as a Medical Intervention

The PMHL classifies psychotherapy under the umbrella of "medical intervention" rather than as an independent professional practice. Indeed, the concept of medical intervention in Article 2/ö of the PMHL is defined as bodily and mental interventions, such as psychotherapy, performed by persons authorized to practice the medical profession. Specifically, the handling of psychotherapy legally as a medical intervention constitutes, in our opinion, the biggest legal obstacle for non-medical professionals to use this authority.

On the other hand, Article 10 of the PMHL regulates that alongside psychiatrists, psychologists and clinical psychologists can also perform psychotherapy applications under specified conditions. However, this authorization does not eliminate the reality that psychotherapy practices have been placed under the hierarchy and supervision of medicine. This is because the authority to diagnose mental illness is exclusively granted to physicians via Article 12/1 of the PMHL. This situation leaves the initiation and referral authority, which is legally mandatory for non-physician authorized professional groups to conduct a curative process like psychotherapy, always to the medical profession. Therefore, the psychotherapy process legally begins and continues under the hierarchy of the physician's diagnostic authority.

Professional Groups Authorized to Practice Psychotherapy

The PMHL limits the authority to practice psychotherapy with a rigid hierarchy shaped around the power to diagnose mental illness and the legal definition of the profession. In this framework, primary and undisputed authority in mental health services is allocated to mental health and diseases specialist physicians (psychiatrists). The PMHL explicitly grants the authority to diagnose mental illness solely to mental health and diseases specialist physicians (or child and adolescent mental health specialists in child cases) pursuant to Article 12/1 of the PMHL. From a legal perspective, since the definition of mental illness in Article 2/I of the PMHL covers temporary or permanent disabilities requiring medical intervention, the legal starting point and final authority of all treatment processes inevitably become the physician. Therefore, psychiatrists are positioned as the primary authorized practitioners at the center of treatment, both because they possess the monopoly on diagnosis and because they harbor psychotherapy competence as a natural part of their specialty training.

The PMHL grants the authority to practice psychotherapy to clinical psychologists and psychologists meeting certain training criteria alongside physicians. However, this authority is tied to the strict training conditions specified in Article 10 of the PMHL. Accordingly, it is mandatory for the practitioner to have completed at least a master's education in clinical/applied fields related to mental health and to have practiced under supervision during this education. In this context, pursuant to the PMHL, for non-physician professionals to have the authority to practice psychotherapy, it is mandatory to meet the detailed education conditions specified in Article 10 of the PMHL. These conditions require having completed at least a master's education in clinical/applied fields related to mental health. Furthermore, during the graduate education process, it is mandatory to fulfill the compulsory practical and theoretical conditions determined by clauses a, b, and c of Article 10/1 of the PMHL. These conditions must include a minimum of 200 hours of theoretical education, a total of 750 hours of clinical psychotherapy practice (150 hours of which being supervision education), and additionally a practice containing 500 hours of clinical experience and education. These rigid academic requirements reflect the PMHL's aim to reserve the authority of psychotherapy only for highly specialized individuals.

Consequently, clinical psychologists and psychologists meeting the necessary criteria have been rendered possessors of conditional autonomy and practice authority, albeit in the shadow of the physician's diagnostic authority, thanks to their professional definitions including psychological intervention and meeting the graduate education requirement (Master's/PhD and supervision) sought by the law.

The Authority Status of Nurses: The Legal Firewall and Exclusion.

The PMHL has formally recognized advanced academic specialization within the nursing profession. Indeed, the Proposal defines professionals who have graduated from nursing or equivalent undergraduate programs of universities, received the title of nurse, and completed master's and/or doctoral programs in the field of mental health and diseases or psychiatric nursing as "Expert Psychiatric Nurses" via Article 9/2-a of the PMHL. Despite this, it introduces a structural restriction preventing this academic specialization from transforming into actual authority. Therefore, the autonomous practice of psychotherapy by the said experts is absolutely prohibited in the PMHL. The fundamental legal basis for this situation is the insurmountable legal firewall the PMHL builds between "support and care," which constitutes the legal domain of nursing, and the concepts of "treatment and cure" allocated to the disciplines of medicine and psychology.

One of the most important regulations eliminating nurses' authority to practice psychotherapy constitutes Article 10 of the PMHL. This is because nurses are not included among the professionals authorized to practice psychotherapy in the relevant provision. On the other hand, Article 2/m of the PMHL, while defining mental intervention, mentions "interventions applied within the scope of their authorities by members of the profession serving in the field." However, the legal and traditional definition of nursing services is limited to "care and support" services, not "medical treatment." As a natural consequence of this, a nurse, even if possessing a doctoral degree in the field of psychiatry and completing necessary therapy trainings, cannot possess the authority to practice psychotherapy, which is legally classified in the "treatment" category. Therefore, the PMHL possesses a barrier that makes it impossible to exceed the legal boundaries (scope of practice) brought by the professional title, no matter how high the academic competence is. In this aspect, the PMHL puts forth a model completely diverging from the model adopted in Anglo-Saxon legal systems based on competence.

In its current form, the PMHL, in our opinion, completely excludes the "Advanced Practice Nurse Psychotherapist" model, which is becoming increasingly widespread and accepted internationally, from the Turkish legal system. Indeed, regarding psychotherapeutic interventions, the role of nurses is removed from being an autonomous clinician and reduced to a secondary and complementary position within the team, dependent on the directives of the physician who is the final decision-maker in diagnosis and treatment processes. Thus, even in the institutions where they receive education, nurses can only be included in the process under physician supervision and provided they remain within the scope of "nursing services." Furthermore, penal sanctions are envisaged in Article 18 of the PMHL in the event that psychotherapy is practiced by professional groups other than authorized persons. When viewed from this aspect, generally, a model falling within the Continental European legal model has been adopted.

Comparative Synthesis: Turkey as a "Restricted" Jurisdiction

In Turkish law, considering the current approach within the PMHL, it is possible to state that the "Delegated Medical Act" model, prevalent in conservative Continental European Law jurisdictions, has been adopted. Indeed, Turkish law accepts that authority stems primarily from professional title and the pre-existing medical hierarchy, unlike the US or the UK, where competence and educational attainment (such as a Master's degree) determine clinical authority. In this aspect, the PMHL maintains a stance that rejects the concept of full practice authority.

Indeed, the PMHL has not accepted the nurse as an independent health professional regarding the execution of diagnostic and treatment activities. Rather, it accepts them as auxiliary personnel utilized in the execution of health services. In this respect, the understanding adopted in Turkish law has essentially been maintained as is. The same situation applies regarding the Nursing Law, the fundamental regulation concerning the nursing profession. Therefore, in our opinion, the PMHL possesses an approach that follows the fundamental legal regulations at this point. In this aspect, nurses in Turkey are positioned as "functional auxiliaries" with limited therapeutic potential. Indeed, although the legislation emphasizes that services are provided by a "team" for a holistic approach, the structure of this team is not horizontal and collaborative. On the contrary, a vertical and hierarchical structure is in question.

The fact that legal regulations possess this approach is criticized in the literature. The existence of a contradiction with the "Task Shifting" recommendations by the World Health Organization also lies at the source of the criticisms (Agyapong et al., 2016; Efendi et al., 2022). In this context, it is stated that closing health workforce shortages and treatment gaps becomes difficult as a result of such legal approaches. In the literature in Turkey as well, the confinement of psychiatric and mental health nurses within the boundaries of physician-led care, instead of being liberated for the needs of the population in this field, is criticized (Bilkay et al., 2025). It is stated that what should happen is the adoption of policies officially recognizing the roles of nurses in offering psychotherapy under appropriate supervision (Bilkay et al., 2025). Indeed, studies conducted in different geographical contexts such as Indonesia show that delegating psychosocial intervention tasks to nurses is feasible and acceptable when necessary political and legal regulations exist and appropriate supervision is provided, and also that nurses can deliver these services effectively (Aurizki & Wilson, 2022).

In our opinion, regarding psychotherapy practices, the primary issue in determining the scope of authorized persons is not the scope of authorized persons itself. The important issue is that the competency conditions for practicing psychotherapy are determined correctly. This is because the problem currently questioned and existing in Turkey is not who practices psychotherapies. The real problem is whether what is being practiced is technically a psychotherapy. Here, the PMHL in Turkish law is a cornerstone precisely to solve this problem. Because in Turkey, even individuals who have merely completed a four-year psychology education open a private place, conduct so-called psychological counseling, and offer so-called psychotherapy services. Within the scope of existing legal regulations in Turkish law, these practices cannot be definitively prevented. Here, the PMHL solves precisely this problem and offers a solution path to at least eliminate "what should not be" by revealing what psychotherapy and practice conditions are. In other words, the basic competency standard in psychotherapy practices will at least be determined. After this, discussing the authority problem of other mental health professionals such as expert psychiatric nurses is, in our view, a subsequent matter. At least in the proceeding process, the authority issue is a situation that can be reviewed again according to the needs of the time with changes that can be made along with new legislative activities. However, at this point, our opinion is also that expert psychiatric nurses meeting basic competency standards (PMHL Art. 9/2-a) should be able to conduct psychotherapy practices, at least under the supervision and control of a physician, within the framework of the task shifting model via legislative changes to be made in the future, despite the current rigid legal limitation.

ETHICAL STANDARDS AND DILEMMAS IN PSYCHOTHERAPY PRACTICE

The integration of psychotherapy into mental health nursing does not merely signify an expansion of clinical skills. It simultaneously brings about a radical shift in the ethical dimension of practice. While the legal frameworks discussed in previous sections define what a nurse *can* do, ethical standards establish what a nurse *should* do.

In Turkey and some EU countries where legal authority lags behind professional competence, nurses frequently confront the concept of “moral distress.” Moral distress arises when an individual knows the correct course of action but cannot carry it out due to institutional or legal constraints (Haines et al., 2024; Kornaros et al., 2018; Larsman et al., 2024). This distress becomes particularly pronounced at moments when a nurse is compelled to restrict a patient's freedom. This situation conflicts directly with the nurse's obligation to promote the patient's self-recovery (Bífárìn et al., 2024). Therefore, ethical reasoning is a fundamental and continuous necessity for mental health nurses, especially in ambiguous and rapidly changing clinical situations (Bífárìn et al., 2024). This section analyzes these dilemmas within the comparative context of Anglo-Saxon and Continental European legal systems through the lens of four fundamental biomedical ethics principles: beneficence, non-maleficence, autonomy, and justice.

The Conflict Between Competence and Licensure: Beneficence vs. Non-Maleficence

At the root of the ethical dilemmas frequently encountered in modern psychiatric nursing lies a deep disconnect between the nurse's clinical capability and their legal authority. This situation is fueled by the conflict between two fundamental ethical principles. The first is the principle of beneficence, which mandates that the health-care professional act in the patient's best interest to alleviate suffering. The second is the principle of non-maleficence, which involves the duty to adhere to legal limits designed to protect public safety (Almotiry et al., 2023; Manderius et al., 2023).

The critical conflict between these two principles becomes particularly evident in "restricted" jurisdictions like Turkey. In these systems, even if the nurse possesses the skill to treat, they do not hold the legal license to practice it. However, although professional ethics education generally emphasizes simply obeying the law, the reality that legality and ethics do not always overlap is ignored at this point (Wilkenfeld & Durmis, 2022). For example, consider an expert nurse in a public hospital in Turkey who holds a master's degree in psychotherapy. Suppose this nurse identifies that a patient in acute distress would benefit from Cognitive Behavioral Therapy (CBT). However, in the face of the strict provisions of the PMHL, it is unlawful for the expert psychiatric nurse to initiate CBT, even under a physician's order or supervision. The PMHL even envisages criminal sanctions at this point. Conversely, if the physician is unavailable or lacks CBT training, the nurse's refraining from using their skills amounts to withholding evidence-based treatment from the patient. This is a clear violation of the principle of beneficence (Almotiry et al., 2023). Consequently, the nurse falls into deep "moral distress," knowing the right action to take but being unable to execute it due to institutional or legal barriers (Kornaros et al., 2018). Ultimately, such legal restrictions on the scope of practice contribute significantly to "ethical value conflicts" for nurses (Larsman et al., 2024). In addition to ethical dilemmas, the sensory and emotional burden of providing care to trauma victims in complex clinical environments can lead to professional traumatization and identity loss, necessitating robust institutional support to protect nurses' well-being (Albayrak Günday & Gülırmak Güler, 2026).

In the US, however, the legal clarity provided by Nurse Practice Acts appears to resolve this tension. Indeed, the PMHNP in the US has both the duty and the authority to act. In contrast, in Continental European legal systems, the nurse is forced to make a difficult choice between "ethical illegality" (providing the therapy the patient needs but violating the statute) or "legal unethicality" (withholding treatment to comply with the law). Whereas, the International Council of Nurses Code of Ethics emphasizes that the nurse's primary responsibility is to people requiring nursing care. In this respect, it possesses content that supports human rights and patient advocacy (Stievano & Tschudin, 2019). Otherwise, the nurse's primary loyalty is not to laws or institutions. Theoretically, this principle creates a universal and "supranational" ethical obligation above the restrictions imposed by national laws. However, the practical problem is that a nurse's defense of "I acted in accordance with universal ethics for my patient's benefit" holds no weight in a trial conducted in a court of law. This legal and ethical disconnect drives nurses into a serious ethical impasse between the ideal of protecting patient safety and autonomy and the obligation to comply with legal boundaries (Bífárìn et al., 2024).

Informed Consent and the Ambiguity of Professional Identity

The principle of autonomy, one of the cornerstones of biomedical ethics, mandates that patients fully understand not only the nature, risks, and benefits of the treatment to be administered to them, but also the qualifications and professional boundaries of the provider offering this treatment. This obligation constitutes the heart of the "Informed Consent" doctrine (Baptista et al., 2022; Beauchamp & Childress, 2019). Indeed, an ethically valid consent process requires transparency and veracity. Consequently, psychotherapists are both ethically and legally obliged to clearly declare their professional identities and competency levels to patients (Blease et al., 2020; Trachsel & Holtforth, 2019).

In jurisdictions such as the US and the UK, where titles like "Advanced Practice Nurse" or PMHNP are under legal protection, it is observed that the consent process is relatively transparent. In this way, the patient has the opportunity to consent to treatment knowing that the professional before them is a psychotherapist with a nursing background and understanding the scope and legal limits of this role. This situation ensures that the therapeutic alliance is established on a foundation of trust (Halter et al., 2021). However, in jurisdictions where the nurse's role is left legally ambiguous or restricted, the declaration of professional identity poses a quite serious problem.

In the context of Turkey, the PMHL prohibits nurses from using the title of "psychotherapist" or introducing themselves in a way that implies psychotherapeutic authority, and prescribes severe penal sanctions. This confronts nurses in Turkey with a deep "transparency paradox" between professional ethics and legal obligations. A similar situation applies regarding EU countries that adopt the same stance.

At the first dimension of the said paradox lies the criminalization of transparency. If a competent expert psychiatric nurse acts honestly towards their patient and states, "The treatment I will apply to you is psychotherapy and I am a nurse," this declaration will virtually carry the nature of a confession to an unlawful intervention. Furthermore, since the act would not be a medical intervention by nature, patient consent would not be evaluated as a ground for justification. Because the consent is now an invalid consent. Conversely, in the opposite case, the administration of the treatment would already not be legally possible. This impasse pushes the nurse into a process of "forced deception" in order to meet the patient's clinical need and observe the principle of beneficence. To avoid legal sanction, the nurse is forced to present structured treatments they apply, such as Cognitive Behavioral Therapy (CBT), under legal guises such as "psychosocial support," "counseling," or "education." This situation causes the patient to be misled regarding the true nature of the service received, thereby violating the "truth-telling" condition of informed consent (Gallagher, 2020).

Finally, the ethical confusion gains an even more systemic dimension with the practice of working "in the physician's shadow," which emerges as a common workaround in restrictive systems. Showing the psychotherapy service actually administered by the nurse as if it were performed by a physician in official records and billing constitutes a "systemic deception." Although this practical application bureaucratically facilitates the patient's access to care, it deprives the patient of the right to know who is actually treating them (Trachsel & Holtforth, 2019). In such a scenario, the therapeutic relationship is virtually forced to be built upon a lie. This is incompatible with the principle of authenticity in psychotherapy ethics (Khanahmadi, 2020). Consequently, the current legal regulation drags the nurse into an insoluble ethical impasse, forcing them to either violate the principle of beneficence by not treating the patient or to violate the principles of autonomy and veracity by conducting treatment secretly and under misleading names.

Confidentiality, The Duty to Warn, and Vicarious Liability

Psychotherapy is a process uniquely dependent on absolute confidentiality by its very nature. In this respect, it is impossible to build and maintain the therapeutic process without this foundation of privacy (Khanahmadi, 2020). In this context, nurses have both an ethical and legal duty to protect patient privacy and respect confidentiality unless there is a clear legal mandate or an imminent and serious threat to the safety of the patient or third parties (Albayrak Günday & Gülırmak Güler, 2026; Almotiry et al., 2023; Conlon et al., 2024). However, in situations where a patient poses a serious danger to themselves or others, the "Duty to Warn," known as the obligation to breach confidentiality, comes into play. This situation creates a distinct ethical responsibility area that is quite difficult for nurses to manage (Conlon et al., 2024).

In the US, following the *Tarasoff v. Regents of the University of California* decision, which was a turning point in legal literature, mental health professionals, including nurses, have a distinct and undisputed legal obligation to warn potential victims of violence (Anfang & Appelbaum, 1996; Bersoff, 2014; Herbert & Young, 2002; Günday, 2015). This precedent provides a clear ethical roadmap to clinicians by ruling that public safety outweighs patient privacy. Similarly, in the UK, the NMC Code permits the breach of confidentiality with legal assurance in risky situations where public interest is at stake (Bífárìn et al., 2024). However, the situation in Turkey has a much more complex appearance due to the existing hierarchical legal structure and the uncertainties introduced by the PMHL. Although there is a general "notification obligation" in risk situations in Turkish law (Günday, 2015), in legal systems where decision-making authority is ultimately concentrated in the physician within the medical hierarchy, this leads to the diffusion of responsibility (Conlon et al., 2024). This hierarchical structure confronts nurses with a serious "ethical trap."

Indeed, regarding this issue, for example, a scenario should be considered where a nurse evaluates a patient as dangerous during a therapy session, but the supervisor psychiatrist disagrees with this view and decides not to warn the authorities. In this scenario, the nurse remains in an insoluble dilemma. Indeed, while reporting independently carries the risk of violating the chain of institutional hierarchy and patient confidentiality for the nurse; remaining silent pushes the nurse to virtually become a partner in the legal and ethical liability of a potential incident of violence.

The concept of "Vicarious Liability" in the UK offers a safety net that encourages nurses to report risks without fear of personal litigation, thanks to the institution (NHS) assuming liability arising from the employee's actions (Tingle, 2022). In Turkey, although a general framework regarding the malpractice liability of a psychiatrist exists (Günday, 2015), there is no legal regulation regulating specific liability cases, particularly regarding psychotherapeutic interventions. In this framework, the legal solution to specific issues that may occur in professional and patient relationships in the field of mental health, such as privacy in psychotherapies or the duty to warn third parties, is uncertain in Turkish law. Although the PMHL attempts to solve the issue by introducing certain regulations on these matters, there is currently no enacted legal regulation available. Therefore, while the situation is legally uncertain even for authorized mental health professionals; attempting to interpret the issue and offer a solution proposal for nurses is, in our opinion, nothing more than optimism. However, it must be said that general liability law principles are ultimately valid in the legal relationship with mental patients in Turkish law.

Boundary Violations in the "Hands-On" Tradition

The historical and ontological foundations of the nursing profession are based on physical proximity, touch, and inclusive care. In contrast, the professional psychotherapy process traditionally requires a rigid structural distance demanding the rule of "abstinence" and neutrality. While the "therapeutic use of self" approach in nursing encourages closeness and intimacy (Zur, 2007); psychotherapy necessitates the maintenance of a distinct boundary where the therapist refrains from gratifying the patient's desires, particularly to manage transference and counter-transference processes healthily. This principle, termed the "distance protection duty" in legal doctrine and psychotherapy ethics (Günday, 2015), commands the therapist to limit their relationship with the patient solely to the purpose of professional treatment (Boemke, 2011; Dammann, 2004; Günday, 2015). In this framework, the relationship between the therapist and the patient is by nature a relationship of trust; it must be separated from friendship, companionship, or romantic intimacies with sharp lines (Appelbaum & Gutheil, 2007; Günday, 2015; Laufs et al., 2002). Furthermore, this separation must continue not only during the therapy but also in the process after the completion of the therapy (Günday, 2015; Gründel, 2000).

Professional boundaries are vital lines protecting both the vulnerable patient and the healthcare provider, especially considering the asymmetric power difference in therapeutic relationships (Baca, 2011; Unhjem & Hem, 2025). The therapist's use of the trust the patient places in them or the feelings directed through transference to satisfy their own personal, social, or sexual needs is a clear violation of both the "distance protection duty" and the "duty of care" (Günday, 2015; LeBoeuf, 1988). Of course, not every boundary crossing is an absolute violation; some out-of-office encounters managed transparently in the informed consent process or humane gestures made in a cultural context should be able to be therapeutically beneficial (Amaglo, 2022; Crowden, 2008). However, it is necessary to accept boundary violations where boundaries become blurred and the patient is exploited as absolutely unethical and to handle them within the scope of legal liability.

The reflection of this theoretical framework in practice creates a serious "role conflict," especially for nurses working in inpatient treatment institutions. While ward nurses assume the role of the "authoritarian figure" administering the patient's medications, regulating daily life, and enforcing ward rules; on the other hand, they assume the role of the "empathic figure" providing psychological support to the same patient. This "dual relationship" carries the risk of blurring the boundaries in the patient's mind (Afolabi, 2015; Baca, 2011). While APNs in the US can separate these roles by working within their legal authorities; nurses in Turkey, whose authority to practice psychotherapy is taken away by the Art. 10 of PMHL, are in a paradoxical vulnerability because they are not legally considered "therapists."

The real ethical dilemma for nurses in Turkey is the intense transference and counter-transference dynamics they are inevitably exposed to due to the physical proximity brought by care, even though they are legally considered "not practicing psychotherapy." Since the system does not legally recognize the nurse as a "therapist," it deems the clinical supervision support that would enable them to manage these complex boundaries unnecessary and does not offer it. Whereas, clinical supervision is an indispensable safety mechanism for professionals working in the field of mental health, whether they have authority or not, to establish a safe relationship with the patient without violating the "distance protection duty" (Barnett & Molzon, 2014; Falender, 2020). Therefore, the prohibitive approach in Turkish law not only leaves the nurse without authority; it also leaves them open to ethical risks by depriving them of supervision, which is the most important shield protecting them against boundary violations.

Suicide Risk Assessment and the "Standard of Care"

The clinical management of suicidal patients constitutes one of the highest-risk ethical and legal challenges for mental health professionals. In this context, there is a fundamental principle accepted in legal doctrine and clinical practice. That is, liability stems not from the suicide itself, which is an act of the patient's free will and sometimes unforeseeable; but from the failure to conduct an adequate, comprehensive, and standard-compliant "suicide risk assessment" (Günday, 2015; Sabé et al., 2020). Indeed, as Simon and Sadoff (2005) accurately emphasized, a clinician is not the absolute guarantor of the patient's life. However, regarding a "rigorous assessment process," the situation is the opposite. Therefore, legal and ethical liability depends not on whether the result (death) could be prevented, but on whether the risk was foreseeable and whether necessary "protective measures" were taken in light of this foresight (Günday, 2015; Stanley et al., 2019).

A claim of ethical failure and malpractice against a nurse or therapist generally arises from ignoring "red flags" (e.g., previous suicide attempts, concrete and detailed plans, farewell behaviors, or giving away possessions). However, there is, of course, no single universally accepted "gold standard" method for suicide risk assessment. Nevertheless, judicial decisions and scientific doctrine stipulate at this point that assessments be made within the measure of "reasonable care" (Günday, 2015). In this context, the assessment process should never rely solely on the patient's verbal declaration of "I will not kill myself" or unilateral information. Because suicidal individuals may have a tendency to hide their plans (Günday, 2015). Therefore, clinical judgment should be supported by structured risk assessment tools, anamnesis information obtained from patient relatives, and examination of previous medical records (Grant & Lusk, 2015; Hawton et al., 2022). When risk is detected, implementing proportional clinical actions such as increasing session frequency, including the family in the process, or initiating involuntary hospitalization procedures constitutes a requirement of the "standard of care" (Günday, 2015).

The concept of the "No-Suicide Contract," frequently resorted to in clinical practice, is subject to serious criticism in current literature. This method, where the patient signs a written document stating they will not kill themselves, has no significance alone in both legal and ethical terms, even if it creates a "false sense of security" in the clinician (Egan, 1997; Garvey et al., 2009; Rudd et al., 2005). Because empirical studies do not provide evidence that such contracts are effective in preventing suicide. On the contrary, excessive reliance on these contracts can cause negligence by replacing comprehensive clinical judgment and supervision (Range et al., 2002). Moreover, obtaining such a signature from a patient whose judgment is impaired or who is in acute crisis is a situation that can be considered unethical even in terms of informed consent capacity (Egan, 1997; Garvey et al., 2009). As a result of this, the modern approach envisages conducting a collaborative "Safety Planning" that includes who to contact in a moment of crisis, how to manage triggers, and how to ensure a safe environment, instead of bargaining (contracting) with the patient (Stanley & Brown, 2012; Wortzel et al., 2013).

REFERENCES

Afolabi, O. E. (2015). Dual relationships and boundary crossing: A critical issues in clinical psychology practice. *International Journal of Psychology and Counselling, 7*(2), 29–39.

Agyapong, V. I. O., Farren, C., & McAuliffe, E. (2016). Improving Ghana's mental healthcare through task-shifting—Psychiatrists and health policy directors perceptions about government's commitment and the role of community mental health workers. *Globalization and Health, 12*, 57. Advance online publication. DOI: 10.1186/s12992-016-0199-z PMID: 27716339

Albayrak, E., & Asi Karakaş, S. (2022). An investigation of internalized stigma and recovery levels of patients registered in a Community Mental Health Center. *Perspectives in Psychiatric Care, 58*(4), 1940–1948. DOI: 10.1111/ppc.13011 PMID: 34973035

Albayrak Günday, E., & Gülırmak Güler, K. (2025). Psychosocial therapies in psychiatry. In M. Aydın (Ed.), *Fundamentals of Psychiatric Nursing* (pp. [PDF'deki Sayfa Aralığı]). BZT Turan Publishing House.

Albayrak Günday, E., & Gülırmak Güler, K. (2026). Artificial intelligence through the eyes of psychiatric nurses: An in-depth investigation of thought, anxiety and readiness. *Issues in Mental Health Nursing*. Advance online publication. DOI: 10.1080/01612840.2025.2596210 PMID: 41504220

Albayrak Günday, E., & Gülırmak Güler, K. (2026). Examining the construction of sensory balance and well-being in psychiatric nurses caring for trauma victims: A qualitative study. *Journal of Nursing Scholarship, 58*, e70053. DOI: 10.1111/jnu.70053 PMID: 41199426

Almotiry, M. B., Alqahtani, A. A., Al Nime, A. M., Alonezi, B. F., Alotaibi, N. G., Khubrani, H. A. M., & Alotaibi, N. N. S. (2023). Assessment of nurses' knowledge about ethical and legal issues of mental health nursing at psychiatric teaching hospitals. *Journal of Survey in Fisheries Sciences, 10*(6), Articles. https://doi.org/DOI: 10.53555/sfs.v10i6.2247

Amaglo, E. (2022). Managing boundaries and multiple relationships in counselling and psychotherapy. *Global Journal of Psychology, 2*(1), Articles. https://doi.org/DOI: 10.51594/gjp.v2i1.361

American Nurses Association (ANA). (2014). *Scope and Standards of Practice: Psychiatric-Mental Health Nursing* (2nd ed.). Silver Spring, MD: Nursesbooks.org.

American Nurses Credentialing Center (ANCC). (2020). *PMHNP-BC Test Content Outline*.

American Psychiatric Nurses Association (APNA). (2019). *Psychiatric-Mental Health Nursing: Scope and Standards of Practice* (3rd ed.). American Nurses Association.

Anfang, S. A., & Appelbaum, P. S. (1996). Twenty years after Tarasoff: Reviewing the duty to protect. *Harvard Review of Psychiatry, 4*(2), 67–76. DOI: 10.3109/10673229609030526 PMID: 9384976

Antão, C., Santos, B. P. J. dos, Santos, N. R. dos, Fernandes, H., Barroso, B., Mărginean, C. O., & Pimentel, M. H. (2025). Nursing Degree Curriculum: Differences and Similarities Between 15 European Countries. *Nursing Reports, 15*(3), 112. Multidisciplinary Digital Publishing Institute. https://doi.org/DOI: 10.3390/nursrep15030112

Appelbaum, P. S., & Gutheil, T. G. (2007). *Clinical Handbook of Psychiatry & Law* (4th ed.). Lippincott Williams & Wilkins.

Aurizki, G. E., & Wilson, I. (2022). Nurse-led task-shifting strategies to substitute for mental health specialists in primary care: A systematic review. *International Journal of Nursing Practice, 28*(5), e13046. Wiley. https://doi.org/DOI: 10.1111/ijn.13046

Baptista, K., Walbridge, G. B., Marks, J. A., & Knoll, J. L. (2022). Ethics in Psychotherapy: Informed Consent, Digital Professionalism, and Sexual Misconduct. *Focus - American Psychiatric Publishing, 20*(3), 313–317. DOI: 10.1176/appi.focus.20220043 PMID: 37205024

Barker, P. (2009). *Psychiatric and Mental Health Nursing: The Craft of Caring* (2nd ed.). Hodder Arnold.

Barnett, J. E., & Molzon, C. H. (2014). Clinical Supervision of Psychotherapy: Essential Ethics Issues for Supervisors and Supervisees. *Journal of Clinical Psychology, 70*(11), 1051–1061. DOI: 10.1002/jclp.22126 PMID: 25220636

Beauchamp, T. L., & Childress, J. F. (2019). *Principles of Biomedical Ethics* (8th ed.). Oxford University Press.

Beis, P., Graf, M., & Hachtel, H. (2022). Impact of legal traditions on forensic mental health treatment worldwide. *Frontiers in Psychiatry, 13*, 876619. Frontiers Media. https://doi.org/DOI: 10.3389/fpsyt.2022.876619

Bersoff, D. N. (2014). Protecting victims of violent patients while protecting confidentiality. *The American Psychologist, 69*(5), 461–467. DOI: 10.1037/a0037198 PMID: 25046702

Bifarin, O., Collier-Sewell, F., Smith, G., Moriarty, J., Shepherd, H., Andrews, L., Pearson, S., & Kasperska, M. (2024). Standards of proficiency for registered nurses—To what end? A critical analysis of contemporary mental health nursing within the United Kingdom context. *Nursing Inquiry*, *31*(3), e12630. DOI: 10.1111/nin.12630 PMID: 38436620

Bilkay, H. İ., Öztürk, C., Şirin, B., & Bozkurt, A. (2025). Investigation of psychiatric nurses' views on psychotherapy implementation processes: A qualitative study. *BMC Nursing*, *24*(1), 785–796. DOI: 10.1186/s12912-025-03460-8 PMID: 40597100

Blease, C., Arnott, T., Kelley, J. M., Proctor, G., Kube, T., Gaab, J., & Locher, C. (2020). Attitudes About Informed Consent: An Exploratory Qualitative Analysis of UK Psychotherapy Trainees. *Frontiers in Psychiatry, 11*, 183. Frontiers Media. https://doi.org/DOI: 10.3389/fpsyt.2020.00183

Boemke, B. (2011). Haftung des Psychotherapeuten (Einzelbeitrag). *MHP (Medizinrecht, Haftung und Prozess), 45.*

Bolton, P., West, J., Whitney, C., Jordans, M. J. D., Bass, J., Thornicroft, G., & Raviola, G. (2023). Expanding mental health services in low- and middle-income countries: A task-shifting framework for delivery of comprehensive, collaborative, and community-based care. *Cambridge Prisms: Global Mental Health*, *10*, e16. DOI: 10.1017/gmh.2023.5 PMID: 37854402

Broeck, N. V., & Lietaer, G. (2008). Psychology and Psychotherapy in Health Care. *European Psychologist*, *13*(1), 53. DOI: 10.1027/1016-9040.13.1.53

Buppert, C. (2017). *Nurse Practitioner's Business Practice and Legal Guide*. Jones & Bartlett Learning.

Burgi, M., & Igl, G. (2021). *Rechtliche Voraussetzungen und Möglichkeiten der Etablierung von Community Health Nursing (CHN) in Deutschland.* Nomos Verlag., DOI: 10.5771/9783748924319

Cahill, M., Alexander, M., & Gross, L. (2014). The 2014 NCSBN Consensus Report on APRN Regulation. *Journal of Nursing Regulation*, *4*(4), 5–12. DOI: 10.1016/s2155-8256(15)30111-3

Coffey, M., & Hannigan, B. (2013). New roles for nurses as approved mental health professionals in England and Wales. *International Journal of Nursing Studies*, *50*(10), 1423–1430. DOI: 10.1016/j.ijnurstu.2013.02.014 PMID: 23522939

Cohen, I., Gal, ali, & Enosh, G. (2022). Two Roads Converge: The Interchange Between the Mental Health and Legal Discourses in Sexual Assault Trials. *Social & Legal Studies*, *32*(3), 441–463. DOI: 10.1177/09646639221117388

Conlon, D., Raeburn, T., & Wand, T. (2024). Nurses' understanding of their duty of confidentiality to patients in mental health care: A qualitative exploratory study. *Collegian Journal of the Royal College of Nursing Australia, 31*(3), 144–153. DOI: 10.1016/j.colegn.2024.02.002

Crowden, A. (2008). Professional boundaries and the ethics of dual and multiple overlapping relationships in psychotherapy. *Monash Bioethics Review, 27*, 10–27. DOI: 10.1007/bf03351302 PMID: 19760852

Dammann, O. (2004). *Medizinrecht: Zivilrecht, Versicherungsrecht, Arzneirecht, Berufsrecht, Vertragsarzttecht, Krankenhausrecht*. Nomos Verlag.

Davis, W. D., Stanley, J., Buck, M., Walters, E., & DeGarmo, S. (2024). LACE and the APRN Consensus Model: Implications for Advancing Nursing Practice. *AACN Advanced Critical Care, 35*(1), 20–28. DOI: 10.4037/aacnacc2024956 PMID: 38457622

Debout, C., Eterstein, C., & Greiner, D. (2012). Advanced practice nursing in France: A perspective. *International Nursing Review, 59*(4), 466–467. PMID: 23134129

Decock, N., Friganović, A., Kurtović, B., Oomen, B., Crombez, P., & Willems, C. (2022). Temper the Specialist Nurses Heterogeneity in the Interest of Quality Practice and Mobility—18 EU Countries Study. *Health Care, 10*(3), 435–444. DOI: 10.3390/healthcare10030435 PMID: 35326913

Delaney, K. R. (2023). Inclusion of Psychiatric–Mental Health Advanced Practice Nurses in Federal Behavioral Workforce Planning. *Psychiatric Services (Washington, D.C.), 75*(6), 594–596. DOI: 10.1176/appi.ps.20230321 PMID: 38088040

Devictor, J., Burnet, E., Henriot, T., Leclercq, A., Ganne-Carrié, N., Kilpatrick, K., & Jović, L. (2022). Implementing advanced practice nursing in France: A country-wide survey 2 years after its introduction. *Nursing Open, 10*(3), 1437–1448. DOI: 10.1002/nop2.1394 PMID: 36168185

Dimond, B. (2015). *Legal Aspects of Nursing* (7th ed.). Pearson.

Directive 2005/36/EC of the European Parliament and of the Council of 7 September 2005 on the recognition of professional qualifications. *Official Journal of the European Union*, L 255/22.

Doody, O., Graham, M., Hegarty, O., Sloane, A. M., Walsh, P., Synnott, M., Russell, M., Dunworth, T., Sheridan, J., & Murphy, L. (2025). Identifying the landscape and contribution of advanced nurse practitioners in supporting healthcare provision in Ireland in the 21st century: An integrative review. *International Journal of Nursing Studies Advances, 8*, 100304. DOI: 10.1016/j.ijnsa.2025.100304 PMID: 40018051

Dury, C., Hall, C. L., Danan, J., Mondoux, J., Barbieri-Figueiredo, M. C. A., Costa, M. A., & Debout, C. (2014). Specialist nurse in Europe: Education, regulation and role. *International Nursing Review, 61*(4), 454–462. DOI: 10.1111/inr.12123 PMID: 25214392

Efendi, F., Aurizki, G. E., Yusuf, A., & McKenna, L. (2022). "Not shifting, but sharing": Stakeholders' perspectives on mental health task-shifting in Indonesia. *BMC Nursing, 21*(1), 165. DOI: 10.1186/s12912-022-00945-8 PMID: 35751061

Egan, M. P. (1997). Contracting for Safety: A Concept Analysis. *Crisis, 18*(1), 17. DOI: 10.1027/0227-5910.18.1.17 PMID: 9141775

Escardívol, R. B. i, Mateo-Viladomat, E., Galbany-Estragués, P., Vilar-Pont, M., Solé, M. A. C. i, Lopez, G., Flores-Montoya, R., Vicente-Belis, M., Escoda-Geli, N., Molina-Nadal, A., Vélez, O. C., & Solà, G. J. i. (2024). Implementation of Nurse Prescriptions throughout the Public Health System in Catalonia (2021–2022). *Health Care, 12*(12), 1232. DOI: 10.3390/healthcare12121232 PMID: 38921348

European Commission. (2005). *User Guide: Directive 2005/36/EC*. Brussels: DG Internal Market.

European Federation of Nurses Associations (EFN). (2015). *EFN Competency Framework for General Care Nurses*. EFN.

European Union. (2012). *Consolidated Version of the Treaty on the Functioning of the European Union*. Article 168.

Falender, C. A. (2020). Ethics of Clinical Supervision: An International Lens. *Psychology in Russia : State of the Art, 13*(1), 42. DOI: 10.11621/pir.2020.0105

Forchuk, C. (2021). *Overview ofPeplau's Theory*., DOI: 10.4324/9781003000853-21

Fulton, J. S. (2019). Fulfilling Our Social Mandate. *Clinical Nurse Specialist CNS, 33*(2), 61. DOI: 10.1097/nur.0000000000000430 PMID: 30730448

Gaebel, W., Zielasek, J., & Kowitz, S. (2020). Psychiatric training in Germany. *International Review of Psychiatry (Abingdon, England), 32*(2), 133–138. PMID: 31689126

Gallagher, A. (2020). *Slow Ethics for Nursing Practice: Reclaiming the Value of Time*. Oxford University Press. (Hemşirelikte dürüstlük ve rol çatışmaları üzerine).

García-Sastre, M., Castro-Molina, F. J., Cabanillas, R. C., Corrales, C. S., Golmar, L. J., Román, J. C., & Aguilera-Serrano, C. (2024). Psychotherapeutic nursing as Advanced Clinical Practice for the promotion of mental health in Spain. *International Nursing Review, 71*(2), 244. DOI: 10.1111/inr.12935 PMID: 38191271

Garvey, K. A., Penn, J. V., Campbell, A. L., Esposito-Smythers, C., & Spirito, A. (2009). Contracting for safety with patients: clinical practice and forensic implications. *PubMed, 37*(3), 363. https://pubmed.ncbi.nlm.nih.gov/19767501

Glarcher, M., & Lex, K. M. (2020). Advanced Nursing Practice in Austria under consideration of outcome measurement. *Zeitschrift für Evidenz, Fortbildung und Qualität im Gesundheitswesen, 155*, 11. DOI: 10.1016/j.zefq.2020.06.012 PMID: 32811773

Grant, C., & Lusk, J. (2015). A multidisciplinary approach to therapeutic risk management of the suicidal patient. *Journal of Multidisciplinary Healthcare, 8*, 291–298. DOI: 10.2147/jmdh.s50529 PMID: 26150725

Gründel, M. (2000). *Psychotherapeutisches Haftungsrecht (Die zivilrechtliche Haftung des Psychologischen Psycotherapeuten bei Verletzung seiner Berufspflichten)*. Springer.

Gülırmak Güler, K., Güleç Keskin, S., & Albayrak, E. (2024). The power of virtual connections: A randomized controlled trial of online positive psychotherapy training on effective communication skills of nursing students. *Nurse Education in Practice, 77*, 103967. DOI: 10.1016/j.nepr.2024.103967 PMID: 38615450

Günday, H. M. (2015). *Psikiyatristin Hukukî Sorumluluğu*. Yetkin Yayınları.

Günday, H. M., & Albayrak Günday, E. (2025). Artificial intelligence in mental health practices: Legal liability analysis under Turkish, European, and Common Law frameworks. *Psikiyatride Güncel Yaklaşımlar-Current Approaches in Psychiatry, 17*(4), 806–821. DOI: 10.18863/pgy.1620119

Haines, S. G., Stanton, R., Anderson, C., & Welch, A. (2024). Ethical challenges for nurses delivering coercive interventions in community mental health settings: A scoping review. *International Journal of Mental Health Nursing, 33*(4), 750–759. DOI: 10.1111/inm.13290 PMID: 38205562

Halter, M. J., Rolin, D., Adamaszek, M., & Russell, B. (2021). Professional Identity and Scope of Practice for the Psychiatric Mental Health Nurse Practitioner [Mesleki kimlik ve yetki sınırları için]. *Journal of the American Psychiatric Nurses Association.*

Hawton, K., Lascelles, K., Pitman, A., Gilbert, S., & Silverman, M. M. (2022). Assessment of suicide risk in mental health practice: Shifting from prediction to therapeutic assessment, formulation, and risk management. *The Lancet. Psychiatry, 9*(11), 922–928. DOI: 10.1016/s2215-0366(22)00232-2 PMID: 35952701

Hein, L. C., & Schärer, K. (2014). A Modern History of Psychiatric–Mental Health Nursing. *Archives of Psychiatric Nursing*, *29*(1), 49–55. DOI: 10.1016/j.apnu.2014.10.003 PMID: 25634875

Herbert, P. B., & Young, K. A. (2002). Tarasoff at twenty-five. *PubMed, 30*(2), 275. https://pubmed.ncbi.nlm.nih.gov/12108565

Hoffmeister, L., Huebner, J., Keinki, C., & Muenstedt, K. (2021). Education of non-medical practitioners in Germany—An analysis of course subjects of specialized schools. *Wiener Medizinische Wochenschrift*, *174*, 189. DOI: 10.1007/s10354-021-00896-w PMID: 34902098

Horatio: European Psychiatric Nurses. (2018). *The Role of the Psychiatric Nurse in Europe.*

Hurley, J., Lakeman, R., Linsley, P., Ramsay, M., & Lawson, S. (2022). Utilizing the mental health nursing workforce: A scoping review of mental health nursing clinical roles and identities. *International Journal of Mental Health Nursing, 31*(4), 796-822. Wiley. https://doi.org/DOI: 10.1111/inm.12983

Jones, B. D. M., Umer, M., Kittur, M. E., Finkelstein, O., Xue, S., Dimick, M. K., Ortiz, A., Goldstein, B. I., Mulsant, B. H., & Husain, M. I. (2023). A systematic review on the effectiveness of dialectical behavior therapy for improving mood symptoms in bipolar disorders. *International Journal of Bipolar Disorders*, *11*, 6. DOI: 10.1186/s40345-023-00288-6 PMID: 36739574

Júnior, J. M. P., Clementino, F. de S., Santos, R. C. de A., Vítor, A. F., & Miranda, F. A. N. de. (2017). Enfermagem e o processo de desinstitucionalização no âmbito da saúde mental: revisão integrativa Nursing and the deinstitutionalization process in the mental health scope: integrative review. *Revista de Pesquisa Cuidado é Fundamental Online, 9*(3), 893. https://doi.org/DOI: 10.9789/2175-5361.2017.v9i3.893-898

Khanahmadi, M. (2020). Ethical Codes and Psychotherapy. *International Journal of Ethics & Society*, *1*(4). https://ijethics.com/article-1-62-en.html

Kornaros, K., Zwedberg, S., Nissen, E., & Salomonsson, B. (2018). A hermeneutic study of integrating psychotherapist competence in postnatal child health care: Nurses' perspectives. *BMC Nursing*, *17*(1). Advance online publication. DOI: 10.1186/s12912-018-0311-1 PMID: 30258284

Krug, K., Kraus, K., Herrmann, K., & Joos, S. (2016). Complementary and alternative medicine (CAM) as part of primary health care in Germany–comparison of patients consulting general practitioners and CAM practitioners: A cross-sectional study. *BMC Complementary and Alternative Medicine*, *16*(1), 409. DOI: 10.1186/s12906-016-1402-8 PMID: 27776512

Ladd, E., Miller, M., Wheeler, K., Wainaina, S., Aguirre, F., McGrath, H., Lee, S., Nashwan, A. J., Neary, A., & Core, K. (2020). A Global SWOT Analysis of Advanced Practice Nursing: Policy, Regulation, and Practice. *Research Square (Research Square)*. https://doi.org/DOI: 10.21203/rs.3.rs-113320/v1

Laireiter, A., & Weise, C. (2019). The Heterogeneity of National Regulations in Clinical Psychology and Psychological Treatment in Europe. *Clinical Psychology in Europe*, *1*(1). Advance online publication. DOI: 10.32872/cpe.v1i1.34406

Lange, K. W. (2021). Task sharing in psychotherapy as a viable global mental health approach in resource-poor countries and also in high-resource settings. *Global Health Journal (Amsterdam, Netherlands)*, *5*(3), 120. DOI: 10.1016/j.glohj.2021.07.001

Larsman, P., Pousette, A., Nilsson, M. S., Gadolin, C., & Törner, M. (2024). Ethical value conflicts in healthcare and their effects on nurses' health, turnover intent, team effectiveness, and patient safety: A longitudinal questionnaire study. *Scandinavian Journal of Work, Environment & Health*, *50*(2), 113. DOI: 10.5271/sjweh.4138 PMID: 38232184

Laufs, A., & Uhlenbruck, W. (2002). *Handbuch des Arztrechts*. (3. Aufl.). München: C.H.

LeBoeuf, D. (1988). Psychiatric Malpractice: Exploitation of Women Patients. *Harvard Women's Law Journal*, *11*, 83–116.

Légifrance. (2010). *Décret n° 2010-534 du 20 mai 2010 relatif à l'usage du titre de psychothérapeute*. Journal Officiel de la République Française.

Maier, C. B. (2019). Nurse prescribing of medicines in 13 European countries. *Human Resources for Health*, *17*(1). Advance online publication. DOI: 10.1186/s12960-019-0429-6 PMID: 31815622

Manderius, C., Clintståhl, K., Sjöström, K., & Örmon, K. (2023). The psychiatric mental health nurse's ethical considerations regarding the use of coercive measures – a qualitative interview study. *BMC Nursing*, *22*(1). Advance online publication. DOI: 10.1186/s12912-023-01186-z PMID: 36698105

Martin, B., Phoenix, B. J., & Chapman, S. A. (2020). How collaborative practice agreements impede the provision of vital behavioral health services. *Nursing Outlook, 68*(5), 581. DOI: 10.1016/j.outlook.2020.04.002 PMID: 32402393

Melcop, N., von Werder, T., Sarubin, N., & Benecke, A. (2019). The Role of Psychotherapy in the German Health Care System: Training Requirements for Psychological Psychotherapists and Child and Adolescent Psychotherapists, Legal Aspects, and Health Care Implementation. *Clinical Psychology in Europe*, *1*(4). Advance online publication. DOI: 10.32872/cpe.v1i4.34304

Možina, M. (2024). Psychotherapy regulation in European countries. *Psychotherapie-Wissenschaft, 14*(2), 93. DOI: 10.30820/1664-9583-2024-2-93

Niles, C. (2013). Examining the Deinstitutionalization Movement in North America. *Deleted Journal, 1*(1). Advance online publication. DOI: 10.25071/2564-4033.37273

Nursing and Midwifery Board of Ireland (NMBI). (2017). *Advanced Practice (Nursing) Standards and Requirements*. NMBI.

Nursing and Midwifery Council (NMC). (2018). *Future Nurse: Standards of Proficiency for Registered Nurses*. NMC.

O'Brien, A. J. (2001). The therapeutic relationship: Historical development and contemporary significance. *Journal of Psychiatric and Mental Health Nursing, 8*(2), 129–137. PMID: 11882118

Oleck, L., Retano, A., Tebaldi, C., McGuinness, T. M., Weiss, S., Carbray, J. A., Rodgers, L. S., Donelson, E. E., Ashton, L. L., Koehn, D., & McCoy, P. (2011). Advanced Practice Psychiatric Nurses Legislative Update: State of the States, 2010. *Journal of the American Psychiatric Nurses Association, 17*(2), 171. DOI: 10.1177/1078390311402331 PMID: 21659307

Oliphant, S. (2023). Navigating advanced nurse practitioner roles in UK mental health services: A scoping review. *International Journal for Advancing Practice, 1*(2), 65–71. DOI: 10.12968/ijap.2023.1.2.65

Palese, A., Zabalegui, A., Sigurðardóttir, Á. K., Bergin, M., Dobrowolska, B., Gasser, C., Pajnkihar, M., & Jackson, C. (2014). Bologna Process, More or Less: Nursing Education in the European Economic Area: A Discussion Paper. *International Journal of Nursing Education Scholarship, 11*(1), 63. https://doi.org/DOI: 10.1515/ijnes-2013-0022

Paul, D. R., M., D., Patricia, Jochen, B., Michelle, P., M., J., Susan, Adriana, C.-A., Andreas, X., & Wendy, P. (2023). Advanced practice nursing in Europe—Results from a pan-European survey of 35 countries. *Journal of Advanced Nursing*, *80*(1), 377. DOI: 10.1111/jan.15775 PMID: 37458267

Pedersen, M. L., Gildberg, F. A., & Birkeland, S. (2022). The Danish Court Case Database: A data source in forensic mental health? *Scandinavian Journal of Forensic Science*, *28*(1), 1. DOI: 10.2478/sjfs-2022-0011

Pepfar. (2007). *Task shifting : rational redistribution of tasks among health workforce teams : global recommendations and guidelines*. https://pesquisa.bvsalud.org/portal/resource/pt/who-43821

Peplau, H. E. (1952). *Interpersonal Relations in Nursing*. G.P. Putnam's Sons.

Phoenix, B. J., & Chapman, S. A. (2020). Effect of state regulatory environments on advanced psychiatric nursing practice. *Archives of Psychiatric Nursing*, *34*(5), 370. DOI: 10.1016/j.apnu.2020.07.001 PMID: 33032760

Poghosyan, L., & Maier, C. B. (2022). Advanced practice nurses globally: Responding to health challenges, improving outcomes. *International Journal of Nursing Studies*, *132*, 104262. DOI: 10.1016/j.ijnurstu.2022.104262 PMID: 35633596

Purgato, M., Uphoff, E., Singh, R., Pachya, A. T., Abdulmalik, J., & van Ginneken, N. (2020). Promotion, prevention and treatment interventions for mental health in low- and middle-income countries through a task-shifting approach. *Epidemiology and Psychiatric Sciences*, *29*. Advance online publication. DOI: 10.1017/s204579602000061x PMID: 32744223

Rae, B. (2024). Medicines management for nurses: Explaining legal governance. *Nursing Standard*, *39*(3), 45. DOI: 10.7748/ns.2024.e12177 PMID: 38186230

Range, L. M., Campbell, C., Kovac, S. H., Marion-Jones, M., Aldridge, H., Kogos, S. C., & Crump, Y. (2002). NO-SUICIDE CONTRACTS: AN OVERVIEW AND RECOMMENDATIONS. *Death Studies*, *26*(1), 51–74. DOI: 10.1080/07481180210147 PMID: 11865883

Rocha, T. I. U., Aschar, S., Hidalgo-Padilla, L., Daley, K., Claro, H. G., Martins, H. C. dos S., dos Santos, D. V. C., Miranda, J. J., Araya, R., & Menezes, P. R. (2020). Recruitment, Training and Supervision of Nurses and Nurse Assistants for a task-shifting depression intervention in two RCTs in Brazil and Peru. *Research Square (Research Square)*. https://doi.org/DOI: 10.21203/rs.3.rs-76085/v1

Rudd, M. D., Mandrusiak, M., & Joiner, T. E. (2005). The case against no-suicide contracts: The commitment to treatment statement as a practice alternative. *Journal of Clinical Psychology*, *62*(2), 243–251. DOI: 10.1002/jclp.20227 PMID: 16342293

Sabé, M., Kaiser, S., & Niveau, G. (2020). Suicide in psychiatry and medical liability: A case series. *International Journal of Law and Psychiatry*, *74*, 101671. DOI: 10.1016/j.ijlp.2020.101671 PMID: 33387984

Sastre-Fullana, P., de Pedro-Gómez, J. E., Bennasar-Veny, M., Serrano-Gallardo, P., & Morales-Asencio, J. M. (2014). Competency frameworks for advanced practice nursing: A literature review. *International Nursing Review*, *61*(4), 534–542. DOI: 10.1111/inr.12132 PMID: 25288021

Scanlon, A. (2006). Humanistic principles in relation to psychiatric nurse education: A review of the literature. *Journal of Psychiatric and Mental Health Nursing*, *13*(6), 758–764. DOI: 10.1111/j.1365-2850.2006.01031.x PMID: 17087680

Scheydt, S., & Hegedüs, A. (2021). Tasks and activities of Advanced Practice Nurses in the psychiatric and mental health care context: A systematic review and thematic analysis. *International Journal of Nursing Studies*, *118*, 103759. DOI: 10.1016/j.ijnurstu.2020.103759 PMID: 32958260

Scheydt, S., Nienaber, A., & Holzke, M. (2025). Task Profiles of Academically Qualified Psychiatric Nurses in Germany: Results of a Cluster Analysis. *Journal of Psychiatric and Mental Health Nursing*, *32*(3), 753. DOI: 10.1111/jpm.13153 PMID: 39918036

Simon, R. I., & Sadoff, R. L. (2005). *Psychiatric Malpractice: Cases and Comments for Clinicians*. American Psychiatric Press.

Slade, E. P., DePriest, K., Commodore-Mensah, Y., Samuel, L., Hanson, G. C., & D'Aoust, R. (2024). State Full Practice Authority Regulations and Nurse Practitioner Practice Autonomy: Evidence From the 2018 National Sample Survey of Registered Nurses. *Medical Care Research and Review : MCRR*, *82*(1), 68. DOI: 10.1177/10775587241282163 PMID: 39470186

Solak, M., & Kayaer, N. (2024). Criminal responsibilities of nurses in Turkish criminal law and determining the awareness levels of senior nursing students regarding this responsibility. *BMC Nursing*, *23*(1), 761. DOI: 10.1186/s12912-024-02418-6 PMID: 39415194

Stanley, B., & Brown, G. K. (2012). Safety Planning Intervention: A Brief Intervention to Mitigate Suicide Risk. *Cognitive and Behavioral Practice*, *19*(2), 256–264.

Stanley, I. H., Simpson, S., Wortzel, H. S., & Joiner, T. E. (2019). Documenting suicide risk assessments and proportionate clinical actions to improve patient safety and mitigate legal risk. *Behavioral Sciences & the Law*, *37*(3), 304. DOI: 10.1002/bsl.2409 PMID: 31063254

Stievano, A., & Tschudin, V. (2019). The ICN code of ethics for nurses: A time for revision. *International Nursing Review*, *66*(2), 154. DOI: 10.1111/inr.12525 PMID: 31124137

Topan, H., Albayrak Günday, E., Sürme, Y., Ceyhan, Ö., Şimşek, N., & Küçük, A. (2025). Guided imagery effects on pain, anxiety, and sleep for lumbar discectomy patients. *Journal of Perianesthesia Nursing*, *40*(1), 56–61. DOI: 10.1016/j.jopan.2024.03.004 PMID: 39023479

Trachsel, M., & grosse Holtforth, M. (2019). How to strengthen patients' meaning response by an ethical informed consent in psychotherapy. *Frontiers in Psychology*, *10*, 1747. Advance online publication. DOI: 10.3389/fpsyg.2019.01747 PMID: 31417470

Travelbee, J. (1971). *Interpersonal Aspects of Nursing*. F.A. Davis.

Unhjem, J. V., & Hem, M. H. (2025). Nurse-patient relationship boundaries and power: A critical discursive analysis. *Nursing Ethics*, *32*(6), 1861. DOI: 10.1177/09697330251314093 PMID: 39828402

Wilkenfeld, D. A., & Durmis, C. (2022). When law and ethics come apart: Constraints versus guidance. *Nursing Ethics*, *29*(6), 1430. DOI: 10.1177/09697330221105640 PMID: 35724321

World Health Organization (WHO). (2008). *Task Shifting: Global Recommendations and Guidelines*. WHO.

World Health Organization (WHO). (2022). *World Mental Health Report: Transforming Mental Health for All*. World Health Organization.

Wortzel, H. S., Matarazzo, B. B., & Homaifar, B. Y. (2013). A Model for Therapeutic Risk Management of the Suicidal Patient. *Journal of Psychiatric Practice*, *19*(4), 323-326. Lippincott Williams & Wilkins. https://doi.org/DOI: 10.1097/01.pra.0000432603.99211.e8

Wright, J. H., Basco, M. R., & Thase, M. E. (2009). *Learning Cognitive-Behavior Therapy: An Illustrated Guide*. American Psychiatric Publishing.

Yoshinaga, N., Tanoue, H., & Hayashi, Y. (2022). Naturalistic outcome of nurse-led psychological therapy for mental disorders in routine outpatient care: A retrospective chart review. *Archives of Psychiatric Nursing*, *40*, 43. DOI: 10.1016/j.apnu.2022.04.008 PMID: 36064244

Ypma, P., M, M. D. G., Pomme, A. O., Drevon, C., & Papadopoulos, I. (2020). Mapping and assessment of developments for one of the sectoral professions under directive 2005/36/EC Nurse responsible for general care: final study. *Middlesex University Research Repository (Middlesex University Of London)*. https://doi.org/ DOI: 10.2873/30

Zhu, Y., Gan, L., Shen, Y., Wang, J., Lu, M., & Wang, J. (2022). Humanistic Nursing Care for Patients in Low-Resourced Clinical Settings from Students' Perspectives: A Participatory Qualitative Study. *International Journal of Environmental Research and Public Health*, *19*(19), 12656. DOI: 10.3390/ijerph191912656 PMID: 36231956

Zur, O. (2007). *Appendix A Examples of Boundary Crossings and Boundary Violations in Psychotherapy*.

Compilation of References

Aafjes-van Doorn, K., Klinar Alfaro, D., Fialová, M., & Kamsteeg, C. (2018). Psychotherapy integration training around the globe: A personal and empirical perspective. *Journal of Psychotherapy Integration*, *28*(4), 505–520. DOI: 10.1037/int0000135

Ababkov, V. A., Isurina, G. L., Kazakovtsev, B. A., Kulakov, S. A., Nazyrov, R. K., Podsadnyi, S. A., et al. (2000). *Psikhoterapiya. Uchebnik dlya studentov meditsinskii vuzov* [Psychotherapy. A textbook for medical students]. Publisher. (In Russian).

Abiri, A., Ferere, A. H., Jordan, J., & Kinuthia, W. (2024). Decolonizing Nursing Education: Promoting Curricula for Community Engagement. In *Transforming Social Determinants to Promote Global Health: Achieving Health Equity through Lived Experiences* (pp. 421–433). Springer Nature Switzerland.

Abramova, G. S. (2003). *Prakticheskaya psikhologiya. Uchebnik dlya studentov vuzov* [Practical psychology. Textbook for university students]. Publisher. (In Russian).

Açıkgöz, S., & Coşkunsever, A. (2025). Bir Yöntem Olarak Pozitif Psikoterapi Yaklaşımının Manevi Danışmanlık ve Rehberlik Uygulamalarında Kullanılabilirliği. *İslami İlimler Dergisi*, (40), 237-253. https://doi.org/.DOI: 10.34082/islamiilimler.1605479

Ackerman, C. E., Warren, M. A., & Donaldson, S. I. (2018). Scaling the heights of positive psychology: A systematic review of measurement scales. *International Journal of Wellbeing*, *8*, 1–21.

Afolabi, O. E. (2015). Dual relationships and boundary crossing: A critical issues in clinical psychology practice. *International Journal of Psychology and Counselling*, *7*(2), 29–39.

Agyapong, V. I. O., Farren, C., & McAuliffe, E. (2016). Improving Ghana's mental healthcare through task-shifting—Psychiatrists and health policy directors perceptions about government's commitment and the role of community mental health workers. *Globalization and Health, 12*, 57. Advance online publication. DOI: 10.1186/s12992-016-0199-z PMID: 27716339

Akiki, T. J., Averill, C. L., & Abdallah, C. G. (2017). A network-based neurobiological model of PTSD: Evidence from structural and functional neuroimaging studies. *Current Psychiatry Reports, 19*, 81. DOI: 10.1007/s11920-017-0840-4

Ak, M., Kırpınar, İ., Atmaca, M., Erkan, A., Güler, Ö., Kesici, Ş., & Kumsar, N. A. (2020). *Cognitive behavioral therapy in clinical practice-2*. Nobel Academic Publishing.

Albayrak Günday, E., & Gülırmak Güler, K. (2025). Psychosocial therapies in psychiatry. In M. Aydın (Ed.), *Fundamentals of Psychiatric Nursing* (pp. [PDF'deki Sayfa Aralığı]). BZT Turan Publishing House.

Albayrak Günday, E., & Gülırmak Güler, K. (2026). Artificial intelligence through the eyes of psychiatric nurses: An in-depth investigation of thought, anxiety and readiness. *Issues in Mental Health Nursing*. Advance online publication. DOI: 10.1080/01612840.2025.2596210 PMID: 41504220

Albayrak Günday, E., & Gülırmak Güler, K. (2026). Examining the construction of sensory balance and well-being in psychiatric nurses caring for trauma victims: A qualitative study. *Journal of Nursing Scholarship, 58*, e70053. DOI: 10.1111/jnu.70053 PMID: 41199426

Albayrak, E., & Asi Karakaş, S. (2022). An investigation of internalized stigma and recovery levels of patients registered in a Community Mental Health Center. *Perspectives in Psychiatric Care, 58*(4), 1940–1948. DOI: 10.1111/ppc.13011 PMID: 34973035

Almotiry, M. B., Alqahtani, A. A., Al Nime, A. M., Alonezi, B. F., Alotaibi, N. G., Khubrani, H. A. M., & Alotaibi, N. N. S. (2023). Assessment of nurses' knowledge about ethical and legal issues of mental health nursing at psychiatric teaching hospitals. *Journal of Survey in Fisheries Sciences, 10*(6), Articles. https://doi.org/DOI: 10.53555/sfs.v10i6.2247

Alpay, H., & Çelik, D. (2022). Complex post-traumatic stress disorder: A review. *Psikiyatride Güncel Yaklasimlar, 14*(4), 589–596. DOI: 10.18863/pgy.1050659

Altschul, S. (1984). Attachment and Loss, Vol. 3. Loss, Sadness and Depression. By John Bowlby. *Journal of the American Psychoanalytic Association, 32*(1), 216–218.

Amaglo, E. (2022). Managing boundaries and multiple relationships in counselling and psychotherapy. *Global Journal of Psychology, 2*(1), Articles. https://doi.org/DOI: 10.51594/gjp.v2i1.361

American Nurses Association (ANA). (2014). *Scope and Standards of Practice: Psychiatric-Mental Health Nursing* (2nd ed.). Silver Spring, MD: Nursesbooks.org.

American Nurses Association. (2001). Code of ethics for nurses with interpretive statements. Nursesbooks. org.

American Nurses Credentialing Center (ANCC). (2020). *PMHNP-BC Test Content Outline.*

American Psychiatric Nurses Association (APNA). (2019). *Psychiatric-Mental Health Nursing: Scope and Standards of Practice* (3rd ed.). American Nurses Association.

Anfang, S. A., & Appelbaum, P. S. (1996). Twenty years after Tarasoff: Reviewing the duty to protect. *Harvard Review of Psychiatry*, *4*(2), 67–76. DOI: 10.3109/10673229609030526 PMID: 9384976

Antão, C., Santos, B. P. J. dos, Santos, N. R. dos, Fernandes, H., Barroso, B., Mărginean, C. O., & Pimentel, M. H. (2025). Nursing Degree Curriculum: Differences and Similarities Between 15 European Countries. *Nursing Reports, 15*(3), 112. Multidisciplinary Digital Publishing Institute. https://doi.org/DOI: 10.3390/nursrep15030112

Antebi-Gruszka, N., & Scheer, J. R. (2021). Associations Between Trauma-Informed Care Components and Multiple Health and Psychosocial Risks Among LGBTQ Survivors of Intimate Partner Violence. *Journal of Mental Health Counseling*, *43*(2), 139–156. DOI: 10.17744/mehc.43.2.04

APA. (2013a). *Diagnostic and statistical manual of mental disorders* (5. baskı). American Psychiatric Association.

APA. (2013b). Diagnostic and Statistical Manual of Mental Disorders DSM-V. Translated by P. D. E. Köroğlu.

Appelbaum, P. S., & Gutheil, T. G. (2007). *Clinical Handbook of Psychiatry & Law* (4th ed.). Lippincott Williams & Wilkins.

Applebaum, A. J., & Breitbart, W. (2013). Care for the cancer caregiver: A systematic review. *Palliative & Supportive Care*, *11*(3), 231–252. DOI: 10.1017/S1478951512000594

Arkhipova, I. V., Kokorina, N. P., & Magarill, Yu. A. (2003). Psikhogennye faktory i rak molochnoi zhelezy [Psychogenic factors and breast cancer]. In *Aktual'nye problemy raka molochnoi zhelezy* (Vol. 7, pp. 7–8). (In Russian).

Arranz, E. B., Olabarrieta, F., Manzano, A., Martín, J. L., Cruz, N., & Etxaniz, A. (2016). Psychosocial Intervention. *Psychosocial Intervention*, *25*(2), 127–134.

Arving, C., Thormodsen, I., & Brekke, G.. (2012). Early rehabilitation of cancer patients – a randomized controlled intervention study. *BMC Cancer*, *12*, 13–19.

Aslan, B. (2025). Cognitive-Behavioral Case Formulation of Panic Disorder. *Turkish Journal of Integrative Psychotherapy*, *8*(15), 89–102.

Assaz, D. A., Roche, B., Kanter, J. W., & Oshiro, C. K. (2018). Cognitive defusion in acceptance and commitment therapy: What are the basic processes of change? *The Psychological Record*, *68*(4), 405–418.

Astin, J. A., Shapiro, J., & Shapiro, D. H. (2013). Psychological control and morbidity/mortality in breast cancer patients: A 20 year follow-up study. *Behavioral Medicine (Washington, D.C.)*, *39*, 7–10.

Ata, E. E., & Doğan, S. (2018). The effect of a brief cognitive behavioral stress management program on mental status, coping with stress attitude, and caregiver burden while caring for schizophrenic patients. *Archives of Psychiatric Nursing*, *32*(1), 112–119. PMID: 29413060

Aurizki, G. E., & Wilson, I. (2022). Nurse-led task-shifting strategies to substitute for mental health specialists in primary care: A systematic review. *International Journal of Nursing Practice, 28*(5), e13046. Wiley. https://doi.org/DOI: 10.1111/ijn.13046

Aypay, A., & Kara, A. (2018). Pozitif Psikoterapi Denge Modeli Bağlamında Dengeli Yaşam Ölçeği ve Dengeli Yaşam Temel Becerileri Ölçeğinin Geliştirilmesi. *Sakarya University Journal of Education*, *8*(3), 63. DOI: 10.19126/suje.408531

Baer, R. (2015). Ethics, values, virtues, and character strengths in mindfulness-based interventions: A psychological science perspective. *Mindfulness*, *6*(4), 956–969.

Bahari, Z., Vosoghi, N., Ramazanzadeh, N., Moshfeghi, S., & Aghamohammadi, M. (2024). Patient trust in nurses: Exploring the relationship with care quality and communication skills in emergency departments. *BMC Nursing*, *23*(1), 595. PMID: 39183274

Balabuha, O. S. (2010). Kachestvo zhizni kak osnova program reabilitacii onkologicheskih bol'nyh [Quality of life as the basis of rehabilitation programs for cancer patients] [In Russian]. *Mezhdunarodnyj Medicinskij Zhurnal*, *4*, 11–13.

Baltrusch, H. J., Stangel, W., & Titze, I. (1991). Stress, cancer and immunity: New developments in biopsychosocial and psychoneuroimmunologic research. *Acta Neurologica, 13*, 315–327.

Banerjee, S. C., Manna, R., Coyle, N., Penn, S., Gallegos, T. E., Zaider, T., Krueger, C. A., Bialer, P. A., Bylund, C. L., & Parker, P. A. (2017). The implementation and evaluation of a communication skills training program for oncology nurses. *Translational Behavioral Medicine*, *7*(3), 615–623. DOI: 10.1007/s13142-017-0473-5

Baptista, K., Walbridge, G. B., Marks, J. A., & Knoll, J. L. (2022). Ethics in Psychotherapy: Informed Consent, Digital Professionalism, and Sexual Misconduct. *Focus - American Psychiatric Publishing, 20*(3), 313–317. DOI: 10.1176/appi.focus.20220043 PMID: 37205024

Baranowsky, A. B., & Gentry, J. E. (2015). *Trauma practice: Tools for stabilization and recovery*. Hogrefe Publishing.

Baranowsky, A. B., & Gentry, J. E. (2023). *Trauma practice: A cognitive behavioral somatic therapy*. Hogrefe Publishing GmbH.

Barker, P. (2009). *Psychiatric and Mental Health Nursing: The Craft of Caring* (2nd ed.). Hodder Arnold.

Barker, P. J., & Buchanan-Barker, P. (2011). Mental Health Nursing and the Politics of Recovery: A Global Reflection. *Archives of Psychiatric Nursing*, *25*(5), 350–358. DOI: 10.1016/j.apnu.2011.03.009

Barnett, J. E., & Molzon, C. H. (2014). Clinical Supervision of Psychotherapy: Essential Ethics Issues for Supervisors and Supervisees. *Journal of Clinical Psychology*, *70*(11), 1051–1061. DOI: 10.1002/jclp.22126 PMID: 25220636

Bartrop, R. W., Luckhurst, E., Lazarus, L., Kiloh, L. G., & Penny, R. (1977). Depressed lymphocyte function after bereavement. *Lancet, 1*(8016), 834–836.

Baysal, E., Rodriguez-Arrastia, M., & Roman, P. (2025). Innovative Game-Based Teaching Methods for Promoting Nursing Students' Cultural Competence and Attitudes Toward Refugees: An Explanatory Sequential Mixed Study. *Journal of Transcultural Nursing*, *36*(3), 290–302. PMID: 39543903

Bazzano, A., Wolfe, C., Zylowska, L., Wang, S., Schuster, E., Barrett, C., & Lehrer, D. (2015). Mindfulness based stress reduction (MBSR) for parents and caregivers of individuals with developmental disabilities: A community-based approach. *Journal of Child and Family Studies*, *24*(2), 298–308.

Beauchamp, T. L., & Childress, J. F. (1994). *Principles of biomedical ethics*. Edicoes Loyola.

Beauchamp, T. L., & Childress, J. F. (2019). *Principles of Biomedical Ethics* (8th ed.). Oxford University Press.

Beauchamp, T., & Childress, J. (2019). Principles of biomedical ethics: Marking its fortieth anniversary. *The American Journal of Bioethics*, *19*(11), 9–12. PMID: 31647760

Beck, A. T., & Dozois, D. J. (2011). Cognitive Therapy: Current Status and Future Directions. *Annual Review of Medicine*, *62*(1), 397–409. PMID: 20690827

Beck, J. S. (2020). *Cognitive behavior therapy: Basics and beyond*. Guilford Publications.

Beis, P., Graf, M., & Hachtel, H. (2022). Impact of legal traditions on forensic mental health treatment worldwide. *Frontiers in Psychiatry, 13*, 876619. Frontiers Media. https://doi.org/DOI: 10.3389/fpsyt.2022.876619

Belisle, J., & Tarbox, J. (2024). Relational frame theory and acceptance and commitment therapy. In Roane, H. S., Craig, A. R., Saini, V., & Ringdahl, J. E. (Eds.), *Behavior analysis: Translational perspectives and clinical practice* (pp. 526–547). The Guilford Press.

Bengisoy, A., Özdemir, M. B., Erkıvanç, F., Şahin, S., & İskifoğlu, T. Ç. (2019). Content analysis of research articles using cognitive behavioral therapy 1997-2018. *Turkish Psychological Counseling and Guidance Journal*, *9*(54), 745–793.

Benjet, C., Bromet, E., Karam, E. G., Kessler, R. C., McLaughlin, K. A., Ruscio, A. M., Shahly, V., Stein, D. J., Petukhova, M., & Hill, E. (2016). The epidemiology of traumatic event exposure worldwide: Results from the World Mental Health Survey Consortium. *Psychological Medicine*, *46*(2), 327–343. DOI: 10.1017/S0033291715001981

Berghoff, C. R., Ritzert, T. R., & Forsyth, J. P. (2018). Value-guided action: Within-day and lagged relations of experiential avoidance, mindful awareness, and cognitive fusion in a non-clinical sample. *Journal of Contextual Behavioral Science*, *10*, 19–23.

Berryhill, M. B., & Lechtenberg, M. M. (2015). Acceptance and commitment therapy with adolescents: Identifying and clarifying values. *Journal of Family Psychotherapy*, *26*(1), 25–30.

Bersoff, D. N. (2014). Protecting victims of violent patients while protecting confidentiality. *The American Psychologist, 69*(5), 461–467. DOI: 10.1037/a0037198 PMID: 25046702

Bhugra, D., & Bhui, K. (Eds.). (2018). *Textbook of cultural psychiatry*. Cambridge University Press.

Bieling, P. J., McCabe, R. E., & Antony, M. M. (2022). *Cognitive-behavioral therapy in groups*. Guilford publications.

Bifarin, O., Collier-Sewell, F., Smith, G., Moriarty, J., Shepherd, H., Andrews, L., Pearson, S., & Kasperska, M. (2024). Standards of proficiency for registered nurses—To what end? A critical analysis of contemporary mental health nursing within the United Kingdom context. *Nursing Inquiry, 31*(3), e12630. DOI: 10.1111/nin.12630 PMID: 38436620

Bilkay, H. İ., Öztürk, C., Şirin, B., & Bozkurt, A. (2025). Investigation of psychiatric nurses' views on psychotherapy implementation processes: A qualitative study. *BMC Nursing, 24*(1), 785–796. DOI: 10.1186/s12912-025-03460-8 PMID: 40597100

Bishop, S. R. (2002). What do we really know about mindfulness-based stress reduction? *Biopsychosocial Science and Medicine, 64*(1), 71–83.

Black, D. S. (2011). A brief definition of mindfulness. *Behavioral Neuroscience, 7*(2), 109.

Black, D. S., Milam, J., & Sussman, S. (2009). Sitting-meditation interventions among youth: A review of treatment efficacy. *Pediatrics, 124*(3), e532–e541.

Blackledge, J. T., & Barnes-Holmes, D. (2009). Core processes in acceptance and commitment therapy. *Acceptance and commitment therapy: Contemporary theory, research, and practice, 1*, 41-58.

Blackledge, J. T. (2007). Disrupting verbal processes: Cognitive defusion in acceptance and commitment therapy and other mindfulness-based psychotherapies. *The Psychological Record, 57*(4), 555–576.

Blanke, E. S., Schmidt, M. J., Riediger, M., & Brose, A. (2020). Thinking mindfully: How mindfulness relates to rumination and reflection in daily life. *Emotion (Washington, D.C.), 20*(8), 1369.

Blease, C., Arnott, T., Kelley, J. M., Proctor, G., Kube, T., Gaab, J., & Locher, C. (2020). Attitudes About Informed Consent: An Exploratory Qualitative Analysis of UK Psychotherapy Trainees. *Frontiers in Psychiatry, 11*, 183. Frontiers Media. https://doi.org/DOI: 10.3389/fpsyt.2020.00183

Boeldt, D., McMahon, E., McFaul, M., & Greenleaf, W. (2019). Using virtual reality exposure therapy to enhance treatment of anxiety disorders: Identifying areas of clinical adoption and potential obstacles. *Frontiers in Psychiatry*, *10*, 773. PMID: 31708821

Boemke, B. (2011). Haftung des Psychotherapeuten (Einzelbeitrag). *MHP (Medizinrecht, Haftung und Prozess), 45.*

Bolier, L., Haverman, M., Westerhof, G. J., Riper, H., Smit, F., & Bohlmeijer, E. (2013). Positive psychology interventions: A meta-analysis of randomized controlled studies. *BMC Public Health*, *13*(1), 119. PMID: 23390882

Bolier, L., Ketelaar, S. M., & Nieuwenhuijsen, K.. (2014). Workplace mental health promotion online to enhance well-being of nurses and allied health professionals: A cluster-randomized controlled trial. *Internet Interventions : the Application of Information Technology in Mental and Behavioural Health*, *1*, 196–204.

Bolton, D. (2023). A revitalized biopsychosocial model: Core theory, research paradigms, and clinical implications. *Psychological Medicine*, *53*(16), 7504–7511. PMID: 37681273

Bolton, P., West, J., Whitney, C., Jordans, M. J. D., Bass, J., Thornicroft, G., & Raviola, G. (2023). Expanding mental health services in low- and middle-income countries: A task-shifting framework for delivery of comprehensive, collaborative, and community-based care. *Cambridge Prisms: Global Mental Health*, *10*, e16. DOI: 10.1017/gmh.2023.5 PMID: 37854402

Boyd, J. E., Lanius, R. A., & McKinnon, M. C. (2018). Mindfulness-based treatments for posttraumatic stress disorder: A review of the treatment literature and neurobiological evidence. *Journal of Psychiatry & Neuroscience : JPN*, *43*(1), 7–25. DOI: 10.1503/jpn.170021

Broeck, N. V., & Lietaer, G. (2008). Psychology and Psychotherapy in Health Care. *European Psychologist*, *13*(1), 53. DOI: 10.1027/1016-9040.13.1.53

Brouzos, A., Vatkali, E., Mavridis, D., Vassilopoulos, S. P., & Baourda, V. C. (2022). Psychoeducation for adults with post-traumatic stress symptomatology: A systematic review and meta-analysis. *Journal of Contemporary Psychotherapy*, *52*(2), 155–164. DOI: 10.1007/s10879-021-09526-3

Buckley, C., Radhakrishnan, A., Boran, L., Brennan, M., & Travers, Á. (n.d.). Barriers and Facilitators of Help-Seeking for LGBTQ+ Survivors of Sexual Violence. *Systematic Reviews*.

Bukharov, Ya. M., & Golubev, M. V. (2007). *Psikhoterapiya v praktike vracha-nepsikhoterapevta* [Psychotherapy in medical practice – neprihotliva]. Publisher. (In Russian).

Buletov, D. A. (n.d.). *Reabilitaciya detej s onkologicheskoj patologiej. Vzglyad onkologa* [Rehabilitation of children with oncological pathology. Oncologist's look]. (In Russian).

Buppert, C. (2017). *Nurse Practitioner's Business Practice and Legal Guide*. Jones & Bartlett Learning.

Burback, L., Brult-Phillips, S., Nijdam, M. J., McFarlane, A., & Vermetten, E. (2024). Treatment of posttraumatic stress disorder: A state-of-the-art review. *Current Neuropharmacology*, *22*(4), 557–635. DOI: 10.2174/1570159X21666230428091433

Burgi, M., & Igl, G. (2021). *Rechtliche Voraussetzungen und Möglichkeiten der Etablierung von Community Health Nursing (CHN) in Deutschland*. Nomos Verlag., DOI: 10.5771/9783748924319

Butler, A. C., Chapman, J. E., Forman, E. M., & Beck, A. T. (2006). The Empirical Status of Cognitive-Behavioral Therapy: A Review of Meta-analyses. *Clinical Psychology Review*, *26*(1), 17–31. PMID: 16199119

Büyükbayram, A., Çam, O., & Turgut, E. Ö. (2016). Mental health and psychiatric nursing approach after trauma. Anadolu Nursing and Health Sciences Journal, 19(3).

Cahill, M., Alexander, M., & Gross, L. (2014). The 2014 NCSBN Consensus Report on APRN Regulation. *Journal of Nursing Regulation*, *4*(4), 5–12. DOI: 10.1016/s2155-8256(15)30111-3

Campinha-Bacote, J. (2002). The process of cultural competence in the delivery of healthcare services: A model of care. *Journal of Transcultural Nursing*, *13*(3), 181–184. PMID: 12113146

Campinha-Bacote, J. (2011). Delivering patient-centered care in the midst of a cultural conflict: The role of cultural competence. *Online Journal of Issues in Nursing*, *16*(2), 1–8. PMID: 22088154

Canivet, D., Delvaux, N., Gibon, A.-S., Brancart, C., Slachmuylder, J.-L., & Razavi, D. (2014). Improving communication in cancer pain management nursing: A randomized controlled study assessing the efficacy of a communication skills training program. *Supportive Care in Cancer*, *22*(12), 3311–3320. DOI: 10.1007/s00520-014-2357-2

Carliner, H., Gary, D., McLaughlin, K. A., & Keyes, K. M. (2017). Trauma exposure and externalizing disorders in adolescents: Results from the National Comorbidity Survey Adolescent Supplement. *Journal of the American Academy of Child and Adolescent Psychiatry*, *56*(9), 755–764.e3. DOI: 10.1016/j.jaac.2017.06.006

Carolan, S., Harris, P. R., & Cavanagh, K. (2017). Improving employee well-being and effectiveness: Systematic review and meta-analysis of web-based psychological interventions delivered in the workplace. *Journal of Medical Internet Research*, *19*, e271. PMID: 28747293

Carr, A., Cullen, K., Keeney, C., Canning, C., Mooney, O., Chinseallaigh, E., & O'Dowd, A. (2021). Effectiveness of positive psychology interventions: A systematic review and meta-analysis. *The Journal of Positive Psychology*, *16*(6), 749–769.

Cavanagh, K., Strauss, C., Forder, L., & Jones, F. (2014). Can mindfulness and acceptance be learnt by self-help?: A systematic review and meta-analysis of mindfulness and acceptance-based self-help interventions. *Clinical Psychology Review*, *34*(2), 118–129.

Chakhssi, F., Kraiss, J. T., Sommers-Spijkerman, M., & Bohlmeijer, E. T. (2018). The effect of positive psychology interventions on well-being and distress in clinical samples with psychiatric or somatic disorders: A systematic review and meta-analysis. *BMC Psychiatry*, *18*(1), 211. PMID: 29945603

Chand, S. P., Kuckel, D. P., & Huecker, M. R. (2023). Cognitive behavior therapy. In *StatPearls* [Internet]. StatPearls Publishing.

Chase, J. A., Houmanfar, R., Hayes, S. C., Ward, T. A., Vilardaga, J. P., & Follette, V. (2013). Values are not just goals: Online ACT-based values training adds to goal setting in improving undergraduate college student performance. *Journal of Contextual Behavioral Science*, *2*(3-4), 79–84.

Cherkasova, E. A., Krom, I. L., & Novichkova, I. Yu. (2013). Mediko-sociologicheskoe obosnovanie reabilitacii onkologicheskih bol'nyh [Medico-sociological substantiation of rehabilitation of oncological patients] [In Russian]. *Sociologicheskie Nauki*, *2*, 10–15.

Chochinov, H. M., Hack, T., Hassard, T., Kristjanson, L. J., McClement, S., & Harlos, M. (2005). Dignity Therapy: A Novel Psychotherapeutic Intervention for Patients Near the End of Life. *Journal of Clinical Oncology*, *23*(24), 5520–5525. DOI: 10.1200/JCO.2005.08.391

Clarke, T. (n.d.). *Exploring the mental health and acculturation needs of sexual and/or gender minority forced migrants*.

Coffey, M., & Hannigan, B. (2013). New roles for nurses as approved mental health professionals in England and Wales. *International Journal of Nursing Studies*, *50*(10), 1423–1430. DOI: 10.1016/j.ijnurstu.2013.02.014 PMID: 23522939

Cohen, I., Gal, ali, & Enosh, G. (2022). Two Roads Converge: The Interchange Between the Mental Health and Legal Discourses in Sexual Assault Trials. *Social & Legal Studies*, *32*(3), 441–463. DOI: 10.1177/09646639221117388

Conlon, D., Raeburn, T., & Wand, T. (2024). Nurses' understanding of their duty of confidentiality to patients in mental health care: A qualitative exploratory study. *Collegian Journal of the Royal College of Nursing Australia*, *31*(3), 144–153. DOI: 10.1016/j.colegn.2024.02.002

Cope, T. A. (2009). Positive Psychotherapy's Theory of the Capacity to Know as Explication of Unconscious Contents. *Journal of Religion and Health*, *48*(1), 79–89. DOI: 10.1007/s10943-008-9225-7 PMID: 19229628

Corso, K. A., & Gage, D. (2016). Nurses and Psychologists Advancing the Patient-Centered Medical Home Model. *Nursing Administration Quarterly*, *40*(3), 192–201. DOI: 10.1097/NAQ.0000000000000176

Coutinho, M., Trindade, I. A., & Ferreira, C. (2021). Experiential avoidance, committed action and quality of life: Differences between college students with and without chronic illness. *Journal of Health Psychology*, *26*(7), 1035–1045.

Crawford, A., Richardson, L., Simmonds, E., Wiljer, D., & Strudwick, G. (2022). Digital compassion, health equity, and cultural safety: from the therapeutic relationship to the organization of virtual care. In *Virtual Mental Health Care for Rural and Underserved Settings* (pp. 55–67). Springer International Publishing.

Cristian, A., Tran, A., & Patel, K. (2012). Patient safety in cancer rehabilitation. *Physical Medicine and Rehabilitation Clinics of North America*, *23*(2), 441–456.

Crowden, A. (2008). Professional boundaries and the ethics of dual and multiple overlapping relationships in psychotherapy. *Monash Bioethics Review*, *27*, 10–27. DOI: 10.1007/bf03351302 PMID: 19760852

Cuijpers, P., Karyotaki, E., de Wit, L., & Ebert, D. D. (2020). The effects of fifteen evidence-supported therapies for adult depression: A meta-analytic review. *Psychotherapy Research*, *30*(3), 279–293. PMID: 31394976

Currid, T. J., Nikčević, A. V., & Spada, M. M. (2011). Cognitive behavioral therapy and its relevance to nursing. *British Journal of Nursing (Mark Allen Publishing)*, *20*(22), 1443–1447. PMID: 22241494

Dahl, J. (2015). Valuing in ACT. *Current Opinion in Psychology, 2*, 43–46.

Dalirirad, H., Seyedfatemi, N., & Najafi, T. (2021). Effect of an Educational Support Programme on Caregiver Burden Among the Family Members of Patients Undergoing Coronary Artery Bypass Graft Surgery. *Sultan Qaboos University Medical Journal, 21*(2), e266–e274. DOI: 10.18295/squmj.2021.21.02.016

Dammann, O. (2004). *Medizinrecht: Zivilrecht, Versicherungsrecht, Arzneirecht, Berufsrecht, Vertragsarzttecht, Krankenhausrecht*. Nomos Verlag.

Danböck, S. K., Duek, O., Ben-Zion, Z., Korem, N., Amen, S. L., Kelmendi, B., Wilhelm, F. H., Levy, I., & Harpaz-Rotem, I. (2024). Effects of a dissociative drug on fronto-limbic resting-state functional connectivity in individuals with posttraumatic stress disorder: A randomized controlled pilot study. *Psychopharmacology, 241*(2), 243–252. DOI: 10.1007/s00213-023-06479-4

David, D., & Montgomery, G. H. (2011). The scientific status of psychotherapies: A new evaluative framework for evidence-based psychosocial interventions. *Clinical Psychology : a Publication of the Division of Clinical Psychology of the American Psychological Association, 18*(2), 89–99.

Davis, W. D., Stanley, J., Buck, M., Walters, E., & DeGarmo, S. (2024). LACE and the APRN Consensus Model: Implications for Advancing Nursing Practice. *AACN Advanced Critical Care, 35*(1), 20–28. DOI: 10.4037/aacnacc2024956 PMID: 38457622

Dawson, K. S., Bryant, R. A., Harper, M., Tay, A. K., Rahman, A., Schafer, A., & Van Ommeren, M. (2015). Problem Management Plus (PM+): A WHO transdiagnostic psychological intervention for common mental health problems. *World Psychiatry; Official Journal of the World Psychiatric Association (WPA), 14*(3), 354. PMID: 26407793

De Carlo, A., Carluccio, F., Rapisarda, S., Mora, D., & Ometto, I. (2020). Three uses of virtual reality in work and organizational psychology interventions. A dialogue between virtual reality and organizational well-being: Relaxation techniques, personal resources, and anxiety/depression treatments. *TPM. Testing, Psychometrics, Methodology in Applied Psychology, 27*(1).

Debout, C., Eterstein, C., & Greiner, D. (2012). Advanced practice nursing in France: A perspective. *International Nursing Review, 59*(4), 466–467. PMID: 23134129

Decock, N., Friganović, A., Kurtović, B., Oomen, B., Crombez, P., & Willems, C. (2022). Temper the Specialist Nurses Heterogeneity in the Interest of Quality Practice and Mobility—18 EU Countries Study. *Health Care*, *10*(3), 435–444. DOI: 10.3390/healthcare10030435 PMID: 35326913

Del Rosario, N., & Beshai, S. (2022). Do you mind? Examining the impact of psychoeducation specificity on perceptions of mindfulness-based programs. *International Journal of Environmental Research and Public Health*, *19*(15), 9621.

Delaney, K. R., Cooper, J. L., & Nshemerewire, S. (n.d.). *THE PRACTICE OF CHILD MENTAL HEALTH NURSES.*

Delaney, H., & Casey, C. (2022). The promise of a four-day week? A critical appraisal of a management-led initiative. *Employee Relations: The International Journal*, *44*(1), 176–190. DOI: 10.1108/ER-02-2021-0056

Delaney, K. R. (2023). Inclusion of Psychiatric–Mental Health Advanced Practice Nurses in Federal Behavioral Workforce Planning. *Psychiatric Services (Washington, D.C.)*, *75*(6), 594–596. DOI: 10.1176/appi.ps.20230321 PMID: 38088040

Delaney, K. R., Naegle, M. A., Valentine, N. M., Antai-Otong, D., Groh, C. J., & Brennaman, L. (2017). The Effective Use of Psychiatric Mental Health Nurses in Integrated Care: Policy Implications for Increasing Quality and Access to Care. *The Journal of Behavioral Health Services & Research*. Advance online publication. DOI: 10.1007/s11414-017-9555-x

Delaney, K. R., & Vanderhoef, D. (2019). The Psychiatric Mental Health Advanced Practice Registered Nurse Workforce: Charting the Future. *Journal of the American Psychiatric Nurses Association*, *25*(1), 11–18. DOI: 10.1177/1078390318806571

Demiralp, M., & Oflaz, F. (2007). Cognitive-behavioral therapy techniques and psychiatric nursing practice. *Anadolu Journal of Psychiatry*, *8*(2), 132–139.

Demirci, H., Bilge, Y., Emiral, E., & Şen, S. (2024). Enhancing recovery in post-earthquake adolescents: Examining the impact of a psychoeducational intervention on traumatic stress symptoms and coping strategies. *Current Psychology (New Brunswick, N.J.)*, *43*(33), 26983–26996. DOI: 10.1007/s12144-024-06333-6

Devictor, J., Burnet, E., Henriot, T., Leclercq, A., Ganne-Carrié, N., Kilpatrick, K., & Jović, L. (2022). Implementing advanced practice nursing in France: A country-wide survey 2 years after its introduction. *Nursing Open*, *10*(3), 1437–1448. DOI: 10.1002/nop2.1394 PMID: 36168185

Dewing, J. (2020). Privilege and the call of the appeal.

Dimond, B. (2015). *Legal Aspects of Nursing* (7th ed.). Pearson.

Dionne-Odom, J. N., Applebaum, A. J., Ornstein, K. A., Azuero, A., Warren, P. P., Taylor, R. A., Rocque, G. B., Kvale, E. A., Demark-Wahnefried, W., Pisu, M., Partridge, E. E., Martin, M. Y., & Bakitas, M. A. (2018). Participation and interest in support services among family caregivers of older adults with cancer. *Psycho-Oncology*, *27*(3), 969–976. DOI: 10.1002/pon.4603

Directive 2005/36/EC of the European Parliament and of the Council of 7 September 2005 on the recognition of professional qualifications. *Official Journal of the European Union*, L 255/22.

Dobkin, P. L., Hickman, S., & Monshat, K. (2014). Holding the heart of mindfulness-based stress reduction: Balancing fidelity and imagination when adapting MBSR. *Mindfulness*, *5*(6), 710–718.

Dobson, K. S., & Dozois, D. J. (Eds.). (2021). *Handbook of cognitive-behavioral therapies*. Guilford Publications.

Dolev-Amit, T., Rubin, A., & Zilcha-Mano, S. (2021). Is awareness of strengths intervention sufficient to cultivate wellbeing and other positive outcomes? *Journal of Happiness Studies*, *22*(2), 645–666.

Doody, O., Graham, M., Hegarty, O., Sloane, A. M., Walsh, P., Synnott, M., Russell, M., Dunworth, T., Sheridan, J., & Murphy, L. (2025). Identifying the landscape and contribution of advanced nurse practitioners in supporting healthcare provision in Ireland in the 21st century: An integrative review. *International Journal of Nursing Studies Advances*, *8*, 100304. DOI: 10.1016/j.ijnsa.2025.100304 PMID: 40018051

Doorley, J. D., Goodman, F. R., Kelso, K. C., & Kashdan, T. B. (2020). Psychological flexibility: What we know, what we do not know, and what we think we know. *Social and Personality Psychology Compass*, *14*(12), 1–11.

Doran, D. M., Haynes, R. B., & Kushniruk, A.. (2010). Supporting evidence-based practice for nurses through information technologies. *Worldviews on Evidence-Based Nursing*, *7*, 4–15. PMID: 20028493

Douglas, M. K., Rosenkoetter, M., Pacquiao, D. F., Callister, L. C., Hattar-Pollara, M., Lauderdale, J., & Purnell, L. (2014). Guidelines for implementing culturally competent nursing care. *Journal of Transcultural Nursing*, *25*(2), 109–121. PMID: 24549502

Dowlatabadi, M. M., Ahmadi, S. M., Sorbi, M. H., Beiki, O., Razavi, T. K., & Bidaki, R. (2016). The effectiveness of group positive psychotherapy on depression and happiness in breast cancer patients: A randomized controlled trial. *Electronic Physician*, *8*(3), 2175. PMID: 27123227

Drew, B. L. (2014). The Evolution of the Role of the Psychiatric Mental Health Advanced Practice Registered Nurse in the United States. *Archives of Psychiatric Nursing*, *28*(5), 298–300. DOI: 10.1016/j.apnu.2014.07.002

Drissi, N., Ouhbi, S., & Marques, G.. (2021). A systematic literature review on e-Mental health solutions to assist health care workers during COVID-19. *Telemedicine Journal and e-Health*, *27*, 594–602. PMID: 32970532

Dryden, W., & Still, A. (2006). Historical aspects of mindfulness and self-acceptance in psychotherapy. *Journal of Rational-Emotive & Cognitive-Behavior Therapy*, *24*(1), 3–28.

Duran, B. (2021). Trauma and dissociation. In Güler, K. (Ed.), *A clinical perspective on trauma* (pp. 94–112). Eğiten Kitap.

Durbin, A., Durbin, J., Hensel, J. M., & Deber, R. (2016). Barriers and Enablers to Integrating Mental Health into Primary Care: A Policy Analysis. *The Journal of Behavioral Health Services & Research*, *43*(1), 127–139. DOI: 10.1007/s11414-013-9359-6

Dursun, P., & Söylemez, İ. (2020). Post-traumatic growth: A comprehensive assessment with the latest revised model. *Turkish Journal of Psychiatry*, *31*(1), 57–68. DOI: 10.5080/u23694

Duru, H. A., & Yılmaz, M. (2023). The role of the psychiatric nurse in cognitive behavioral therapy applied to patients diagnosed with depression: A literature review. *Mersin Üniversitesi Saglik Bilimleri Dergisi*, *16*(1), 131–146.

Dury, C., Hall, C. L., Danan, J., Mondoux, J., Barbieri-Figueiredo, M. C. A., Costa, M. A., & Debout, C. (2014). Specialist nurse in Europe: Education, regulation and role. *International Nursing Review*, *61*(4), 454–462. DOI: 10.1111/inr.12123 PMID: 25214392

Dutton, S., & Kozachik, S. L. (2020). Evaluating the outcomes of a web-based stress management program for nurses and nursing assistants. *Worldviews on Evidence-Based Nursing*, *17*, 32–38. PMID: 31912984

Edwards, D., & Burnard, P. (2003). A systematic review of stress and stress management interventions for mental health nurses. *Journal of Advanced Nursing*, *42*(2), 169–200. PMID: 12670386

Edwards, K. M., Waterman, E. A., Wheeler, L. A., Xu, W., Herrington, R., Trujllo, P., & Hopfauf, S. (2025). Predictors of Child and Caregiver Attendance in a Strengths-Focused, Culturally Grounded, Family-Based Program to Prevent Adverse Childhood Experiences. *Prevention Science*, •••, 1–12. PMID: 40029566

Efendi, F., Aurizki, G. E., Yusuf, A., & McKenna, L. (2022). "Not shifting, but sharing": Stakeholders' perspectives on mental health task-shifting in Indonesia. *BMC Nursing*, *21*(1), 165. DOI: 10.1186/s12912-022-00945-8 PMID: 35751061

Egan, M. P. (1997). Contracting for Safety: A Concept Analysis. *Crisis*, *18*(1), 17. DOI: 10.1027/0227-5910.18.1.17 PMID: 9141775

Egorov, B. E. (2003). *Ratsional'naya psikhoterapiya: teoriya i praktika. Posobie dlya vrachei* [Rational psychotherapy: Theory and practice. Manual for doctors]. Publisher. (In Russian).

Engin, E. (2021). Trauma and stressor-related disorders. In Olcay Çam, E. E. (Ed.), *The art of psychiatric nursing care in mental health and diseases* (3rd ed., pp. 274–287). Istanbul Medical Bookstores.

Engström, M., Scandurra, I., & Ljunggren, B.. (2009). Evaluation of OLD@HOME virtual health record staff opinions of the system and satisfaction with work. *Telemedicine Journal and e-Health*, *15*(1), 53–61. PMID: 19199848

Epping-Jordan, J. E., Harris, R., Brown, F. L., Carswell, K., Foley, C., García-Moreno, C., & van Ommeren, M. (2016). Self-Help Plus (SH+): A new WHO stress management package. *World Psychiatry; Official Journal of the World Psychiatric Association (WPA)*, *15*(3), 295. PMID: 27717271

Eryılmaz, A. (2011). Yetişkin öznel iyi oluşu ile pozitif psikoterapi bağlamında birincil ve ikincil yetenekler arasındaki ilişkilerin incelenmesi. *Klinik Psikiyatri*, *14*, 17–28.

Eryılmaz, A. (2017). Pozitif psikoterapiler. *Psikiyatride Güncel Yaklasimlar*, *9*(3), 346–362. DOI: 10.18863/pgy.288667

Eryılmaz, A. (2020). *Meta teori: Bir gelişim ve psikoterapi kuramı olarak pozitif psikoterapi*. Nobel Akademik Yayıncılık.

Escardívol, R. B. i, Mateo-Viladomat, E., Galbany-Estragués, P., Vilar-Pont, M., Solé, M. A. C. i, Lopez, G., Flores-Montoya, R., Vicente-Belis, M., Escoda-Geli, N., Molina-Nadal, A., Vélez, O. C., & Solà, G. J. i. (2024). Implementation of Nurse Prescriptions throughout the Public Health System in Catalonia (2021–2022). *Health Care*, *12*(12), 1232. DOI: 10.3390/healthcare12121232 PMID: 38921348

Estes, J. M., & Karten, C. (2014). Nursing Expertise and the Evaluation of Psychosocial Distress in Patients With Cancer and Survivors. *Clinical Journal of Oncology Nursing*, *18*(5), 598–600. DOI: 10.1188/14.CJON.598-600

European Commission. (2005). *User Guide: Directive 2005/36/EC*. Brussels: DG Internal Market.

European Federation of Nurses Associations (EFN). (2015). *EFN Competency Framework for General Care Nurses*. EFN.

European Union. (2012). *Consolidated Version of the Treaty on the Functioning of the European Union*. Article 168.

Falender, C. A. (2020). Ethics of Clinical Supervision: An International Lens. *Psychology in Russia : State of the Art*, *13*(1), 42. DOI: 10.11621/pir.2020.0105

Fang, F., Fall, K., & Mittleman, M. A.. (2012). Suicide and cardiovascular death after a cancer diagnosis. *The New England Journal of Medicine*, *366*, 1310–1318.

Feather, J. S., Howson, M., Ritchie, L., Carter, P. D., Parry, D. T., & Koziol-McLain, J. (2016). Evaluation methods for assessing users' psychological experiences of web-based psychosocial interventions: A systematic review. *Journal of Medical Internet Research*, *18*(6), e181.

Federal Law of 21.11.2011 (2011). Nº 323-FZ "On the fundamentals of protecting the health of citizens in the Russian Federation". https://www.rosminzdrav.ru/ (In Russian).

Ferrell, B., & Wittenberg, E. (2017). A review of family caregiving intervention trials in oncology. *CA: a Cancer Journal for Clinicians*, *67*(4), 318–325. DOI: 10.3322/caac.21396

Finkelhor, D., Shattuck, A., Turner, H., & Hamby, S. (2015). A revised inventory of adverse childhood experiences. *Child Abuse & Neglect*, *48*, 13–21. DOI: 10.1016/j.chiabu.2015.07.011

Fitchett, G., Emanuel, L., Handzo, G., Boyken, L., & Wilkie, D. J. (2015). Care of the human spirit and the role of dignity therapy: A systematic review of dignity therapy research. *BMC Palliative Care*, *14*(1), 8. DOI: 10.1186/s12904-015-0007-1

Forchuk, C. (2021). *Overview of Peplau's Theory*., DOI: 10.4324/9781003000853-21

Forchuk, C. (Ed.). (2021). *From therapeutic relationships to transitional care: A theoretical and practical roadmap*. Routledge.

Ford, D. M., Budworth, L., Lawton, R., Teale, E. A., & O'Connor, D. B. (2023). In-hospital stress and patient outcomes: A systematic review and meta-analysis. *PLoS One, 18*(3), e0282789. PMID: 36893099

Fulton, J. S. (2019). Fulfilling Our Social Mandate. *Clinical Nurse Specialist CNS, 33*(2), 61. DOI: 10.1097/nur.0000000000000430 PMID: 30730448

Gaebel, W., Zielasek, J., & Kowitz, S. (2020). Psychiatric training in Germany. *International Review of Psychiatry (Abingdon, England), 32*(2), 133–138. PMID: 31689126

Gál, É., tefan, S., & Cristea, I. A. (2021). The efficacy of mindfulness meditation apps in enhancing users' well-being and mental health related outcomes: A meta-analysis of randomized controlled trials. *Journal of Affective Disorders, 279*, 131–142. PMID: 33049431

Gallagher, A. (2020). *Slow Ethics for Nursing Practice: Reclaiming the Value of Time*. Oxford University Press. (Hemşirelikte dürüstlük ve rol çatışmaları üzerine).

García-Sastre, M., Castro-Molina, F. J., Cabanillas, R. C., Corrales, C. S., Golmar, L. J., Román, J. C., & Aguilera-Serrano, C. (2024). Psychotherapeutic nursing as Advanced Clinical Practice for the promotion of mental health in Spain. *International Nursing Review, 71*(2), 244. DOI: 10.1111/inr.12935 PMID: 38191271

Garvey, K. A., Penn, J. V., Campbell, A. L., Esposito-Smythers, C., & Spirito, A. (2009). Contracting for safety with patients: clinical practice and forensic implications. *PubMed, 37*(3), 363. https://pubmed.ncbi.nlm.nih.gov/19767501

Geller, S. M., & Greenberg, L. S. (2012). *Therapeutic presence: A mindful approach to effective therapy*. American Psychological Association.

Gençtan, E. (1993). *Psychoanalysis and Beyond* (5th ed.). Remzi Kitabevi.

George, D. A. S. (2023). *Addressing India's Healthcare Worker Shortage: Evaluating Strategies to Improve Medical Education and Retention*. https://doi.org/DOI: 10.5281/ZENODO.8370878

Gerges, S., Hallit, R., & Hallit, S. (2023). Stressors in hospitalized patients and their associations with mental health outcomes: Testing perceived social support and spiritual well-being as moderators. *BMC Psychiatry, 23*(1), 323. PMID: 37161403

Ghielen, S. T. S., van Woerkom, M., & Christina Meyers, M. (2018). Promoting positive outcomes through strengths interventions: A literature review. *The Journal of Positive Psychology, 13*(6), 573–585. DOI: 10.1080/17439760.2017.1365164

Giannetta, N., Villa, G., Pennestrì, F., Sala, R., Mordacci, R., & Manara, D. F. (2021). Ethical problems and moral distress in primary care: A scoping review. *International Journal of Environmental Research and Public Health, 18*(14), 7565. PMID: 34300016

Given, B., & Given, C. W. (n.d.). *WHAT KNOWLEDGE AND SKILLS DO CAREGIVERS NEED?* Goldstein, E., Chokshi, B., Melendez-Torres, G., Rios, A., Jelley, M., & Lewis-O'Connor, A. (2024). Effectiveness of Trauma-Informed Care Implementation in Health Care Settings: Systematic Review of Reviews and Realist Synthesis. *The Permanente Journal, 28*(1), 135–150. DOI: 10.7812/TPP/23.127

Glarcher, M., & Lex, K. M. (2020). Advanced Nursing Practice in Austria under consideration of outcome measurement. *Zeitschrift für Evidenz, Fortbildung und Qualität im Gesundheitswesen, 155*, 11. DOI: 10.1016/j.zefq.2020.06.012 PMID: 32811773

Godbee, M., & Kangas, M. (2020). The relationship between flexible perspective taking and emotional well-being: A systematic review of the "self-as-context" component of acceptance and commitment therapy. *Behavior Therapy, 51*(6), 917–932.

Gómez-Penedo, J. M., Babl, A., Dyresen, A., Fernández-Álvarez, J., & Flückiger, C., & grosse Holtforth, M. (2023). Problem mastery and motivational clarification as mechanisms of change in cognitive-behavioral therapy for depression: Secondary analysis of a randomized controlled trial. *Behaviour Research and Therapy, 167*, 104343. PMID: 37307656

Gottlieb, L. N. (2014). CE: Strengths-based nursing. *AJN The American Journal of Nursing, 114*(8), 24–32. DOI: 10.1097/01.NAJ.0000453039.70629.e2 PMID: 25036663

Gowda, P. C., & Premanand, V. (2025). Mindfulness and Differentiation of Self among Adolescents: Mediating Role of Self-as-context. *Indian Journal of Positive Psychology, 16*(1).

Grant, C., & Lusk, J. (2015). A multidisciplinary approach to therapeutic risk management of the suicidal patient. *Journal of Multidisciplinary Healthcare, 8*, 291–298. DOI: 10.2147/jmdh.s50529 PMID: 26150725

Gregg, J. A. (2013). Self-acceptance and chronic illness. In *The strength of self-acceptance: Theory, practice and research* (pp. 247–262). Springer New York.

Grossman, P., Niemann, L., Schmidt, S., & Walach, H. (2004). Mindfulness-based stress reduction and health benefits: A meta-analysis. *Journal of Psychosomatic Research, 57*(1), 35–43.

Gründel, M. (2000). *Psychotherapeutisches Haftungsrecht (Die zivilrechtliche Haftung des Psychologischen Psycotherapeuten bei Verletzung seiner Berufspflichten)*. Springer.

Guest, H., & Miller, C. L. (2024). Trauma-Informed Care in Nursing Curricula: Development of a Simulation-Based Educational Framework to Guide Health Professions. *Nursing Education Perspectives, 45*(5), 271–275. DOI: 10.1097/01.NEP.0000000000001313

Guillaumie, L., Boiral, O., & Champagne, J. (2017). A mixed-methods systematic review of the effects of mindfulness on nurses. *Journal of Advanced Nursing, 73*(5), 1017–1034.

Gülırmak Güler, K. (2023). *Pozitif psikoterapi temelli umut yerleştirme programının multipl skleroz tanılı bireylerde umut ve yaşam amaçları belirleme düzeyine etkisi*. Doktora Tezi, Ondokuz Mayıs Üniversitesi Lisansüstü Eğitim Enstitüsü Hemşirelik Ana Bilim Dalı.

Gülırmak Güler, K. (2025). Hemşirelik Araştırmalarında Pozitif Psikoterapinin Kullanımı: Bibliyometrik Bir Analiz. *Gümüşhane Üniversitesi Sağlık Bilimleri Dergisi, 14*(2), 823–831. DOI: 10.37989/gumussagbil.1611568

Gülırmak Güler, K., Güleç Keskin, S., & Albayrak, E. (2024a). The power of virtual connections: A randomized controlled trial of online positive psychotherapy training on effective communication skills of nursing students. *Nurse Education in Practice, 77*, 103967. PMID: 38615450

Gülırmak Güler, K., Güleç Keskin, S., & Terzi, M. (2024b). Transformative impact of positive psychotherapy-based hope placement program on life goals and hope level of individuals with multiple sclerosis. *Public Health Nursing (Boston, Mass.), 41*(6), 1402–1417. PMID: 39105489

Gumport, N. B., Williams, J. J., & Harvey, A. G. (2015). Learning cognitive behavior therapy. *Journal of Behavior Therapy and Experimental Psychiatry, 48*, 164–169. PMID: 25898288

Günday, H. M. (2015). *Psikiyatristin hukukî sorumluluğu*. Yetkin Yayınları.

Günday, H. M. (2015). *Psikiyatristin Hukukî Sorumluluğu*. Yetkin Yayınları.

Günday, H. M., & Albayrak Günday, E. (2025). Artificial intelligence in mental health practices: Legal liability analysis under Turkish, European, and common law frameworks. *Psikiyatride Güncel Yaklasimlar, 17*(4), 806–821. DOI: 10.18863/pgy.1620119

Guo, Y. F., Zhang, X., Plummer, V., Lam, L., Cross, W., & Zhang, J. P. (2017). Positive psychotherapy for depression and self-efficacy in undergraduate nursing students: A randomized, controlled trial. *International Journal of Mental Health Nursing*, *26*(4), 375–383. DOI: 10.1111/inm.12255 PMID: 27633932

Guru Basava Aradhya, S., Chithambar Gupta, V., Selvakumar, P., Raman, M. S., Singh, J., Manjunath, T. C., & Sharma, M. (2025). Health Crises and Digitalization: Digital Health. In Yıldırım, S. Y., & Kandpal, V. (Eds.), *Sustainable Digitalization Strategies in Business and Healthcare* (pp. 171–198). IGI Global Scientific Publishing., DOI: 10.4018/979-8-3373-5087-5.ch007

Guruge, S., & Khanlou, N. (2004). *Intersectionalities of Influence: Researching the Health of Immigrant and Refugee Women. 36*(3).

Haberlin, S. (2024). Sitting with the data: Experimenting with meditative thematic analysis. *The Qualitative Report*, *29*(7), 1969–1980.

Haines, S. G., Stanton, R., Anderson, C., & Welch, A. (2024). Ethical challenges for nurses delivering coercive interventions in community mental health settings: A scoping review. *International Journal of Mental Health Nursing*, *33*(4), 750–759. DOI: 10.1111/inm.13290 PMID: 38205562

Halm, M. (2017). The role of mindfulness in enhancing self-care for nurses. *American Journal of Critical Care*, *26*(4), 344–348.

Halter, M. J., Rolin, D., Adamaszek, M., & Russell, B. (2021). Professional Identity and Scope of Practice for the Psychiatric Mental Health Nurse Practitioner [Mesleki kimlik ve yetki sınırları için]. *Journal of the American Psychiatric Nurses Association*.

Haribhai-Thompson, J., McBride-Henry, K., Hales, C., & Rook, H. (2022). Understanding of empathetic communication in acute hospital settings: A scoping review. *BMJ Open*, *12*(9), e063375. PMID: 36171029

Harker, R., Pidgeon, A. M., Klaassen, F., & King, S. (2016). Exploring resilience and mindfulness as preventative factors for psychological distress burnout and secondary traumatic stress among human service professionals. *Work (Reading, Mass.)*, *54*(3), 631–637. DOI: 10.3233/WOR-162311

Harnett, N. G., & Lebois, L. A. M. (2022). Leveraging resting-state neurophenotypes to identify susceptibility to and heterogeneity of posttraumatic stress disorder. *Neuropsychopharmacology: Official Publication of the American College of Neuropsychopharmacology*, *47*(1), 403–404. DOI: 10.1038/s41386-021-01134-y

Harris, N., Brazeau, J. N., Rawana, E. P., Brownlee, K., & Mazmanian, D. (2016). A Preliminary Examination of a Strengths-Based Treatment for Adolescent Substance Use Issues Examen préliminaire d'un traitement axé sur les forces destiné aux adolescents ayant des troubles liés à la toxicomanie. Vol. 50 No. 2, 145–163

Harris, R. (2006). Embracing your demons: An overview of acceptance and commitment therapy. *Psychotherapy in Australia*, *12*(4), 70–76.

Hart, P. L., Brannan, J. D., & De Chesnay, M. (2014). Resilience in nurses: An integrative review. *Journal of Nursing Management*, *22*(6), 720–734. PMID: 25208943

Hasanov, R. Sh., Ozol, S. A., Gilyazutdinov, I. A., & Gataullin, I. G. (2013). Sovremennye principy reabilitacii onkologicheskih bol'nyh [Modern principles of rehabilitation of cancer patients] [In Russian]. *Povolzhskij Onkologicheskij Vestnik*, *4*, 49–55.

Havale, D. S., Patole, J., Anute, N., Rane, D. P., Shah, A. H., & Selvakumar, P. (2026). Digital Tools and Resources for Teaching Sustainability. In Hans, E., & Hans, A. (Eds.), *Harnessing E-Learning to Create a Sustainable Future* (pp. 45–74). IGI Global Scientific Publishing., DOI: 10.4018/979-8-3373-0112-9.ch003

Hawkins, P., & Shohet, R. (2012). *Supervision in the Helping Professions* (4th ed.). Open University Press.

Hawton, K., Lascelles, K., Pitman, A., Gilbert, S., & Silverman, M. M. (2022). Assessment of suicide risk in mental health practice: Shifting from prediction to therapeutic assessment, formulation, and risk management. *The Lancet. Psychiatry*, *9*(11), 922–928. DOI: 10.1016/s2215-0366(22)00232-2 PMID: 35952701

Hayes, S. C. (2004). Acceptance and commitment therapy, relational frame theory, and the third wave of behavioral and cognitive therapies. *Behavior Therapy*, *35*(4), 639–665.

Hayes, S. C., Luoma, J. B., Bond, F. W., Masuda, A., & Lillis, J. (2006). Acceptance and commitment therapy: Model, processes and outcomes. *Behaviour Research and Therapy*, *44*(1), 1–25.

Heaney, F., Conway, Y., & Cormack, S. (2023). Principles of trauma care. In *Orthopaedic and trauma nursing: An evidence-based approach to musculoskeletal care* (ss. 215-239).

Hein, L. C., & Schärer, K. (2014). A Modern History of Psychiatric–Mental Health Nursing. *Archives of Psychiatric Nursing*, *29*(1), 49–55. DOI: 10.1016/j.apnu.2014.10.003 PMID: 25634875

Hendriks, T., de Jong, J., Hassankhan, A., & van Woerkom, M. (2024). BAMBOO for Refugees—A culturally sensitive positive psychology intervention: A protocol for a pilot randomized controlled trial. *International Journal of Applied Positive Psychology*, *9*(2), 553–582.

Hendriks, T., Schotanus-Dijkstra, M., Hassankhan, A., De Jong, J., & Bohlmeijer, E. (2020). The efficacy of multi-component positive psychology interventions: A systematic review and meta-analysis of randomized controlled trials. *Journal of Happiness Studies*, *21*(1), 357–390.

Herbert, P. B., & Young, K. A. (2002). Tarasoff at twenty-five. *PubMed, 30*(2), 275. https://pubmed.ncbi.nlm.nih.gov/12108565

Herman, J. L. (1992). *Trauma and recovery*. Basic Books.

Hermaszewska, S., Sweeney, A., Camminga, B., Botelle, R., Elliott, K., & Sin, J. (2022). Lived experiences of transgender forced migrants and their mental health outcomes: Systematic review and meta-ethnography. *BJPsych Open*, *8*(3), e91. DOI: 10.1192/bjo.2022.51

Herringa, R. J. (2017). Trauma, PTSD, and the developing brain. *Current Psychiatry Reports*, *19*, 69. DOI: 10.1007/s11920-017-0825-3

Hersch, R. K., Cook, R. F., & Deitz, D. K.. (2016). Reducing nurses' stress: A randomized controlled trial of a web-based stress management program for nurses. *Applied Nursing Research*, *32*, 18–25. PMID: 27969025

Higgins, J., & Green, S. (2011) Combining groups. In: Cochrane Handbook for Systematic Reviews of Interventions Version 5.1.0, p. 7.7.3.8. Available at: https://training.cochrane.org/handbook/archive/v5.1/ (accessed 11 August 2022).

Higgins, J. P. T., Thompson, S. G., & Deeks, J. J.. (2003). Measuring inconsistency in meta-analyses. *British Medical Journal*, *327*, 557–560. PMID: 12958120

Hirsch, C. R., Beale, S., Grey, N., & Liness, S. (2019). Approaching cognitive behavior therapy for generalized anxiety disorder from a cognitive process perspective. *Frontiers in Psychiatry*, *10*, 796. PMID: 31780964

Hoeve, Y. T., Jansen, G., & Roodbol, P. (2014). The nursing profession: Public image, self-concept and professional identity. A discussion paper. *Journal of Advanced Nursing*, *70*(2), 295–309.

Hoffmeister, L., Huebner, J., Keinki, C., & Muenstedt, K. (2021). Education of non-medical practitioners in Germany—An analysis of course subjects of specialized schools. *Wiener Medizinische Wochenschrift*, *174*, 189. DOI: 10.1007/s10354-021-00896-w PMID: 34902098

Hofmann, S. G., & Asmundson, G. J. (2008). Acceptance and mindfulness-based therapy: New wave or old hat? *Clinical Psychology Review*, *28*(1), 1–16.

Hofstede, G. (2001). *Culture's consequences: Comparing values, behaviors, institutions and organizations across nations*. Sage publications.

Holmes, J. (1995). Supportive Psychotherapy the Search for Positive Meanings. *The British Journal of Psychiatry*, *167*(4), 439–445. PMID: 8829709

Hoppen, T. H., & Morina, N. (2021). Efficacy of positive psychotherapy in reducing negative and enhancing positive psychological outcomes: A meta-analysis of randomised controlled trials. *BMJ Open*, *11*(9), e046017. PMID: 34489269

Horatio: European Psychiatric Nurses. (2012, July). Psychiatric/mental health nurses and psychotherapy: Position document. http://www.horatioweb.eu/downloads/Psychotherapy_position_paper.pdf. Retrieved December 10, 2025.

Horatio: European Psychiatric Nurses. (2018). *The Role of the Psychiatric Nurse in Europe*.

Horvath, A. O., Del Re, A. C., Flückiger, C., & Symonds, D. (2011). Alliance in individual psychotherapy. *Psychotherapy (Chicago, Ill.)*, *48*(1), 9–16. DOI: 10.1037/a0022186

House, J. S., Landis, K. R., & Umberson, D. (1988). Social relationships and health. *Science*, *241*, 540–545.

Hurley, J., Lakeman, R., Linsley, P., Ramsay, M., & Lawson, S. (2022). Utilizing the mental health nursing workforce: A scoping review of mental health nursing clinical roles and identities. *International Journal of Mental Health Nursing, 31*(4), 796-822. Wiley. https://doi.org/DOI: 10.1111/inm.12983

ICN. (2021). The ICN Code of Ethics for Nurses: Revised 2021. In International Council of Nurses. International Council of Nurses. https://www.icn.ch/sites/default/files/inline-files/2012_ICN_Codeofethicsfornurses International Council of Nurses. (2021). ICN code of ethics for nurses. ICN.

Idrisova, L. E., Solopova, A. G., Tabakman, Yu. Yu., Makatsariya, A. D., & Surenkov, A. A. (2016). *Osnovnye napravleniya psihologicheskoj reabilitacii onkoginekologicheskih bol'nyh* [The main directions of psychological rehabilitation of oncogynecologic patients]. *Akusherstvo* [In Russian]. *Ginekologiya i Reprodukcija, 4*, 94–104.

İlgar, M. Z., & İlgar, S. C. (2019). Cognitive behavioral change and motivational interviewing. *Theory and Practice in Education, 15*(1), 47–73.

Imel, Z., Baldwin, S., Bonus, K., & MacCoon, D. (2008). Beyond the individual: Group effects in mindfulness-based stress reduction. *Psychotherapy Research, 18*(6), 735–742.

Ingstad, K., Pedersen, M. K., Uhrenfeldt, L., & Pedersen, P. U. (2023). Patients' expectations of and experiences with psychosocial care needs in perioperative nursing: A descriptive study. *BMC Nursing, 22*(1), 304. PMID: 37670261

International Council of Nurses (ICN). (2021). Guidelines on Mental Health Nursing and Well-Being Support. Geneva: ICN. https://www.icn.ch/resources/publications-and-reports/guidelines-mental-health-nursing

Jacobsen, P. B., & Jim, H. S. (2008). Psychosocial interventions for anxiety and depression in adult cancer patients: Achievements and challenges. *CA: a Cancer Journal for Clinicians, 58*(4), 214–230.

Jakel, P., Kenney, J., & Ludan, N.. (2016). Effects of the use of the provider resilience mobile application in reducing compassion fatigue in oncology nursing. *Clinical Journal of Oncology Nursing, 20*, 611–616. PMID: 27857259

Javadzade, N., Esmaeili, S. V., Omranifard, V., & Zargar, F. (2024). Effect of mindfulness-based stress reduction (MBSR) program on depression, emotion regulation, and sleep problems: A randomized controlled trial study on depressed elderly. *BMC Public Health, 24*(1), 271.

Jeffreys, M. R. (2015). *Teaching cultural competence in nursing and health care: Inquiry, action, and innovation*. Springer Publishing Company.

Jessen, S., Mirkovic, J., Brendmo, E. H., & Nes, L. S. (2021). Evaluating a strengths-based mHealth tool (MyStrengths): Explorative feasibility trial. *JMIR Formative Research, 5*(11), e30572. DOI: 10.2196/30572 PMID: 34787580

Joaquim, S. B., Simões de Almeida, R., & Marques, A. J. (2023). Transdiagnostic cognitive behavioral group interventions: A systematic review. *Cognitive Therapy and Research, 47*(3), 303–326.

Jones, B. D. M., Umer, M., Kittur, M. E., Finkelstein, O., Xue, S., Dimick, M. K., Ortiz, A., Goldstein, B. I., Mulsant, B. H., & Husain, M. I. (2023). A systematic review on the effectiveness of dialectical behavior therapy for improving mood symptoms in bipolar disorders. *International Journal of Bipolar Disorders*, *11*, 6. DOI: 10.1186/s40345-023-00288-6 PMID: 36739574

Júnior, J. M. P., Clementino, F. de S., Santos, R. C. de A., Vítor, A. F., & Miranda, F. A. N. de. (2017). Enfermagem e o processo de desinstitucionalização no âmbito da saúde mental: revisão integrativa Nursing and the deinstitutionalization process in the mental health scope: integrative review. *Revista de Pesquisa Cuidado é Fundamental Online*, *9*(3), 893. https://doi.org/DOI: 10.9789/2175-5361.2017.v9i3.893-898

Justice, L., Brems, C., & Ehlers, K. (2018). Bridging body and mind: Considerations for trauma-informed yoga. *International Journal of Yoga Therapy*, *28*(1), 39–50. DOI: 10.17761/2018-00017R2

Kaas, M. J. (2020). Will We Be Ready? Preparing Psychiatric-Mental Health Nurses for Future Practice. *Journal of the American Psychiatric Nurses Association*, *26*(1), 112–119. DOI: 10.1177/1078390319878767

Kabat-Zinn, J. (2016). Sitting meditations. *Mindfulness*, *7*(6), 1441–1444.

Kague, J. (n.d.). *Addressing Mental Health Challenges in Pediatric Nursing: Strategies for Comprehensive Care.*

Kahler, C. W., Spillane, N. S., Day, A. M., Cioe, P. A., Parks, A., Leventhal, A. M., & Brown, R. A. (2015). Positive psychotherapy for smoking cessation: A pilot randomized controlled trial. *Nicotine & Tobacco Research: Official Journal of the Society for Research on Nicotine and Tobacco*, *17*(11), 1385–1392. DOI: 10.1093/ntr/ntv011 PMID: 25646352

Kalaycı, T., Aygün, Ü., & Sayir, F. (2023). Multiple trauma approach in earthquake. *Ağrı Medical Faculty Journal*, *1*(2), 22–25.

Karanci, A. N., Işıklı, S., Aker, A. T., Gül, E. İ., Erkan, B. B., Özkol, H., & Güzel, H. Y. (2012). Personality, posttraumatic stress and trauma type: Factors contributing to posttraumatic growth and its domains in a Turkish community sample. *European Journal of Psychotraumatology*, *3*(1), 17303. DOI: 10.3402/ejpt.v3i0.17303

Kaya, H. (2017). Psychological traces of terrorism: A review of direct and indirect exposure. Master's Thesis, Ankara University Institute of Health Sciences, Department of Interdisciplinary Forensic Sciences.

Keng, S. L., Smoski, M. J., & Robins, C. J. (2011). Effects of mindfulness on psychological health: A review of empirical studies. *Clinical Psychology Review, 31*(6), 1041–1056.

Keser Özcan, N. (2020). Depressive disorder. In F. Oflaz & N. Yıldırım (Eds.), *Psychiatric nursing certification topics* (pp. 417–431). Psychiatric Nursing Association Publications No:1, Akademisyen Nobel Medical Bookstores.

Khanahmadi, M. (2020). Ethical Codes and Psychotherapy. *International Journal of Ethics & Society, 1*(4). https://ijethics.com/article-1-62-en.html

Kiliç, N., & Eryilmaz, A. (2019). Investigating narcissistic personality traits in the context of positive psychotherapy. *Archives of Neuropsychiatry, 56*(1), 40–46. PMID: 30911236

King, N. J., & Ollendick, T. H. (2008). The elegant psychosocial intervention: A heuristic conceptual framework for clinicians and researchers. *Behavioural and Cognitive Psychotherapy, 36*(3), 253–261.

Kirmayer, L. J. (2012). Cultural competence and evidence-based practice in mental health: Epistemic communities and the politics of pluralism. *Social Science & Medicine, 75*(2), 249–256. PMID: 22575699

Kissane, D. W., Clarke, D. M., & Street, A. F. (2001). Demoralization syndrome – a relevant psychiatric diagnosis for palliative care. *Journal of Palliative Care, 17*, 12–21.

Kittler, M. G., Rygl, D., & Mackinnon, A. (2011). Special Review Article: Beyond culture or beyond control? Reviewing the use of Hall's high-/low-context concept. *International Journal of Cross Cultural Management, 11*(1), 63–82.

Kleinman, A. (1988). *Rethinking psychiatry: from cultural category to personal experience The Free Press.*

Kloos, N., Drossaert, C. H. C., & Bohlmeijer, E. T.. (2019). Online positive psychology intervention for nursing home staff: A cluster-randomized controlled feasibility trial of effectiveness and acceptability. *International Journal of Nursing Studies, 98*, 48–56. PMID: 31295708

Kluft, R. (2014). Stabilization basics. In M. L. Brand, R. A. Lanius, U. Schnyder, & R. P. Frewen (Eds.), *Neurobiology and treatment of traumatic dissociation: Towards an embodied self* (ss. 319-338).

Ko, A. H., Dollinger, M., & Rosenbaum, E. (2008). *Everyone's guide to cancer therapy: How cancer is diagnosed, treated and managed day to day* (5th ed., Vol. 2). Publisher.

Köbler, P., Krauss-Köstler, E. K., Stein, B., Ficker, J. H., Wilhelm, M., Dechêne, A., & Waller, C. (2022). Specialized biopsychosocial care in inpatient somatic medicine units—A pilot study. *Frontiers in Public Health, 10*, 844874. PMID: 35493384

Kornaros, K., Zwedberg, S., Nissen, E., & Salomonsson, B. (2018). A hermeneutic study of integrating psychotherapist competence in postnatal child health care: Nurses' perspectives. *BMC Nursing, 17*(1). Advance online publication. DOI: 10.1186/s12912-018-0311-1 PMID: 30258284

Köroğlu, E. (2015). *Klinik Psikiyatri*. Boylam Psikiyatri Enstitüsü.

Kostanski, M., & Hassed, C. (2008). Mindfulness as a concept and a process. *Australian Psychologist, 43*(1), 15–21.

Ko, Y. S., & Hyun, M. Y. (2015). Effects of a positive psychotherapy program on depression, self-esteem, and hope in patients with major depressive disorders. *Journal of Korean Academy of Psychiatric and Mental Health Nursing, 24*(4), 246–256.

Krug, K., Kraus, K., Herrmann, K., & Joos, S. (2016). Complementary and alternative medicine (CAM) as part of primary health care in Germany–comparison of patients consulting general practitioners and CAM practitioners: A cross-sectional study. *BMC Complementary and Alternative Medicine, 16*(1), 409. DOI: 10.1186/s12906-016-1402-8 PMID: 27776512

Kul, A., & Türk, F. (2020). Kabul ve adanmışlık terapisi (ACT) üzerine bir derleme çalışması. *OPUS International Journal of Society Researches, 16*(29 Ekim Özel Sayısı), 3773-3805.

Kulakov, A. A., Chuchkov, V. M., & Matyakin, Ye. G.. (2012). Reabilitaciya onkologicheskih bol'nyh s defektom i polnoj vtorichnoj adentiej posle udaleniya obeih verhnih chelyustej [Rehabilitation of cancer patients with a defect and a complete secondary adentia after removal of both upper jaws] [In Russian]. *Opuholi Golovy i Shei, 4*, 34–40.

Kump, B., & Scholz, M. (2022). Organizational routines as a source of ethical blindness. *Organization Theory, 3*(1), 26317877221075640.

Lackner, R. (2023). *Stabilization in trauma treatment: A holistic cross-method practical guide*. Springer Nature.

Ladd, E., Miller, M., Wheeler, K., Wainaina, S., Aguirre, F., McGrath, H., Lee, S., Nashwan, A. J., Neary, A., & Core, K. (2020). A Global SWOT Analysis of Advanced Practice Nursing: Policy, Regulation, and Practice. *Research Square (Research Square)*. https://doi.org/DOI: 10.21203/rs.3.rs-113320/v1

Laireiter, A., & Weise, C. (2019). The Heterogeneity of National Regulations in Clinical Psychology and Psychological Treatment in Europe. *Clinical Psychology in Europe*, *1*(1). Advance online publication. DOI: 10.32872/cpe.v1i1.34406

Lange, K. W. (2021). Task sharing in psychotherapy as a viable global mental health approach in resource-poor countries and also in high-resource settings. *Global Health Journal (Amsterdam, Netherlands)*, *5*(3), 120. DOI: 10.1016/j.glohj.2021.07.001

Larmar, S., Wiatrowski, S., & Lewis-Driver, S. (2014). Acceptance & commitment therapy: An overview of techniques and applications. *Journal of Service Science and Management*, *7*, 216–221.

Larsman, P., Pousette, A., Nilsson, M. S., Gadolin, C., & Törner, M. (2024). Ethical value conflicts in healthcare and their effects on nurses' health, turnover intent, team effectiveness, and patient safety: A longitudinal questionnaire study. *Scandinavian Journal of Work, Environment & Health*, *50*(2), 113. DOI: 10.5271/sjweh.4138 PMID: 38232184

Laufs, A., & Uhlenbruck, W. (2002). *Handbuch des Arztrechts*. (3. Aufl.). München: C.H.

LeBoeuf, D. (1988). Psychiatric Malpractice: Exploitation of Women Patients. *Harvard Women's Law Journal*, *11*, 83–116.

Lee, C. Y., Fang, C. K., & Yang, Y. C.. (2012). Demoralization syndrome among cancer outpatients in Taiwan. *Supportive Care in Cancer*, *20*, 2259–2267.

Légifrance. (2010). *Décret n° 2010-534 du 20 mai 2010 relatif à l'usage du titre de psychothérapeute*. Journal Officiel de la République Française.

Leininger, M. M., & McFarland, M. R. (2006). *Culture care diversity and universality: A worldwide nursing theory*. Jones & Bartlett Learning.

LeMoult, J., Humphreys, K. L., Tracy, A., Hoffmeister, J.-A., Ip, E., & Gotlib, I. H. (2020). Meta-analysis: Exposure to early life stress and risk for depression in childhood and adolescence. *Journal of the American Academy of Child and Adolescent Psychiatry*, *59*(7), 842–855. DOI: 10.1016/j.jaac.2019.10.011

Levenson, J. S., Craig, S. L., & Austin, A. (2023). Trauma-informed and affirmative mental health practices with LGBTQ+ clients. *Psychological Services*, *20*(Suppl 1), 134–144. DOI: 10.1037/ser0000540

Levi-Belz, Y., Krysinska, K., & Andriessen, K. (2021). "Turning personal tragedy into triumph": A systematic review and meta-analysis of studies on posttraumatic growth among suicide-loss survivors. *Psychological Trauma: Theory, Research, Practice, and Policy*, *13*(3), 322–335. DOI: 10.1037/tra0000977

Levin, M., & Hayes, S. C. (2011). Mindfulness and acceptance: The perspective of acceptance and commitment therapy. *Acceptance and mindfulness in cognitive behavior therapy: Understanding and applying the new therapies*, 291-316.

Levin, T., & Kissane, W. D. (2006). Psychooncology – the state of its development in 2006. *European Journal of Psychiatry*, *20*(2).

Lewis, C., Roberts, N. P., Andrew, M., Starling, E., & Bisson, J. I. (2020). Psychological therapies for post-traumatic stress disorder in adults: Systematic review and meta-analysis. *European Journal of Psychotraumatology*, *11*(1), 1729633. DOI: 10.1080/20008198.2020.1729633

Lewis, C., Roberts, N. P., Gibson, S., & Bisson, J. I. (2020). Dropout from psychological therapies for post-traumatic stress disorder (PTSD) in adults: Systematic review and meta-analysis. *European Journal of Psychotraumatology*, *11*(1), 1709709. DOI: 10.1080/20008198.2019.1709709

Lianos, G. D., Mangano, A., Cho, W. C., Dionigi, G., & Roukos, D. H. (2015). Circulating tumor DNA: New horizons for improving cancer treatment. *Future Oncology (London, England)*, *11*(4), 545–548.

Ličen, S., & Prosen, M. (2023). The development of cultural competences in nursing students and their significance in shaping the future work environment: A pilot study. *BMC Medical Education*, *23*(1), 819. DOI: 10.1186/s12909-023-04800-5

Lichko, A. E. (1980). Zhurnal nevrologii i psikhiatrii im. [In Russian]. *S. S. Korsakova*, *8*, 1195–1198.

Lim, W. L., & Tierney, S. (2023). The effectiveness of positive psychology interventions for promoting well-being of adults experiencing depression compared to other active psychological treatments: A systematic review and meta-analysis. *Journal of Happiness Studies*, *24*(1), 249–273. PMID: 36373089

Liu, A., Yazdani, Y., Elias, M., Patel, K., Budzi, D., Saad, A., & Pottie, K. (2025). Transition in care interventions for Refugee, Immigrant and other Migrant (RIM) populations: A health equity-oriented scoping review. *Globalization and Health*, *21*(1), 25. PMID: 40307839

Lu, J., Chen, Y., & Mudathir, D. (2025). Mindfulness and stress among undergraduate students: Examining the mediation roles of self-as-context and cognitive defusion as decentering facets. *Journal of American College Health*, •••, 1–8.

Luoma, J. B., & Platt, M. G. (2015). Shame, self-criticism, self-stigma, and compassion in acceptance and commitment therapy. *Current Opinion in Psychology*, *2*, 97–101.

Luxton, D. D. (Ed.). (2015). *Artificial intelligence in behavioral and mental health care*.

Lyons, P., Edwardes, A., Bladon, L., & Abel, K. M. (2025). Culturally sensitive mental health research: A scoping review. *BMC Psychiatry*, *25*(1), 190. PMID: 40033264

Lyu, X.-C., Jiang, H.-J., Lee, L.-H., Yang, C.-I., & Sun, X.-Y. (2024). Oncology nurses' experiences of providing emotional support for cancer patients: A qualitative study. *BMC Nursing*, *23*(1), 58. DOI: 10.1186/s12912-024-01718-1

Magidson, J. F., & Weisberg, R. B. (2014). Implementing Cognitive Behavioral Therapy in Specialty Medical Settings. *Cognitive and Behavioral Practice*, *21*(4), 367–371. DOI: 10.1016/j.cbpra.2014.08.003

Magill, M., Ray, L., Kiluk, B., Hoadley, A., Bernstein, M., Tonigan, J. S., & Carroll, K. (2019). A meta-analysis of cognitive-behavioral therapy for alcohol or other drug use disorders: Treatment efficacy by contrast condition. *Journal of Consulting and Clinical Psychology*, *87*(12), 1093. PMID: 31599606

Mahdavi, M., Emadian, S. O., & Hassanzade, R. (2022). Comparıson Of The Effectıveness Of Mındfulness-Based Cognıtıve Therapy And Acceptance And Commıtment Therapy On Health-Promotıng Behavıors In Patıents Wıth Ulceratıve Colıts. *Journal of Positive School Psychology*, *6*(7).

Maier, C. B. (2019). Nurse prescribing of medicines in 13 European countries. *Human Resources for Health*, *17*(1). Advance online publication. DOI: 10.1186/s12960-019-0429-6 PMID: 31815622

Malik, A., & Sinha, N. (2025). Integrating positive psychology into nursing education: A strengths-based intervention. *Journal of Applied Research in Higher Education*, •••, 1–21. DOI: 10.1108/JARHE-12-2024-0738

Malkina-Pykh, I. G. (2005). *Moskovskii psikhologicheskii zhurnal, 12*. (In Russian).

Manderius, C., Clintståhl, K., Sjöström, K., & Örmon, K. (2023). The psychiatric mental health nurse's ethical considerations regarding the use of coercive measures – a qualitative interview study. *BMC Nursing*, *22*(1). Advance online publication. DOI: 10.1186/s12912-023-01186-z PMID: 36698105

Markowitz, J. C. (2015). Interpersonal psychotherapy. *Psychiatry*, •••, 1859–1870. PMID: 25677355

Markowitz, J. C., & Weissman, M. M. (2012). Interpersonal psychotherapy: Past, present and future. *Clinical Psychology & Psychotherapy*, *19*(2), 99–105. PMID: 22331561

Markus, H. R., & Kitayama, S. (2014). Culture and the self: Implications for cognition, emotion, and motivation. In *College student development and academic life* (pp. 264–293). Routledge.

Marseille, A. (2025). Positive Psychotherapy: A Transcultural Approach to Psychotherapy for the Twenty-First Century. In *Psychotherapy in the Third Millennium-Cross-Cutting Themes and Proposals for Reflection*. IntechOpen. DOI: DOI: 10.5772/intechopen.1007778

Martin, B., Phoenix, B. J., & Chapman, S. A. (2020). How collaborative practice agreements impede the provision of vital behavioral health services. *Nursing Outlook*, *68*(5), 581. DOI: 10.1016/j.outlook.2020.04.002 PMID: 32402393

Martínez, M., Arantzamendi, M., Belar, A., Carrasco, J. M., Carvajal, A., Rullán, M., & Centeno, C. (2017). 'Dignity therapy', a promising intervention in palliative care: A comprehensive systematic literature review. *Palliative Medicine*, *31*(6), 492–509. DOI: 10.1177/0269216316665562

Marvaldi, M., Mallet, J., & Dubertret, C.. (2021). Anxiety, depression, trauma-related, and sleep disorders among healthcare workers during the COVID-19 pandemic: A systematic review and meta-analysis. *Neuroscience and Biobehavioral Reviews*, *126*, 252–264. PMID: 33774085

Maslach, C. (2018). Burnout: A multidimensional perspective. In Professional burnout (pp. 19-32). CRC Press.

Mattheß, C., Farrell, D., Mattheß, M., Bumke, P., Sodemann, U., & Mattheß, H. (2019). The therapeutic value of trauma stabilisation in the treatment of post-traumatic stress disorder – A Southeast Asian study. *Asian Journal of Psychiatry*, *41*, 45–49. DOI: 10.1016/j.ajp.2018.09.010

McCabe, C. (2004). Nurse–patient communication: An exploration of patients' experiences. *Journal of Clinical Nursing*, *13*(1), 41–49. PMID: 14687292

McDonough, J., Rhodes, K., & Procter, N. (2025). The Impact of Clinical Supervision on the Mental Health Nursing Workforce: A Scoping Review. *International Journal of Mental Health Nursing*, *34*(1), e13463. PMID: 39462993

McFarland, M. R., & Wehbe-Alamah, H. B. (2015). *Leininger's culture care diversity and universality: A worldwide nursing theory*. Jones & Bartlett Publishers.

McLaughlin, K. A., Koenen, K. C., Hill, E. D., Petukhova, M., Sampson, N. A., Zaslavsky, A. M., & Kessler, R. C. (2013). Trauma exposure and posttraumatic stress disorder in a national sample of adolescents. *Journal of the American Academy of Child and Adolescent Psychiatry*, *52*(8), 815–830.e14. DOI: 10.1016/j.jaac.2013.05.011

Meibodi, R. P., Meftagh, S. D., & Shahangian, S. S. (2021). The effect of positive psychotherapy on happiness and character strength in cancer patients. *Journal of Education and Health Promotion*, *10*, 97. DOI: 10.4103/jehp.jehp_595_20 PMID: 34084844

Melcop, N., von Werder, T., Sarubin, N., & Benecke, A. (2019). The Role of Psychotherapy in the German Health Care System: Training Requirements for Psychological Psychotherapists and Child and Adolescent Psychotherapists, Legal Aspects, and Health Care Implementation. *Clinical Psychology in Europe*, *1*(4). Advance online publication. DOI: 10.32872/cpe.v1i4.34304

Melton, L. (2017). Brief introduction to cognitive behavioral therapy for the advanced practitioner in oncology. *Journal of the Advanced Practitioner in Oncology*, *8*(2), 188. DOI: 10.6004/jadpro.2017.8.2.6

Menon, V. (2011). Large-scale brain networks and psychopathology: A unifying triple network model. *Trends in Cognitive Sciences*, *15*(10), 483–506. DOI: 10.1016/j.tics.2011.08.003

Mercin, L. (2005). Comparison of the Characteristics of Piaget and Kohlberg's Theories of Moral Development. *Dicle University Journal of Education*, *5*, 73–86.

Meyer, P. S., Johnson, D. P., Parks, A., Iwanski, C., & Penn, D. L. (2012). Positive living: A pilot study of group positive psychotherapy for people with schizophrenia. *The Journal of Positive Psychology*, *7*(3), 239–248. DOI: 10.1080/17439760.2012.677467

Moore, C. A. (2025). Early-Career Nurses' Mindfulness and Its Association With Anxiety, Burnout, Perceived Stress, Job Satisfaction, and Intent to Stay: A Descriptive Cross-Sectional Study (Doctoral dissertation, The Ohio State University).

Moran, M., & Yılmaz, S. (2024). The use of cognitive behavioral therapy in psychiatric nursing studies. *YOBÜ Health Sciences Faculty Journal*, *5*(1), 91–100.

Motamed-Jahromi, M., Fereidouni, Z., & Dehghan, A. (2017). Effectiveness of positive thinking training program on nurses' quality of work life through smartphone applications. *International Scholarly Research Notices, 2017*, 1–6. PMID: 28589174

Možina, M. (2024). Psychotherapy regulation in European countries. *Psychotherapie-Wissenschaft, 14*(2), 93. DOI: 10.30820/1664-9583-2024-2-93

Munn, Z., Tufanaru, C., & Aromataris, E. (2014). Data extraction and synthesis. *The American Journal of Nursing, 114*, 49–54. PMID: 25742352

Murphy, S. T., Cheavens, J. S., & Strunk, D. R. (2022). Framing an intervention as focused on one's strength: Does framing enhance therapeutic benefit? *Journal of Clinical Psychology, 78*(6), 1046–1057. DOI: 10.1002/jclp.23302 PMID: 34978712

Myslivtseva, A. V., & Zaika, V. G. (2014). *Zhurnal fundamental'noi meditsiny i biologii, 3*, 37–40. (In Russian).

Nakao, M., Shirotsuki, K., & Sugaya, N. (2021). Cognitive–behavioral therapy for management of mental health and stress-related disorders: Recent advances in techniques and technologies. *BioPsychoSocial Medicine, 15*(1), 16. PMID: 34602086

Nguyen, O. T., Shah, S., & Gartland, A. J.. (2021). Factors associated with nurse well-being in relation to electronic health record use: A systematic review. *Journal of the American Medical Informatics Association : JAMIA, 28*, 1288–1297. PMID: 33367819

Nievergelt, C. M., Maihofer, A. X., Atkinson, E. G., Chen, C. Y., Choi, K. W., Coleman, J. R. I., & Koenen, K. C. (2024). Genome-wide association analyses identify 95 risk loci and provide insights into the neurobiology of post-traumatic stress disorder. *Nature Genetics, 56*(5), 792–808. DOI: 10.1038/s41588-024-01707-9

Niles, C. (2013). Examining the Deinstitutionalization Movement in North America. *Deleted Journal, 1*(1). Advance online publication. DOI: 10.25071/2564-4033.37273

Norcross, J. C., & Lambert, M. J. (2018). Psychotherapy relationships that work III. *Psychotherapy (Chicago, Ill.), 55*(4), 303–315. DOI: 10.1037/pst0000193

Northouse, L., Williams, A., Given, B., & McCorkle, R. (2012). Psychosocial Care for Family Caregivers of Patients With Cancer. *Journal of Clinical Oncology, 30*(11), 1227–1234. DOI: 10.1200/JCO.2011.39.5798

Nursing and Midwifery Board of Ireland (NMBI). (2017). *Advanced Practice (Nursing) Standards and Requirements*. NMBI.

Nursing and Midwifery Council (NMC). (2018). *Future Nurse: Standards of Proficiency for Registered Nurses*. NMC.

O'Brien, A. J. (2001). The therapeutic relationship: Historical development and contemporary significance. *Journal of Psychiatric and Mental Health Nursing*, *8*(2), 129–137. PMID: 11882118

O'Brien, W. H., Singh, R., Horan, K., Moeller, M. T., Wasson, R., & Jex, S. M. (2019). Group-based acceptance and commitment therapy for nurses and nurse aides working in long-term care residential settings. *Journal of Alternative and Complementary Medicine (New York, N.Y.)*, *25*(7), 753–761.

O'Hayer, C. V. F., O'Hayer, K. M., & Sama, A. (2018). Acceptance and commitment therapy with pancreatic cancer: An integrative model of palliative care-a case report. *Journal of Pancreatic Cancer*, *4*(1), 1–3.

OECD. (2023). *Artificial Intelligence and the Health Workforce*. OECD Publishing., DOI: 10.1787/9a31d8af-

Oleck, L., Retano, A., Tebaldi, C., McGuinness, T. M., Weiss, S., Carbray, J. A., Rodgers, L. S., Donelson, E. E., Ashton, L. L., Koehn, D., & McCoy, P. (2011). Advanced Practice Psychiatric Nurses Legislative Update: State of the States, 2010. *Journal of the American Psychiatric Nurses Association*, *17*(2), 171. DOI: 10.1177/1078390311402331 PMID: 21659307

Oliphant, S. (2023). Navigating advanced nurse practitioner roles in UK mental health services: A scoping review. *International Journal for Advancing Practice*, *1*(2), 65–71. DOI: 10.12968/ijap.2023.1.2.65

Ong, C. W., Barthel, A. L., & Hofmann, S. G. (2024). The relationship between psychological inflexibility and well-being in adults: A meta-analysis of the acceptance and action questionnaire. *Behavior Therapy*, *55*(1), 26–41.

Orang, T. M., Missmahl, I., Gardisi, M., & Kluge, U. (2023). Rethinking mental health care provided to migrants and refugees; a randomized controlled trial on the effectiveness of Value Based Counseling, a culturally sensitive, strength-based psychological intervention. *PLoS One*, *18*(3), e0283889. PMID: 37000817

Osman, F. E. S., Sherif, Z. A. E. G., Shalaby, M., & Shaheen, S. H. A. M. (2018). Evaluate the effect of empathy-based training program on psychiatric nurses' communication skills. IOSR Journal of Nursing and Health Science (IOSR-JNHS), 7(3), 32-41.

Osmancevic, S., Steiner, L. M., Großschädl, F., Lohrmann, C., & Schoberer, D. (2025). The effectiveness of cultural competence interventions in nursing: A systematic review and meta-analysis. *International Journal of Nursing Studies*, •••, 105079.

Özcan, Ö., & Çelik, G. G. (2017). Cognitive behavioral therapy. *Turkey Clinics, 3*(2), 115–120.

Özdel, K. (2015). Cognitive Behavioral Therapies from Past to Present: Theory and Practice. *Türkiye Klinikleri, 8*(2), 10–20.

Özden, M. Ş. (2018). Trauma and dissociative disorders: A general overview. *Bartın University Faculty of Literature Journal, 3*(3), 71–76.

Özen, Y., & Türkmen, İ. (2023). How Positive Is Positive Psychotherapy? (Examination of Positive Psychotherapy). *Innovare Journal Of Social Sciences, 11*(2), 7–11.

Page, M. J., McKenzie, J. E., & Bossuyt, P. M.. (2021). The PRISMA 2020 statement: An updated guideline for reporting systematic reviews. *BMJ (Clinical Research Ed.), 372*(71). PMID: 33782057

Palese, A., Zabalegui, A., Sigurðardóttir, Á. K., Bergin, M., Dobrowolska, B., Gasser, C., Pajnkihar, M., & Jackson, C. (2014). Bologna Process, More or Less: Nursing Education in the European Economic Area: A Discussion Paper. *International Journal of Nursing Education Scholarship, 11*(1), 63. https://doi.org/DOI: 10.1515/ijnes-2013-0022

Panter-Brick, C., & Eggerman, M. (2011). Understanding culture, resilience, and mental health: The production of hope. In *The social ecology of resilience: A handbook of theory and practice* (pp. 369–386). Springer New York.

Pan, Y., Li, F., Liang, H., Shen, X., Bing, Z., Cheng, L., & Dong, Y. (2024). Effectiveness of Mindfulness-Based Stress Reduction on Mental Health and Psychological Quality of Life among University Students: A GRADE-Assessed Systematic Review. *Evidence-Based Complementary and Alternative Medicine : eCAM, 2024*(1), 8872685.

Papadopoulos, I. (Ed.). (2006). *Transcultural health and social care: development of culturally competent practitioners*. Elsevier Health Sciences.

Paul, D. R., M., D., Patricia, Jochen, B., Michelle, P., M., J., Susan, Adriana, C.-A., Andreas, X., & Wendy, P. (2023). Advanced practice nursing in Europe—Results from a pan-European survey of 35 countries. *Journal of Advanced Nursing, 80*(1), 377. DOI: 10.1111/jan.15775 PMID: 37458267

Payson, H. (2023). Reconnecting: Trauma, addiction, and group EMDR therapy. In Luber, M. (Ed.), *EMDR group therapy: Emerging principles and protocols to treat trauma and beyond* (p. 233).

Pedersen, M. L., Gildberg, F. A., & Birkeland, S. (2022). The Danish Court Case Database: A data source in forensic mental health? *Scandinavian Journal of Forensic Science*, *28*(1), 1. DOI: 10.2478/sjfs-2022-0011

Pepfar. (2007). *Task shifting : rational redistribution of tasks among health workforce teams : global recommendations and guidelines*. https://pesquisa.bvsalud.org/portal/resource/pt/who-43821

Peplau, H. E. (1952). *Interpersonal Relations in Nursing*. G.P. Putnam's Sons.

Peplau, H. E. (1997). Peplau's theory of interpersonal relations. *Nursing Science Quarterly*, *10*(4), 162–167. PMID: 9416116

Peseschkian, H. (2023). Positive psychotherapy: Core principles: Emphasizing capacities and balance can give patients a new perspective on their disorder. *Current Psychiatry*, *22*(1), 5–10. DOI: 10.12788/cp.0317

Peseschkian, H., & Remmers, A. (2025a). Life balance with positive psychotherapy. In *Positive Psychiatry, Psychotherapy and Psychology: Clinical Applications for Positive Mental Health* (pp. 91–99). Springer Nature Switzerland.

Peseschkian, N. (1987). *Positive Psychotherapy: Theory and Practice of a New Method*. Springer-Verlag.

Peseschkian, N. (2002). *Günlük yaşamın psikoterapisi (Çev. K. Teksöz)*. Beyaz Yayınları.

Peseschkian, N. (2005). *Pozitif aile terapisi (Çev. M. Naim)*. Beyaz Yayınları.

Peseschkian, N. (2007). *Eğer hiç sahip olmadığın bir şeye sahip olmak istiyorsan, o zaman hiç yapmadığın bir Şey yap (Çev. S. Köseoğlu)*. Beyaz Yayınları.

Phoenix, B. J., & Chapman, S. A. (2020). Effect of state regulatory environments on advanced psychiatric nursing practice. *Archives of Psychiatric Nursing*, *34*(5), 370. DOI: 10.1016/j.apnu.2020.07.001 PMID: 33032760

Pirhofer, J., Bükki, J., Vaismoradi, M., Glarcher, M., & Paal, P. (2022). A qualitative exploration of cultural safety in nursing from the perspectives of Advanced Practice Nurses: Meaning, barriers, and prospects. *BMC Nursing*, *21*(1), 178. PMID: 35787799

Pletnev, S. D. (1996). Lasers in clinical medicine. *Meditsina = Medicine*.

Poghosyan, L., & Maier, C. B. (2022). Advanced practice nurses globally: Responding to health challenges, improving outcomes. *International Journal of Nursing Studies*, *132*, 104262. DOI: 10.1016/j.ijnurstu.2022.104262 PMID: 35633596

Popay, J., Roberts, H., Sowden, A., ... (2006) Guidance on the conduct of narrative synthesis in systematic reviews – a product from the ESRC Methods Programme. https://www.lancaster.ac.uk/media/lancaster-university/content-assets/documents/fhm/dhr/chir/NSsynthesisguidanceVersion1-April2006.pdf

Porter, M., & Wang, J. (2022). Personal resources and work engagement: A literature review. *Journal of Continuing Education in Nursing*, *53*, 115–121. PMID: 35244461

Powers, M. B., Zum Vörde Sive Vörding, M. B., & Emmelkamp, P. M. (2009). Acceptance and commitment therapy: A meta-analytic review. *Psychotherapy and Psychosomatics*, *78*(2), 73–80.

Praissman, S. (2008). Mindfulness-based stress reduction: A literature review and clinician's guide. *Journal of the American Association of Nurse Practitioners*, *20*(4), 212–216.

Punkanen, M., & Buckley, T. (2021). Embodied safety and bodily stabilization in the treatment of complex trauma. *European Journal of Trauma & Dissociation = Revue Européenne du Trauma et de la Dissociation*, *5*(3), 100156. DOI: 10.1016/j.ejtd.2020.100156

Purgato, M., Uphoff, E., Singh, R., Pachya, A. T., Abdulmalik, J., & van Ginneken, N. (2020). Promotion, prevention and treatment interventions for mental health in low- and middle-income countries through a task-shifting approach. *Epidemiology and Psychiatric Sciences*, *29*. Advance online publication. DOI: 10.1017/s204579602000061x PMID: 32744223

Purnell, L. D. (2016). The Purnell model for cultural competence. In *Intervention in mental health-substance use* (pp. 57–78). CRC Press.

Rae, B. (2024). Medicines management for nurses: Explaining legal governance. *Nursing Standard*, *39*(3), 45. DOI: 10.7748/ns.2024.e12177 PMID: 38186230

Rahal, G. M., & Gon, M. C. C. (2020). A systematic review of values interventions in acceptance and commitment therapy. *International Journal of Psychology & Psychological Therapy*, *20*(3), 355–372.

Rahman, A., Khan, M. N., Hamdani, S. U., Chiumento, A., Akhtar, P., Nazir, H., & van Ommeren, M. (2019). Effectiveness of a brief group psychological intervention for women in a post-conflict setting in Pakistan: A single-blind, cluster, randomised controlled trial. *Lancet*, *393*(10182), 1733–1744. PMID: 30948286

Ramaci, T., Bellini, D., Presti, G., & Santisi, G. (2019). Psychological flexibility and mindfulness as predictors of individual outcomes in hospital health workers. *Frontiers in Psychology*, *10*, 1302.

Range, L. M., Campbell, C., Kovac, S. H., Marion-Jones, M., Aldridge, H., Kogos, S. C., & Crump, Y. (2002). NO-SUICIDE CONTRACTS: AN OVERVIEW AND RECOMMENDATIONS. *Death Studies*, *26*(1), 51–74. DOI: 10.1080/07481180210147 PMID: 11865883

Rangel, A., Camerer, C., & Montague, P. R. (2008). A framework for studying the neurobiology of value-based decision making. *Nature Reviews. Neuroscience*, *9*(7), 545–556.

Rashid, T. (2015). Positive psychotherapy: A strength-based approach. *The Journal of Positive Psychology*, *10*(1), 25–40. DOI: 10.1080/17439760.2014.920411

Raval, V. V., Gopal, B., Aggarwal, P., Mohan, M. P., Padmakumari, P., Thomas, E., & Hay, M. C. (2024). Training in Cultural Competence for Mental Health Care: A Mixed-Methods Study of Students, Faculty, and Practitioners from India and USA. *Culture, Medicine and Psychiatry*, *48*(4), 699–730. PMID: 38954183

Ravitz, P., Watson, P., Lawson, A., Constantino, M. J., Bernecker, S., Park, J., & Swartz, H. A. (2019). Interpersonal psychotherapy: A scoping review and historical perspective (1974–2017). *Harvard Review of Psychiatry*, *27*(3), 165–180. PMID: 30883446

Reddemann, L., & Piedfort-Marin, O. (2017). Stabilization in the treatment of complex post-traumatic stress disorders: Concepts and principles. *European Journal of Trauma & Dissociation = Revue Européenne du Trauma et de la Dissociation*, *1*(1), 11–17. DOI: 10.1016/j.ejtd.2017.01.009

Robinson, L. K., Sterling, L., Jackson, J., Gentry, E., Araujo, F., LaFond, C., Jacobson, K. C., & Lee, R. (2022). A secondary traumatic stress reduction program in emergency room nurses. *SAGE Open Nursing*, *8*, 23779608221094530. DOI: 10.1177/23779608221094530

Rocha, T. I. U., Aschar, S., Hidalgo-Padilla, L., Daley, K., Claro, H. G., Martins, H. C. dos S., dos Santos, D. V. C., Miranda, J. J., Araya, R., & Menezes, P. R. (2020). Recruitment, Training and Supervision of Nurses and Nurse Assistants for a task-shifting depression intervention in two RCTs in Brazil and Peru. *Research Square (Research Square)*. https://doi.org/DOI: 10.21203/rs.3.rs-76085/v1

Rodriguez, V. H., Medrano, C. T., & Plaza, I. (2018). Wearable sensors for measuring movement in short sessions of mindfulness sitting meditation: A pilot study. *Journal of Healthcare Engineering*, *2018*(1), 7275049.

Roepke, A. M. (2015). Psychosocial interventions and posttraumatic growth: A meta-analysis. *Journal of Consulting and Clinical Psychology, 83*(1), 129–142. DOI: 10.1037/a0036872

Rokach, A. (2016). Psychological, emotional and physical experiences of hospitalized children. *Clinical Case Reports and Reviews, 2*(4), 399–401.

Ross, C. A., & Haley, C. (2004). Acute stabilization and three-month follow-up in a trauma program. *Journal of Trauma & Dissociation, 5*(1), 103–112. DOI: 10.1300/J229v05n01_06

Rotenberg, V. S. (2001). *Snovideniya, gipnoz i deyatel'nost' mozga* [Dreams, hypnosis and brain activity]. RON. (In Russian)

Rothschild, B. (2021). *Revolutionizing trauma treatment: Stabilization, safety, & nervous system balance*. W. W. Norton & Company.

Roussel, J., Lehwaldt, D., & Rogers, M. (2024). The International Council of Nurses Nurse Practitioner/Advanced Practice Nurse Network. In *Advanced Practice Nurse Networking to Enhance Global Health* (pp. 43–57). Springer International Publishing.

Rudd, M. D., Mandrusiak, M., & Joiner, T. E. (2005). The case against no-suicide contracts: The commitment to treatment statement as a practice alternative. *Journal of Clinical Psychology, 62*(2), 243–251. DOI: 10.1002/jclp.20227 PMID: 16342293

Ruppert, F. (2011). *Travma, bağlanma ve aile konstelasyonları: Ruhun yaralarını anlamak ve iyileştirmek*. Kaknüs Yayınları.

Sabé, M., Kaiser, S., & Niveau, G. (2020). Suicide in psychiatry and medical liability: A case series. *International Journal of Law and Psychiatry, 74*, 101671. DOI: 10.1016/j.ijlp.2020.101671 PMID: 33387984

Saimonton, K., & Saimonton, S. (2001). *Psikhoterapiya raka* [Psychotherapy cancer]. Publisher. (In Russian).

Sakai, S., An, J., Kang, M., & Kwak, H. (2025). Somatic in the East, Psychological in the West?: Investigating Clinically-Grounded Cross-Cultural Depression Symptom Expression in LLMs. arXiv preprint arXiv:2508.03247.

Sakarya, G., & Karaaziz, M. (2025). A Review of Social Anxiety Disorder and Cognitive Behavioral Therapy. *Journal* of *Social. Human, and Administrative Sciences, 8*(8), 638–656.

Salem, G. M. M., Hashimi, W., & El-Ashry, A. M. (2025). Reflective mindfulness and emotional regulation training to enhance nursing students' self-awareness, understanding, and regulation: A mixed method randomized controlled trial. *BMC Nursing*, *24*(1), 478. PMID: 40307764

Saotome, T., Klein, L., & Faux, S. (2015). Cancer rehabilitation: A barometer for survival? *Supportive Care in Cancer*, *23*(10), 3033–3041.

Sarı, T. (2015). Pozitif psikoterapi: Gelişimi, temel ilk eve yöntemleri ve Türk kültürüne uygulanabilirliği. *The Journal of Happiness & Well-Being*, *3*(2), 182–203.

Sasikala, K., Dahiya, R., Selvakumar, P., Sudheer, P., Rajagopalan, K. K., Manjunath, T. C., & Sharma, M. (2026). Reducing Carbon Footprint With AI-Driven Logistics Planning. In Chahal, B., David, A., Singh, A., Madaan, G., & Singh, G. (Eds.), *Impact of Generative AI on Food Supply Chain Management* (pp. 189–216). IGI Global Scientific Publishing., DOI: 10.4018/979-8-3693-9856-2.ch007

Sastre-Fullana, P., de Pedro-Gómez, J. E., Bennasar-Veny, M., Serrano-Gallardo, P., & Morales-Asencio, J. M. (2014). Competency frameworks for advanced practice nursing: A literature review. *International Nursing Review*, *61*(4), 534–542. DOI: 10.1111/inr.12132 PMID: 25288021

Satyanarayana, P., Anute, N., Ghewari, A., Chahande, S., Sharma, A., Selvakumar, P., & Manjunath, T. C. (2026). Interdisciplinary Applications of AI and AR in Research. In Vrba, J., & Huynh, T. (Eds.), *Revolutionizing Academic Research With AI and Augmented Reality* (pp. 283–310). IGI Global Scientific Publishing., DOI: 10.4018/979-8-3373-1414-3.ch009

Scanlon, A. (2006). Humanistic principles in relation to psychiatric nurse education: A review of the literature. *Journal of Psychiatric and Mental Health Nursing*, *13*(6), 758–764. DOI: 10.1111/j.1365-2850.2006.01031.x PMID: 17087680

Scheel, M., Davis, C. K., & Henderson, J. D. (2012). Therapist Use of Client Strengths. *The Counseling Psychologist*, *41*(3), 392. DOI: 10.1177/0011000012439427

Scheydt, S., & Hegedüs, A. (2021). Tasks and activities of Advanced Practice Nurses in the psychiatric and mental health care context: A systematic review and thematic analysis. *International Journal of Nursing Studies*, *118*, 103759. DOI: 10.1016/j.ijnurstu.2020.103759 PMID: 32958260

Scheydt, S., Nienaber, A., & Holzke, M. (2025). Task Profiles of Academically Qualified Psychiatric Nurses in Germany: Results of a Cluster Analysis. *Journal of Psychiatric and Mental Health Nursing*, *32*(3), 753. DOI: 10.1111/jpm.13153 PMID: 39918036

Schiraldi, G. R. (2016). *The self-esteem workbook* (2nd ed.). New Harbinger Publications.

Schrank, B., Brownell, T., Tylee, A., & Slade, M. (2014). Positive psychology: An approach to supporting recovery in mental illness. *East Asian Archives of Psychiatry, 24*(3), 95–103. PMID: 25316800

Seligman, M. E. P. (1975). *Helplessness: On depression, development, and death.* W. H. Freeman.

Seligman, M. E., & Csikszentmihalyi, M. (2000). Positive psychology. *The American Psychologist, 55*(1), 5–14. PMID: 11392865

Seshadri, A., Orth, S. S., Adaji, A., Singh, B., Clark, M. M., Frye, M. A., & Fuller-Tyszkiewicz, M. (2021). Mindfulness-based cognitive therapy, acceptance and commitment therapy, and positive psychotherapy for major depression. *American Journal of Psychotherapy, 74*(1), 4–12. DOI: 10.1176/appi.psychotherapy.20200006 PMID: 32985916

Shadi, A. Z., Zohreh, V., Eesa, M., & Anoshirvan, K. (2024). Moral sensitivity of nursing students: A systematic review. *BMC Nursing, 23*(1), 99. PMID: 38321462

Sheard, T., & Maguire, P. (1999). The effect of psychological interventions on anxiety and depression in cancer patients: Results of two meta-analyses. *British Journal of Cancer, 80*, 1770–1780.

Shore, J. H., Yellowlees, P., Caudill, R., Johnston, B., Turvey, C., Mishkind, M., & Hilty, D. (2018). Best practices in videoconferencing-based telemental health April 2018. *Telemedicine Journal and e-Health, 24*(11), 827–832. PMID: 30358514

Shortland, A. (2016). Working with trauma. In ... *Clinical practice at the edge of care: Developments in working with at-risk children and their families* (ss. 153-174).

Siddiq, H., Elhaija, A., & Wells, K. (2023). An integrative review of community-based mental health interventions among resettled refugees from Muslim-majority countries. *Community Mental Health Journal, 59*(1), 160–174. PMID: 35751790

Siegel, R., Naishadham, D., & Jemal, A. (2013). Cancer statistics, 2013. *CA: a Cancer Journal for Clinicians, 63*(1), 11–30.

Silver, J. K., Baima, J., & Mayer, R. S. (2013). Impairment-driven cancer rehabilitation: An essential component of quality care and survivorship. *CA: a Cancer Journal for Clinicians, 63*(5), 295–317.

Simon, R. I., & Sadoff, R. L. (2005). *Psychiatric Malpractice: Cases and Comments for Clinicians*. American Psychiatric Press.

Slade, E. P., DePriest, K., Commodore-Mensah, Y., Samuel, L., Hanson, G. C., & D'Aoust, R. (2024). State Full Practice Authority Regulations and Nurse Practitioner Practice Autonomy: Evidence From the 2018 National Sample Survey of Registered Nurses. *Medical Care Research and Review : MCRR, 82*(1), 68. DOI: 10.1177/10775587241282163 PMID: 39470186

Slade, M. (2010). Mental illness and well-being: The central importance of positive psychology and recovery approaches. *BMC Health Services Research, 10*(1), 26. PMID: 20102609

Slatyer, S., Craigie, M., Heritage, B., Davis, S., & Rees, C. (2018). Evaluating the effectiveness of a brief mindful self-care and resiliency (MSCR) intervention for nurses: A controlled trial. *Mindfulness, 9*(2), 534–546.

Slepkov, V. A., Suhovolskiy, V. G., & Hhlebopros, Z. G. (2007). Populjacionnaja dinamika v modelirovanii rosta rakovyh opuholej [Population dynamics in the modelling of the growth of cancerous tumors] [In Russian]. *Biophysics, 52*(4), 733–740.

Smith, B. M., Smith, G. S., & Dymond, S. (2020). Relapse of anxiety-related fear and avoidance: Conceptual analysis of treatment with acceptance and commitment therapy. *Journal of the Experimental Analysis of Behavior, 113*(1), 87–104.

Smith-Coggins, R., Howard, S. K., Mac, D. T., Wang, C., Kwan, S., Rosekind, M. R., Sowb, Y., Balise, R., Levis, J., & Gaba, D. M. (2006). Improving Alertness and Performance in Emergency Department Physicians and Nurses: The Use of Planned Naps. *Annals of Emergency Medicine, 48*(5), 596–604.e3. DOI: 10.1016/j.annemergmed.2006.02.005

Smulevich, A. B., Andryushchenko, A. B., & Beskova, D. A. (2009). *Psikhicheskie rasstroistva v obshchei meditsine, 1*, 4–9. (In Russian).

Soares, M. R., Cameira, M. P., Abreu, P., & Pereira, M. (2024). Cultural Diversity and Mental Health Care: A Case Study. *European Psychiatry : the Journal of the Association of European Psychiatrists, 67*(S1), S522–S522.

Solak, M., & Kayaer, N. (2024). Criminal responsibilities of nurses in Turkish criminal law and determining the awareness levels of senior nursing students regarding this responsibility. *BMC Nursing, 23*(1), 761. DOI: 10.1186/s12912-024-02418-6 PMID: 39415194

Son, C., Forsgren, E., Öhlén, J., & Sawatzky, R. (2025). Person-centred care for migrants: A narrative review of health care literature. *Frontiers in Health Services, 5*, 1573813. PMID: 40740479

Sotirov, S., Vankova, D., Vasilev, V., & Sotirova, E. (2019). Clustering of intercriteria analysis data using a health-related quality of life data. In *International Conference on Flexible Query Answering Systems* (pp. 242–249). Springer.

Sousa, L., Ribeiro, C., & Rodrigues, S. (2006). Intervention with multi-problem poor clients: Towards a strengths-focused perspective. *Journal of Social Work Practice*, *20*(2), 189–204. DOI: 10.1080/02650530600776913

Soyer, M. K., Şenol, A., & Tümerdem, B. Ç. (2021). An examination of childhood trauma experiences in a group of adults in terms of various variables. *Humanistic Perspective*, *3*(2), 324–343.

Spiegel, D. (2013). Minding the body: Psychotherapy and cancer survival. *British Journal of Health Psychology*, *19*(3), 1–21.

Spiegel, D., Bloom, J. R., Kraemer, H. C., & Gottheil, E. (1989). Effect of psychosocial treatment on survival of patients with metastatic breast cancer. *Lancet*, *334*(8668), 888–891.

Sreekanthaswamy, N., Chib, S., Maddel, M., Khande, R., Kalshetti, P., Selvakumar, P., & Manjunath, T. C. (2026). AI Smart-Enabled and Machine Learning Intensifies Smart Multimedia Platforms. In van Wyk, M. (Ed.), *AI Smart-Enabled Architecture and Infrastructure for Higher Education* (pp. 29–54). IGI Global Scientific Publishing., DOI: 10.4018/979-8-3693-8915-7.ch002

Stanley, B., & Brown, G. K. (2012). Safety Planning Intervention: A Brief Intervention to Mitigate Suicide Risk. *Cognitive and Behavioral Practice*, *19*(2), 256–264.

Stanley, I. H., Simpson, S., Wortzel, H. S., & Joiner, T. E. (2019). Documenting suicide risk assessments and proportionate clinical actions to improve patient safety and mitigate legal risk. *Behavioral Sciences & the Law*, *37*(3), 304. DOI: 10.1002/bsl.2409 PMID: 31063254

Stepanova, N. V., & Chernavsky, D. S. (1983). A mathematical model of immunosuppression by malignant growth. *Mathematical Modelling*, •••, 379–386.

Stern, D. N. (2004). The present moment as a critical moment. *Negotiation Journal*, *20*(2), 365–372.

Stevens, M. W., King, D. L., Dorstyn, D., & Delfabbro, P. H. (2019). Cognitive–behavioral therapy for Internet gaming disorder: A systematic review and meta-analysis. *Clinical Psychology & Psychotherapy*, *26*(2), 191–203. PMID: 30341981

Stewart, T. M. (2004). Light on body image treatment: Acceptance through mindfulness. *Behavior Modification*, *28*(6), 783–811.

Stievano, A., & Tschudin, V. (2019). The ICN code of ethics for nurses: A time for revision. *International Nursing Review*, *66*(2), 154. DOI: 10.1111/inr.12525 PMID: 31124137

Stige, S. H., & Binder, P.-E. (2017). From painstaking work to a new way of meeting the world—Trauma clients' experiences with skill training in a stabilization group approach. *Psychotherapy Research*, *27*(5), 571–582.

Stige, S. H., Rosenvinge, J. H., & Træen, B. (2013). A meaningful struggle: Trauma clients' experiences with an inclusive stabilization group approach. *Psychotherapy Research*, *23*(4), 419–429. DOI: 10.1080/10503307.2013.778437

Stingl, M., & Hanewald, B. (2025). Culturally sensitive psychotherapy-technique or attitude? *Frontiers in Psychology*, *16*, 1599855. PMID: 41112539

Stuart, G. W. (2014). *Principles and practice of psychiatric nursing* [E-book]. Elsevier Health Sciences.

Suzuki, K. (n.d.). *COLLEGE OF SOCIAL AND BEHAVIORAL SCIENCES*.

Taherkhani, Z., Kaveh, M. H., Mani, A., Ghahremani, L., & Khademi, K. (2023). The effect of positive thinking on resilience and life satisfaction of older adults: A randomized controlled trial. *Scientific Reports*, *13*(1), 3478. PMID: 36859479

Tarbi, E. C., Broden, E. G., Rosa, W. E., Hayden, A., & Morgan, B. E. (2023). Existential Care in Daily Nursing Practice. *AJN. The American Journal of Nursing*, *123*(10), 42–48. DOI: 10.1097/01.NAJ.0000979092.39243.d4

Tarbox, J., Szabo, T. G., & Aclan, M. (2022). Acceptance and commitment training within the scope of practice of applied behavior analysis. *Behavior Analysis in Practice*, *15*(1), 11–32.

Taute, C. (2023). Learning to cope with trauma and moving forward. *Psychology (Irvine, Calif.)*, *14*(6), 1033–1037. DOI: 10.4236/psych.2023.146055

Terzioğlu, M., & Yavuz, K. F. (2023). İlişkisel Çerçeve Kuramı (İÇK): Dil ve Bilişe Ampirik Bir Yaklaşım. *J Cogn Behav Psychother Res*, 188-200.

Theodosopoulos, L., Fradelos, E. C., Panagiotou, A., Dreliozi, A., & Tzavella, F. (2024). Delivering culturally competent care to migrants by healthcare personnel: A crucial aspect of delivering culturally sensitive care. *Social Sciences*, *13*(10), 530.

Tikhonov, A. N., & Samarsky, A. A. (1977). *Uravnenija matematicheskoj fiziki* [Equations of mathematical physics]. Nauka. (In Russian)

Tol, W. A., Leku, M. R., Lakin, D. P., Carswell, K., Augustinavicius, J., Adaku, A., & van Ommeren, M. (2020). Guided self-help to reduce psychological distress in South Sudanese female refugees in Uganda: A cluster randomised trial. *The Lancet. Global Health*, *8*(2), e254–e263. PMID: 31981556

Topan, H., Albayrak Günday, E., Sürme, Y., Ceyhan, Ö., Şimşek, N., & Küçük, A. (2025). Guided imagery effects on pain, anxiety, and sleep for lumbar discectomy patients. *Journal of Perianesthesia Nursing*, *40*(1), 56–61. DOI: 10.1016/j.jopan.2024.03.004 PMID: 39023479

Topol, E. (2019). *Deep medicine: how artificial intelligence can make healthcare human again.*

Tosun, B., Yılmaz, E. B., Dirgar, E., Şahin, E. B., Hatipoğlu, K. P., & Yava, A. (2024). Evaluating the effectiveness of a new curriculum for transcultural nursing education: A mixed-method study. *BMC Nursing*, *23*(1), 813. PMID: 39511551

Towsend, M. C. (2015). Trauma-and stressor-related disorder. In *Psychiatric mental health nursing: Concepts of care in evidence-based practice* (8. Baskı, ss. 559-578).

Trachsel, M., & grosse Holtforth, M. (2019). How to strengthen patients' meaning response by an ethical informed consent in psychotherapy. *Frontiers in Psychology*, *10*, 1747. Advance online publication. DOI: 10.3389/fpsyg.2019.01747 PMID: 31417470

Travado, L. (2015). *The Role and Challenges of Psycho-Oncology in Improving Cancer care.* Unpublished. https://doi.org/DOI: 10.13140/RG.2.1.2076.8086

Travelbee, J. (1971). *Interpersonal Aspects of Nursing*. F.A. Davis.

Triandis, H. C. (2018). *Individualism and collectivism.* Routledge.

Tripp, T., Potash, J. S., & Brancheau, D. (2019). Safe place collage protocol: Art making for managing traumatic stress. *Journal of Trauma & Dissociation*, *20*(5), 511–525. DOI: 10.1080/15299732.2019.1597813

Tufanaru, C., Munn, Z., Aromataris, E., ... (2020) Chapter 3: Systematic reviews of effectiveness. In: JBI Manual for Evidence Synthesis, pp. 71–133.

Türkçapar, H. (2019). Cognitive Behavioral Therapy: Basic Principles and Application. Epsilon Publications, 13th Edition, Istanbul.

Tzur Bitan, D., Shalev, S., & Abayed, S. (2022). Therapists' views of mechanisms of change in psychotherapy: A mixed-method approach. *Frontiers in Psychology*, *13*, 565800. PMID: 35496206

Ungar, M. (Ed.). (2021). *Multisystemic resilience: Adaptation and transformation in contexts of change*. Oxford University Press.

UNHCR. (2024). Community-based Mental Health and Psychosocial Support (MHPSS) approaches for refugees and migrants.

Unhjem, J. V., & Hem, M. H. (2025). Nurse-patient relationship boundaries and power: A critical discursive analysis. *Nursing Ethics*, *32*(6), 1861. DOI: 10.1177/09697330251314093 PMID: 39828402

Valdez, C. E., & Lilly, M. M. (2012). Thought control: Is it ability, strategies, or both that predicts posttraumatic symptomatology in victims of interpersonal trauma? *Journal of Psychopathology and Behavioral Assessment*, *34*, 531–541. DOI: 10.1007/s10862-012-9300-y

Valdez, C. E., Sherrill, A. M., & Lilly, M. (2016). Present moment contact and non-judgment: Pilot data on dismantling mindful awareness in trauma-related symptomatology. *Journal of Psychopathology and Behavioral Assessment*, *38*(4), 572–581.

Valente, S. M. (2017). Managing Professional and Nurse–Patient Relationship Boundaries in Mental Health. *Journal of Psychosocial Nursing and Mental Health Services*, *55*(1), 45–51. DOI: 10.3928/02793695-20170119-09

Vallières, F., Mcauliffe, E., & van Bavel, B.. (2016). There's no app for that: Assessing the impact of mhealth on the supervision, motivation, engagement, and satisfaction of community health workers in Sierra Leone. *Annals of Global Health*, *82*, 936–949. PMID: 28283148

Van Agteren, J., Iasiello, M., Lo, L., Bartholomaeus, J., Kopsaftis, Z., Carey, M., & Kyrios, M. (2021). A systematic review and meta-analysis of psychological interventions to improve mental wellbeing. *Nature Human Behaviour*, *5*(5), 631–652. PMID: 33875837

van der Meer, C. A. I., Bakker, A., & van Zuiden, M.. (2020). Help in hand after traumatic events: A randomized controlled trial in health care professionals on the efficacy, usability, and user satisfaction of a self-help app to reduce trauma-related symptoms. *European Journal of Psychotraumatology*, *11*, 1717155. PMID: 32284818

Van Dis, E. A., Van Veen, S. C., Hagenaars, M. A., Batelaan, N. M., Bockting, C. L., Van Den Heuvel, R. M., & Engelhard, I. M. (2020). Long-term outcomes of cognitive behavioral therapy for anxiety-related disorders: A systematic review and meta-analysis. *JAMA Psychiatry*, *77*(3), 265–273. PMID: 31758858

Van Hees, M. L., Rotter, T., Ellermann, T., & Evers, S. M. (2013). The effectiveness of individual interpersonal psychotherapy as a treatment for major depressive disorder in adult outpatients: A systematic review. *BMC Psychiatry*, *13*(1), 22. PMID: 23312024

Vindevogel, S., Boumahdi, Y., Alabbas, F., & Magerman, J. (2025). Transcultural mental health and psychosocial support in asylum reception centres: A Delphi review of guidelines for the frontline workforce. *International Journal of Migration, Health and Social Care*.

Viskovich, S., Pakenham, K. I., & Fowler, J. A. (2021). A mixed-methods evaluation of experiential intervention exercises for values and committed action from an Acceptance and Commitment Therapy (ACT) mental health promotion program for university students. *Journal of Contextual Behavioral Science*, *22*, 108–118.

Vlake, J. H., Van Bommel, J., Wils, E. J., Korevaar, T. I., Bienvenu, O. J., Klijn, E., & Van Genderen, M. E. (2021). Virtual reality to improve sequelae of the postintensive care syndrome: A multicenter, randomized controlled feasibility study. *Critical Care Explorations*, *3*(9), e0538. PMID: 34549192

Vowles, K. E., Wetherell, J. L., & Sorrell, J. T. (2009). Targeting acceptance, mindfulness, and values-based action in chronic pain: Findings of two preliminary trials of an outpatient group-based intervention. *Cognitive and Behavioral Practice*, *16*(1), 49–58.

Walser, R. D., & O'Connell, M. (2021). Acceptance and commitment therapy and the therapeutic relationship: Rupture and repair. *Journal of Clinical Psychology*, *77*(2), 429–440.

Walsh, S., Cassidy, M., & Priebe, S. (2017). The application of positive psychotherapy in mental health care: A systematic review. *Journal of Clinical Psychology*, *73*(6), 638–651. DOI: 10.1002/jclp.22368 PMID: 27482845

Watson, C., Wijesuriya, R., & Bhugra, D. (2022). Culture and mental illness. Oxford Textbook of Social Psychiatry, 83.

Weissman, M. M. (2006). A brief history of interpersonal psychotherapy. *Psychiatric Annals*, *36*(8).

Westland, G. (2020). Healing trauma through embodied relating. In *Trauma in the creative and embodied therapies: When words are not enough*.

Wheeler, K. (2020). Advanced psychiatric nursing practices: Evidence-based practice guide (A. Atlı Özbaş & N. Gürhan, Trans. Eds.; 2nd ed.). Ankara Nobel Medical Publishers.

Wheeler, K. (2020). *Psychotherapy for advanced practice in psychiatric nursing* (A. A. Özbaş & N. Gürhan, Çev.; K. Wheeler, Ed.; C. 2). Springer Publishing Company.

Wheeler, K. (2013). *Psychotherapy for the advanced practice psychiatric nurse: A how-to guide for evidence-based practice*. Springer Publishing Company.

White, L. (2014). Mindfulness in nursing: An evolutionary concept analysis. *Journal of Advanced Nursing*, *70*(2), 282–294.

Whitworth, J. D. (2016). The role of psychoeducation in trauma recovery: Recommendations for content and delivery. *Journal of Evidence-Informed Social Work*, *13*(5), 442–451. DOI: 10.1080/23761407.2016.1166852

WHO. (2022a) Mental Health and COVID-19: Scientific brief. Available at: https://www.who.int/publications/i/item/WHO-2019-nCoV-Sci_Brief-Mental_health-2022.1 (accessed 23 April 2022).

WHO. (2023). *Self-Help Plus (SH+) and Problem Management Plus (PM+) Implementation Guidance*. World Health Organization.

WHO/Europe. (2024). *Global competency standards for health workers providing care to refugees and migrants*. World Health Organization Regional Office for Europe.

Wies, B., Landers, C., & Ienca, M. (2021). Digital mental health for young people: A scoping review of ethical promises and challenges. *Frontiers in Digital Health*, *3*, 697072. PMID: 34713173

Wilkenfeld, D. A., & Durmis, C. (2022). When law and ethics come apart: Constraints versus guidance. *Nursing Ethics*, *29*(6), 1430. DOI: 10.1177/09697330221105640 PMID: 35724321

Willi, N., Pancoast, A., Drikaki, I., Gu, X., Gillanders, D., & Finucane, A. (2024). Practitioner perspectives on the use of acceptance and commitment therapy for bereavement support: A qualitative study. *BMC Palliative Care*, *23*(1), 59.

Wiltshire, J. T. (2024). The role of mindfulness and embodiment in group-based trauma treatment. *Psychotherapy and Counselling Journal of Australia*, *12*(1). Advance online publication. DOI: 10.59158/001c.94979

Wing Sue, D., & Sue, D. (2008). *Counseling the culturally diverse: Theory and practice*. John Wiley & Sons, Inc.

Winston, A., & Schaefer, A. (2023). Supportive psychotherapy. In *Tasman's psychiatry* (pp. 1–27). Springer International Publishing.

Wong, P. T. P., & Yu, T. T. F. (2021). Existential Suffering in Palliative Care: An Existential Positive Psychology Perspective. *Medicina, 57*(9), 924. DOI: 10.3390/medicina57090924

World Health Organization (WHO). (2008). *Task Shifting: Global Recommendations and Guidelines*. WHO.

World Health Organization (WHO). (2022). *World Mental Health Report: Transforming Mental Health for All*. World Health Organization.

Wortzel, H. S., Matarazzo, B. B., & Homaifar, B. Y. (2013). A Model for Therapeutic Risk Management of the Suicidal Patient. *Journal of Psychiatric Practice, 19*(4), 323-326. Lippincott Williams & Wilkins. https://doi.org/DOI: 10.1097/01.pra.0000432603.99211.e8

Wright, J. H., Basco, M. R., & Thase, M. E. (2009). *Learning Cognitive-Behavior Therapy: An Illustrated Guide*. American Psychiatric Publishing.

Wu, Y. (2021). Empathy in nurse-patient interaction: A conversation analysis. *BMC Nursing*, *20*(1), 18. PMID: 33435957

Xiao, X., Song, H., Sang, T., Wu, Z., Xie, Y., & Yang, Q. (2021). Analysis of real-world implementation of the biopsychosocial approach to healthcare: Evidence from a combination of qualitative and quantitative methods. *Frontiers in Psychiatry*, *12*, 725596. PMID: 34764895

Xie, H. (2013). Strengths-based approach for mental health recovery. *Iranian Journal of Psychiatry and Behavioral Sciences*, *7*(2), 5. PMID: 24644504

Yamada, A.-M., & Brekke, J. S. (2008). Addressing mental health disparities through clinical competence not just cultural competence: The need for assessment of sociocultural issues in the delivery of evidence-based psychosocial rehabilitation services. *Clinical Psychology Review*, *28*(8), 1386–1399. DOI: 10.1016/j.cpr.2008.07.006

Yang, H. M., & Jang, Y. E. (2025). Ethics of nursing in the digital age: Perceptions and challenges among Korean nursing students. *BMC Medical Ethics*, *26*(1), 143. PMID: 41107902

Yao, W., Gu, L., Sun, D., Ka, W., Wen, Z., & Chien, S. (2003). Wild type p53 gene causes reorganization of cytoskeleton and therefore the impaired deformability and difficult migration of murine erythroleukemia cells. *Cell Motility and the Cytoskeleton*, *56*, 1–12.

Yava, A., Tosun, B., Papp, K., Tóthová, V., Şahin, E., Yılmaz, E. B., & Leyva-Moral, J. M. (2023). Developing the better and effective nursing education for improving transcultural nursing skills cultural competence and cultural sensitivity assessment tool (BENEFITS-CCCSAT). *BMC Nursing*, *22*(1), 331. DOI: 10.1186/s12912-023-01476-6

Yavuz, K. F. (2015). Acceptance and Commitment Therapy (ACT): An Overview. *Turkiye Klinikleri Journal of Psychiatry Special Topics*, *8*(2), 21–27.

Ye, J. (2021). Advancing mental health and psychological support for health care workers using digital technologiesand platforms. *JMIR Formative Research*, *5*, e22075. PMID: 34106874

Yildiz, B., & Yildiz, T. (2022). A systematic review and meta-analytical synthesis of the relationship between work engagement and job satisfaction in nurses. *Perspectives in Psychiatric Care*, *58*, 3062–3078. PMID: 35383388

Yılmaz, S. (2016). Trauma and stressor-related disorders. In Gürhan, N. (Ed.), *Mental health and psychiatric nursing* (1st ed., pp. 815–843). Nobel Medical Bookstore.

Yoshinaga, N., Tanoue, H., & Hayashi, Y. (2022). Naturalistic outcome of nurse-led psychological therapy for mental disorders in routine outpatient care: A retrospective chart review. *Archives of Psychiatric Nursing*, *40*, 43. DOI: 10.1016/j.apnu.2022.04.008 PMID: 36064244

Ypma, P., M, M. D. G., Pomme, A. O., Drevon, C., & Papadopoulos, I. (2020). Mapping and assessment of developments for one of the sectoral professions under directive 2005/36/EC Nurse responsible for general care: final study. *Middlesex University Research Repository (Middlesex University Of London)*. https://doi.org/DOI: 10.2873/30

Yüksel, A. (2024). Cognitive Behavioral Therapy Case Formulation for Social Phobia. *Turkey Journal of Integrative Psychotherapy*, *7*(14), 65–71.

Yule, W. (2006). Theory, training and timing: Psychosocial interventions in complex emergencies. *International Review of Psychiatry (Abingdon, England)*, *18*(3), 259–264.

Zarvijani, S. A. H., Moghaddam, L. F., & Parchebafieh, S. (2021). Acceptance and commitment therapy on perceived stress and psychological flexibility of psychiatric nurses: A randomized control trial. *BMC Nursing*, *20*(1), 239.

Zhou, H. (2025). Relationship between empathy and burnout as well as potential affecting and mediating factors from the perspective of clinical nurses: A systematic review. *BMC Nursing*, *24*(1), 38. PMID: 39794782

Zhukova, I. V., & Kolpak, E. P. (2013). *Matematicheskaja model' solidnoj opuholi* /Mathematical model of solid tumor/. *Natural and Mathematical Science in the Modern World, 13*, 18–25.

Zhu, Y., Gan, L., Shen, Y., Wang, J., Lu, M., & Wang, J. (2022). Humanistic Nursing Care for Patients in Low-Resourced Clinical Settings from Students' Perspectives: A Participatory Qualitative Study. *International Journal of Environmental Research and Public Health, 19*(19), 12656. DOI: 10.3390/ijerph191912656 PMID: 36231956

Zur, O. (2007). *Appendix A Examples of Boundary Crossings and Boundary Violations in Psychotherapy.*

About the Contributors

Kübra Gülırmak Güler holds a PhD in Mental Health and Psychiatric Nursing and currently works as a Research Assistant at Ondokuz Mayıs University. She is also a postdoctoral researcher. She holds international certifications in Positive Psychotherapy, Existential Psychotherapy, and Play Therapy, and her doctoral dissertation focused on Positive Psychotherapy. She has published numerous international peer-reviewed articles with diverse populations and has contributed to research projects and book chapters. Her research interests focus on innovative and contemporary issues in nursing, including climate change and mental health, artificial intelligence and digital nursing, existential psychotherapies, trauma, and ambiguous loss. She is places strong emphasis on interdisciplinary collaboration. Her research is predominantly grounded in qualitative methodologies, particularly phenomenological approaches aiming to explore lived experiences and meaning-making processes in mental health care.

***

Vesile Adıgüzel completed her undergraduate studies at Dicle University, her master's degree at Gaziantep University, and her doctorate in Psychiatric Nursing at Istanbul Medeniyet University. She provides counseling in the field of Interpersonal Relationships Psychotherapy and has research in mood disorders, schizophrenia, women's mental health, child and adolescent mental health, and addiction. She served on the board of directors of the Psychiatric Nurses Association from 2022 to 2025. She has been working as an assistant professor at Yalova University since 2023.

Eda Albayrak Günday is a Research Assistant at Erciyes University, Faculty of Health Sciences, specializing in Mental Health and Diseases Nursing. She holds a Ph.D. in Mental Health and Diseases Nursing and has focused her academic career on psychosocial health, mental wellness, and innovative therapeutic interventions. Dr.

Albayrak Günday is an expert in Positive Psychotherapy, and her research primarily investigates psychotherapeutic interventions, the application of balance models, and psychotherapy. Throughout her academic journey, she has been recognized for her contributions to the field, notably receiving the Young Researcher Award at the 8th International & 12th National Psychiatric Nursing Congress. Her work is characterized by an interdisciplinary approach, integrating psychological theories with nursing science to enhance health outcomes. Dr. Albayrak Günday has been the recipient of research support from prestigious institutions, including TÜBİTAK (The Scientific and Technological Research Council of Turkey), and has presented her findings on the use of positive psychotherapy in psychiatric nursing at various international congresses. Beyond her research, she contributes to the academic community through peer-reviewing for scientific journals and stays active in the development of mental health nursing standards.

Elif Güzide Emirza is a research assistant in the Department of Nursing, Division of Psychiatric Nursing, Faculty of Health Sciences, Ondokuz Mayıs University. She completed her undergraduate nursing education at Ordu University and received her master's degree in Nursing from Gazi University. She completed her PhD in Psychiatric Nursing within the Department of Nursing at the Institute of Health Sciences, Gazi University. Her research interests include psychiatric nursing, psychosocial interventions, violence against women, trauma, post-disaster mental health, substance addiction awareness, and digital health applications. Emirza has published numerous articles in international peer-reviewed journals and has served as a principal investigator and researcher in national projects, as well as a contributing author to several scientific book chapters.

SudhaAnanthi G is a dedicated academician with a strong passion for education and continuous learning. Known for her excellent communication skills and ability to inspire others, she excels in both teaching and collaborative environments. As a motivating presence in her team, SudhaAnanthi consistently fosters a positive and productive atmosphere. Her strengths as a team player and her commitment to academic excellence make her a valuable asset in any educational setting.

Marin Georgiev is an Associate Professor from Georgi Rakovski Military Academy, Sofia, Bulgaria. Ph.D. in Organisation and Management at Vasil Levski National Military University, Veliko Tarnovo, Bulgaria. Assoc. Prof. Georgiev has over 200 scientific papers, articles, and reports in Bulgarian, Russian, and English published in scientific journals and proceedings of international conferences, 2 monographs in Bulgarian, and 1 textbook. There are more than 40 publications in the referenced systems of Web of Science and Scopus. His research interests are in the areas of Economics, Education, and National security.

Harun Mirsad Günday is an Assistant Professor of Law at Erciyes University, Faculty of Law, specializing in Medical Law and Comparative Civil Law. He holds a Ph.D. in Private Law and has dedicated a significant portion of his academic career to the legal dimensions of mental health and healthcare provider liability. Dr. Günday is the author of the influential monograph Psikiyatristin Hukukî Sorumluluğu (Legal Liability of the Psychiatrist), which examines the intersection of psychiatric practice and legal responsibility. In addition to his monograph, he has published extensively in the field of health law, contributing to the academic discourse on patient rights and medical ethics. His research expertise lies in comparative analysis, specifically bridging the gap between Continental European, Anglo-Saxon, and Turkish legal frameworks. Throughout his career, Dr. Günday has been the recipient of several prestigious research fellowships and grants from prominent institutions, including TÜBİTAK (The Scientific and Technological Research Council of Turkey) and DAAD (German Academic Exchange Service), enabling him to conduct advanced legal research in Europe. Currently, he leads an interdisciplinary research project investigating the impact of digital behaviors on legal capacity and discernment, while also serving as an editor for the Erciyes University Faculty of Law Journal.

Teodora Petrova received her Master's degree in "Communication Technology and Techniques" from the University of Ruse "Angel Kanchev," her PhD in "Radar and Radionavigation" in 2009, and her Doctor of Science degree in "National Security" in 2024. Since 2014, she has held the academic position of Associate Professor in the professional field 5.2 "Electrical Engineering, Electronics, and Automation." She is the author of five monographs, three books, one textbook, and more than 90 articles, of which 32 are indexed in the Scopus and Web of Science databases. She holds two registered utility models and has filed two patent applications. Her research interests include image processing, the use of unmanned aerial vehicles, and the application of lasers in medicine.

Kübra Tan is an Assistant Professor at Artvin Çoruh University, where she conducts academic work in the field of psychiatric nursing. Her research interests focus on mental health and psychiatric nursing, psychological resilience, stress coping processes, health literacy, therapy-based interventions, emotional regulation, and nursing practices aimed at promoting individuals' mental well-being. In her studies, she particularly concentrates on topics that influence the prevention, promotion, and treatment of mental health, including anxiety disorders, digital addiction, mindfulness-based approaches, and violence. She adopts a comprehensive methodological framework by integrating both quantitative and qualitative research methods. Dr. Tan has published scientific articles in national and international peer-reviewed journals in the field of psychiatric nursing, presented her research findings at academic conferences, and actively participates in interdisciplinary research projects. In addition to her academic activities, she is involved in various scientific and social responsibility initiatives aimed at enhancing mental health within the scope of community service.

Venelin Terziev is a Professor from Angel Kanchev Rousse University – Bulgaria, Vasil Levski National Military University, Veliko Tarnovo, Bulgaria, and University of Telecommunications and Post, Sofia, Bulgaria. D.Sc. in Economics – "Organization and management in the sphere of immaterial production (defence and national security)" at the Vasil Levski National Military University – Veliko Tarnovo, Bulgaria; D.Sc. in Economics – "Finance, currency, credit, and insurance (social security)" at Dimitar Tzenov Academy of Economics – Svishtov, Bulgaria; D.Sc. in Social Activities – "Organization and management of social activities" at Burgas Free University – Burgas, Bulgaria; Ph.D. in Political economy at Chernorisets Hrabar Varna Free University – Bulgaria. Full Member of the Russian Academy of Natural History, Moscow, Russia. Prof. Terziev has over 2000 scientific papers, articles, and reports in Bulgarian, Russian, English, and French published in scientific journals and proceedings of international conferences; 40 monographs in English and Russian; 4 monographs in Bulgarian and 4 textbooks and handbooks.

Ercan Tunç holds a Ph.D. in nursing and is currently working as a research assistant in the Department of Psychiatric Nursing, Faculty of Health Sciences, Ondokuz Mayıs University, Türkiye. His research interests focus on psychological flexibility, acceptance and commitment therapy–based interventions, mindfulness-based approaches, psychoeducation programs, therapeutic communication, and mental health nursing education. He has conducted experimental and qualitative studies examining psychosocial outcomes among individuals with chronic illnesses, psychiatric disorders, and nursing students. Dr. Tunç has published extensively in national and international peer-reviewed journals indexed in SCI-Expanded, SSCI, ESCI, and Scopus, and has authored and co-authored several book chapters in the field of psychiatric nursing. He actively serves as a reviewer for high-impact international journals and contributes to interdisciplinary research addressing mental health, psychosocial adaptation, and nursing education. In addition to his research activities, he is involved in undergraduate and graduate nursing education and participates in projects aimed at strengthening mental health services.

Index

P

R

S

T

W

www.ingramcontent.com/pod-product-compliance
Lightning Source LLC
LaVergne TN
LVHW080903300926
849162LV00003B/533
9798337365268